Orthopaedic Clinical Examination

Orthopaedic Clinical Examination

An Evidence-Based Approach
for Physical Therapists

Joshua Cleland, DPT, OCS

Assistant Professor of Physical Therapy

Franklin Pierce College

Illustrations by Frank H. Netter, MD

Contributing Illustrators

Kip Carter

John Craig, MD

Carlos Machado, MD

James A. Perkins, MS, MFA

Icon Learning Systems · Carlstadt, New Jersey

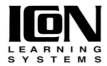

Published by Icon Learning Systems LLC, a subsidiary of MediMedia USA, Inc.
Copyright © 2005 MediMedia, Inc.

FIRST EDITION

ISBN 1-929007-87-6
Library of Congress Catalog No.: 2005920965

Printed in the U.S.A.

NOTICE

Executive Editor: Paul Kelly
Editorial Director: Greg Otis
Managing Editor: Jennifer Surich
Editorial Assistant: Marybeth Thiel
Art Director: Jonathan Dimes
Graphic Design: Colleen Quinn
Director of Manufacturing: Mary Ellen Curry
Senior Production Editor: Melanie Peirson Johnstone
Digital Asset Manager: Karen Oswald
Text Design: Dan Wong
Cover Design: Joanie Krupinski

Binding and Printing by Banta Book Group
Composition and Layout by Maryland Comp

10   9   8   7   6   5   4   3   2   1

I would like to dedicate this book to my father, Robert Cleland, who has provided guidance and unconditional support for 35 years. Dad, thanks for instilling a strong work ethic and for always encouraging me to bring passion into my professional life.

Love,
Josh

" Nothing is really work unless you would rather be doing something else. "

James M. Barrie

Table of Contents

ABOUT THE AUTHOR

Dr. Joshua Cleland, DPT, OCS, earned a Master of Physical Therapy degree from Notre Dame College in Manchester, New Hampshire, and a Doctor of Physical Therapy degree from Creighton University in Omaha, Nebraska. He later received board certification as an Orthopaedic Clinical Specialist (OCS) from the American Physical Therapy Association. Joshua is presently an Assistant Professor in the Physical Therapy Program at Franklin Pierce College in Rindge, New Hampshire; he practices clinically in outpatient orthopaedics at Rehabilitation Services of Concord Hospital in Concord, New Hampshire. He is currently collecting data for his doctoral dissertation project, which he expects to defend early in 2006. In addition, Joshua is a Fellow in the Manual Physical Therapy Fellowship Program at Regis University in Denver, Colorado.

FOREWORD

Until recently, the orthopaedic clinical examination has not kept pace with the development of evidence-based practice. Clinical examination practice patterns have been based largely on what was learned during first professional training programs, continuing education courses, and leisurely browsing in familiar journals. This is not surprising when you consider that there are few high-quality research reports in the peer-reviewed literature elucidating the reliability, diagnostic accuracy, and predictive validity of clinical examination procedures. The paucity of evidence-based information on the diagnostic properties of clinical examination procedures coupled with the general lack of appreciation for the importance of evidence-based decision-making makes the current state of affairs understandable, but not excusable.

Over the past several years, there has been a renewed emphasis in all fields of medicine on defining the accuracy of the clinical examination, including the history, physical examination, and manual testing procedures. To call this a "revolution" might be overstating the case, but nevertheless, interest in the value of the clinical examination is growing, especially as the increase in the cost of health care accelerates. In *Orthopaedic Clinical Examination: An Evidence-Based Approach for Physical Therapists*, Dr. Joshua Cleland has taken the first step toward bringing the orthopaedic clinical examination in line with the principles of evidence-based medicine. The most important feature of this book, which is not found in other texts, is the inclusion of tables containing the measurement properties of clinical examination procedures. Another critical feature is the pertinent study-related information indicating the level of confidence that can be placed in the result of a test or measure when it is applied to a patient in the practice setting. In addition, Dr. Cleland provides clear operational definitions for tests and measures, accompanied by lucid illustrations and figures. Finally, the diagnostic process itself is illustrated in detail, as are key anatomic structures, through the use of classic Netter art. Data from existing studies are used to demonstrate how pre-test probabilities and likelihood ratios can be used to arrive at post-test probabilities. After all, what the practitioner ultimately wants to know is whether a test result increases or decreases the likelihood that a particular patient has the condition being investigated.

A text can capture only information that is contemporary with the text itself. Therefore, this book does not relieve clinicians of the need to know how to search the literature and find current answers to questions about the orthopaedic clinical examination that arise from their work with the patients they see. Rather, the purpose of this book is to give clinicians a rich repository of information on operational definitions and associated diagnostic properties for the most important tests and measures in a framework that can be used to drive clinical decision-making in orthopaedic clinical practice. This information should be viewed as the basis from which up-to-date searches for evidence can be undertaken.

Orthopaedic Clinical Examination: An Evidence-Based Approach for Physical Therapists should find an important place in the education of physical therapists—both students and experienced clinicians.

Lt Col Robert S. Wainner, PT, PhD, OCS, ECS, FAAOMPT
Associate Professor
US Army—Baylor Graduate Program in Physical Therapy
President and Director Research and Practice
Texas Physical Therapy Specialists
Fort Sam Houston, Texas

PREFACE

Over the past several years, evidence-based practice has become the standard of the medical and health care professions. As described by Sackett,[1] evidence-based practice is a combination of three elements: the best available evidence, clinical experience, and patient values. Sackett has further reported that "when these three elements are integrated, clinicians and patients form a diagnostic and therapeutic alliance which optimizes clinical outcomes and quality of life." Unfortunately, the evidence-based approach confronts a number of barriers that may limit the clinician's ability to use the best available evidence to guide decisions about patient care, the most significant being a lack of time and resources. Given the increasing prevalence of new clinical tests in the orthopaedic setting and the frequent omission from textbooks of information about their diagnostic usefulness, the need was clear for a quick reference guide for students and busy clinicians that would enhance their ability to incorporate evidence into clinical decision-making.

This text began as a compilation of references I used to integrate current evidence regarding the diagnostic usefulness of components of the orthopaedic clinical examination for a musculoskeletal evaluation course I was teaching to physical therapy students. As an educator, I felt I had a clear responsibility not only to teach the psychomotor skills required to perform tests and measures, but also to present the evidence for and against the use of various components of the clinical examination.

The purpose of *Orthopaedic Clinical Examination: An Examination-Based Approach for Physical Therapists* is twofold: (1) to serve as a supplement in musculoskeletal evaluation courses in an academic setting, and (2) to provide a quick, user-friendly guide and reference for clinicians who wish to locate evidence related to the diagnostic usefulness of commonly used tests and measures. The first two chapters are intended to introduce the reader to the essential concepts underlying evidence-based practice, including the statistical methods it employs and a critical analysis of research articles. The remainder of the book consists of chapters devoted to body regions. Each chapter begins with a review of the relevant osteology, arthrology, myology, and neurology, and each is liberally illustrated with images by the well-known medical artist, Frank H. Netter, MD. The second portion of each chapter provides data specifically related to the reliability of the historical and physical components of the clinical examination. The remainder is devoted to comprehensive evidence tables that provide information related to the diagnostic accuracy of specific tests and measures that have been investigated in controlled studies; information on each test's sensitivity, specificity, and likelihood ratios is provided. In addition, each evidence table provides the reader with an easy-to-follow guide to the performance and scoring of every test and measure. Tables also contain information regarding the patient population and the reference standard that was used in the corresponding study, along with an overview of the study results and their applicability to the clinician's environment.

I hope that clinicians involved in evaluating patients with musculoskeletal impairments will find this a user-friendly resource for determining the relevance of various components of the orthopaedic examination. I also hope that students and educators will find this a valuable guide to incorporate into courses related to musculoskeletal evaluation and treatment.

Reference

1. Sackett DL, Straws SE, Richardson WS, Rosenberg W, Haynes RB. *Evidence-Based Medicine: How to Practice and Teach EBM*. 2nd ed. London: Harcourt Publishers Limited; 2000.

ACKNOWLEDGMENTS

I would like to acknowledge the many people who have contributed so greatly to the creation of this text.

- I would first like to thank Icon Learning Systems for providing me with the opportunity to write my first book.

- I send my gratitude to the staff at Franklin Pierce College Library, including Jill Wixom, Mary Ley, Lisa Wiley, Beth Pollock, Tim Bigelow, and Anne Power, who spent so much time during the spring and summer of 2004 acquiring interlibrary loans for this project.

- I would like to thank the following persons for reviewing the text before its publication and providing thoughtful suggestions for improvement: Anne Harrison, PT, PhD; Debbie Heiss, PT, PhD, OCS; Mark Erickson, PT, MA, OCS; Burke Gurney, PT, PhD; and Kornelia Kulig, PT, PhD.

- Three former students have earned my gratitude: Jessica Palmer for spending countless hours searching for references and for agreeing to be a model for the figures, and Sara Randall and Lindsey Browne for taking the photographs.

- This text would never have become a reality but for the mentors who have fostered my passion for evidence-based practice: Julie Whitman, PT, DSc, OCS, FAAOMPT; Julie Fritz, PT, PhD, ATC; John Childs, PT, PhD, MBA, OCS, FAAOMPT; Tim Flynn, PT, PhD, OCS, FAAOMPT; Matt Garber, PT, DSc, OCS, FAAOMPT; and Rob Wainner, PT, PhD, OCS, ECS, FAAOMPT.

- I am grateful for ongoing support from Jane Walter Venzke, PT, EdD, FAPTA, Associate Dean of Graduate Studies and Director of the Physical Therapy Program at Franklin Pierce College, and Diane Olimpio, PT, Director of Physical Therapy Rehabilitation Services at Concord Hospital, who have given me the opportunity to continue working toward my professional goals while remaining in New Hampshire.

- I would like to send a special thank you to Cathy Schult for sticking by me over the past 4 years as I worked, worked, and worked. Thanks for everything!

Joshua

The Reliability and Diagnostic Utility of the Orthopaedic Clinical Examination

Chapter 1

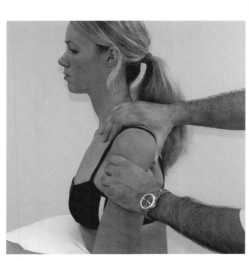

INTRODUCTION   The health sciences and medical professions are undergoing a paradigm shift toward evidence-based practice (EBP), defined as the integration of the best available research evidence and clinical expertise with the patient's values.[1, 2] Evidence should be incorporated into all aspects of physical therapy in patient and client management, including examination, evaluation, diagnosis, prognosis, and intervention. Perhaps the most crucial component is a careful, succinct clinical examination that can lead to an accurate diagnosis, the selection of appropriate interventions, and determination of a prognosis. Thus, the importance of incorporating evidence of the ability of clinical tests and measures to distinguish between patients who do and do not present with specific musculoskeletal disorders cannot go unrecognized.[1, 2]

The diagnostic process entails obtaining a patient history, developing a working hypothesis, and selecting specific tests and measures to confirm or refute the formulated hypothesis. The clinician must determine the pretest (before the evaluation) probability that the patient has a particular disorder. Based on this information, the clinician selects appropriate tests and measures that will help determine the posttest (after the evaluation) probability of the patient having the disorder, until a degree of certainty has been reached such that patient management can begin (the *treatment threshold*). The purpose of clinical tests is not to attain diagnostic certainty but rather to reduce the level of uncertainty until the treatment threshold is reached.[2] The concepts of pretest and posttest probability and treatment threshold will be elaborated later in this chapter. Valuable information can be obtained during each step in the examination process if the tests and measures that are selected exhibit diagnostic utility. Test results should be helpful to the clinician in determining the probability that the patient has a particular disorder. How do we know if a clinical test produces useful information? Determining this requires that the clinician understand the operating characteristics of individual clinical tests and measures.

Historically, textbooks that focus on the orthopaedic clinical examination have ignored the concept of diagnostic accuracy and have simply listed a multitude of tests. This implies that a positive result indicates that the patient has the disorder without consideration of the utility of specific tests. Many of these purportedly effective clinical tests exhibit such poor diagnostic accuracy that only 50% of patients who have a positive test result are found to have the disorder. Exaggerated results from poorly designed clinical tests can lead clinicians to make incorrect treatment decisions.[3] With the number of reported clinical tests and measures continuing to grow, it is essential that a test's diagnostic properties be thoroughly evaluated before it is incorporated into clinical practice.[4] Integration of the best evidence available for the diagnostic utility of each clinical test is essential in determining an accurate diagnosis and implementing effective, efficient treatment. It seems only sensible that clinicians and students should be aware of the diagnostic properties of tests and measures and should know which have clinical utility. The purpose of this text is to assist clinicians in selecting tests and measures that will ensure the appropriate classification of patients and will allow for quick implementation of effective management strategies.

With increased focus on EBP, studies undertaken to investigate the reliability and diagnostic utility of tests are becoming more common. However, the volume of literature makes it difficult for the busy clinician to obtain and analyze all the evidence necessary to guide the clinical examination. A recent study[5] revealed that in a sample of nearly 500 physical therapists, 90% strongly agreed that evidence-based perspectives are necessary for successful practice, 79% strongly agreed that EBP improves quality of care, and 72% believed that EBP assists in decision making. The primary barrier that restricts the integration of EBP was identified as insufficient time to locate the evidence. Poor access to evidence was also reported as a barrier.[6, 7]

The assessment of diagnostic tests involves examination of a number of properties, including reliability and diagnostic accuracy. A test is considered reliable if it produces precise, accurate, and reproducible information. A test is considered to have diagnostic accuracy if it has the ability to discriminate between patients with and without a specific disorder.[8] Scientific evaluation of the clinical utility of physical therapy tests and measures involves comparison of the examination results with reference standards such as radiographic studies (which represent the closest measure of the truth). With the use of statistical methods from the field of epidemiology, the diagnostic accuracy of the test—that is, its ability to determine which patients have the disorder and which do not—is then calculated. This chapter focuses on the characteristics that define the reliability and diagnostic accuracy of specific tests and measures. Chapter 2 focuses on educating the reader to enhance the skills needed to critique articles that investigate diagnostic utility.

Pretest probability is the likelihood that a patient exhibits a specific disorder before the clinical examination is performed. Often, prevalence rates are used as an indication of pretest probability, but in circumstances wherein prevalence rates are unknown, pretest probability is based on a combination of the patient's medical history, results of previous tests, and the clinician's experience.[9] Determination of pretest probability is the first step in the decision-making process for clinicians. Pretest probability is an estimate decided by the clinician that can be expressed as a percentage (eg, 75%, 80%) or as a qualitative measure (eg, somewhat likely, very likely).[9, 10] Once the pretest probability that a patient has a particular disorder is identified, tests and measures that have the potential to alter this probability should be selected for the physical examination. Posttest probability is the likelihood that a patient has a specific disorder after the clinical examination procedures have been performed.

For a clinical test to provide information that can be used to guide clinical decision making, it must be reliable. Reliability is the degree of consistency with which an instrument or rater measures a particular attribute.[11] When we investigate the reliability of a measurement, we are determining the proportion of that measurement that is a true representation and the proportion that is the result of measurement error.[12] Measurements can be affected by random error, which is a deviation from true measurement that occurs as a result of chance.[11]

Random errors may result from patient lability, instrument error, or human error on the part of the person who performs the test.[12] Error that is directly related to patient lability involves factors that can change the outcome of a measurement but that are not related to the variable of interest; this would include such factors as activity level. Consider what would happen if you were carrying out a research study to investigate the effects of hamstring stretching on straight-leg-raise measurements. During baseline measurements, your

RELIABILITY

subject takes the elevator to the data collection center on the 15th floor. However, at the second measurement, the subject runs up to the data collection center. Running up 15 flights of stairs certainly could result in a different straight-leg-raise measurement.

Errors may be associated with instrumentation or with clinical tests and measures. Tests should have well-established operational definitions so they can be performed in an identical fashion each time.[12] In addition, definitions for positive and negative test findings must be kept consistent. The results of a test may not be reliable if different persons are using different criteria for positive and negative results.

The clinical examination combines cognitive and psychomotor skills and presents numerous opportunities for the introduction of clinician error. For example, if a clinician applies inadequate force during a cervical compression test, the measurement might contain error (no symptom production) and be documented as a negative finding, whereas application of adequate force could produce the opposite result. It is essential that clinicians perform tests and measures exactly as the authors of the studies that have investigated their diagnostic utility have instructed. It is these descriptions that were studied to produce the reported diagnostic accuracy. If these are not followed precisely, random error could alter the outcome of the measurement obtained.

When the clinical examination process is discussed, two forms of reliability must be considered: intra-examiner and inter-examiner reliability. Intra-examiner reliability is a measure of the ability of a single rater to obtain the identical measurement during separate performances of the same test. Inter-examiner reliability is a measure of the ability of two or more raters to obtain identical results with the same test.

STATISTICAL CALCULATIONS

The statistical test selected to analyze data and determine the reliability of a measurement will vary according to the level of the measurement obtained from the test that is being investigated. Measurements can be applied on four levels: nominal, ordinal, interval, and ratio.

Nominal scale measurements are simply groupings in which no particular category has a greater value than any other. For example, a group of patients with low back and radicular pain may be categorized the same way as those with a herniated nucleus pulposus and those with lateral foraminal stenosis.

Ordinal measurements are also categorical, but they involve an ordering of the groups with a value placed on group assignments. In addition, ordinal levels do not include categories that are spaced equal distances apart. For example, it is better to have a manual muscle-testing grade of 5/5 than it is to have one of 3/5, and the difference in strength between a 5/5 and a 3/5 is not necessarily the same as that between a 3/5 and a 1/5 (unequal intervals between values).[12]

Interval levels of measurement have order with equal intervals, but they do not have an absolute zero point (the complete absence of a variable). The primary example of an interval scale would be degrees Celsius or Fahrenheit, wherein a zero on the scale does not equal the absence of temperature.[12, 13]

Ratio scales, by contrast, have order, equal distance between variables, and an absolute zero. An example of this would be the Kelvin scale, in which zero represents the absence of heat.[13] A common physical therapy example of a ratio scale would be range of motion, wherein zero indicates the absence of motion.[12] For a more detailed description of the scales of measurement, readers are referred to a text by Rothstein and Echternach entitled *Primer on Measurement: An Introductory Guide to Measurement Issues.*[12]

In the case of nominal or ordinal levels of measurement, percentage agreement is frequently used to calculate the percentage of time that clinicians agree on the results of a test or measure. However, calculation of percentage agreement does not take into account the proportion of agreement that may have occurred simply through chance. The kappa coefficient (κ) is a measure of the proportion of potential agreement after chance has been removed[1, 11, 13]; it is the reliability coefficient most often used for categorical data (positive or negative).[11] A statistic known as *weighted kappa* is frequently used if more than two categories exist, such as with a test that can be scored as hypomobile, normal, or hypermobile. In this instance, the investigator must also analyze disagreement because more possibilities of disagreement exist than in a test that is simply scored as either positive or negative.[14] It should be noted that kappa is not an optimal test because, although observed agreement is independent of prevalence, chance agreement is not. Hence, if the prevalence of disease is either very high or very low, the kappa value may be deflated.[15]

If data collected with the use of a test or measure involve interval or ratio measurements, then correlation coefficients are most often used to determine reliability. The two correlation coefficients commonly used are the Pearson and intraclass correlation coefficients (ICCs).[13] The Pearson correlation coefficient (r) is typically used when the investigator is trying to determine if an association exists between two measurements. More often, the appropriate statistic is the ICC, which is used to investigate the amount of variance between two or more repeated measurements.[16] A number of different ICC formulas can be used.[16] The formula selected varies according to the number of raters and the specific measurements obtained.

The following scale is often used to determine the strength of the coefficients (kappa and ICC) when reliability is calculated: below .50 represents poor reliability, .50 to .75 moderate reliability, and greater than .75 good reliability.[11] "Acceptable reliability" must be decided by the clinician who is using the specific test or measure.[15] This should be based on which variable is being tested, why a particular test is important, and on whom the test will be used.[12] When the strength of a relationship between two measures that have been analyzed with the Pearson correlation coefficient is evaluated, the scale ranges from -1 to 1. Negative values indicate an inverse relationship, positive values indicate a direct relationship, and zero demonstrates that no relationship exists.[17]

Many factors determine which tests a clinician selects; however, before a test is selected or implemented in clinical practice, an understanding of the test's operating characteristics must be attained. Is the measurement captured by the test useful? Does it alter the probability that a person has a particular disorder? The following section describes pretest and posttest probabilities, test characteristics that can shift probability (either negatively or positively), and epidemiologic statistics that assist the clinician in determining magnitude and direction in probability shifts.

Clinical tests and measures can never absolutely confirm or exclude the presence of a specific disease.[18] However, clinical tests can be used to alter the clinician's estimate of the probability that a patient has a specific musculoskeletal disorder. The accuracy of a test is

DIAGNOSTIC ACCURACY

assessed by determination of the measure of agreement between the clinical test and a reference standard.[10, 19] A reference standard is the criterion considered the closest representation of the truth that a disorder is present.[1] Results obtained with the reference standard are compared with those obtained with the use of the test under investigation; in this way, the percentage of people correctly diagnosed, or diagnostic accuracy, can be determined.[20] Diagnostic accuracy is often expressed in terms of positive and negative predictive values (PPVs and NPVs), sensitivity and specificity, and likelihood ratios (LRs).[1, 21]

2×2 Contingency Table

For determination of the clinical utility of a test or measure, the results of the reference standard are directly compared with those of the test under investigation with the use of a 2×2 contingency table.[22] This allows for the calculation of values associated with diagnostic accuracy that may assist the clinician in determining the utility of the clinical test under investigation *(Table 1–1)*.

The 2×2 contingency table is divided into four cells (a, b, c, d); this division allows for a determination of the test's ability to correctly identify true-positives (cell a) and rule out true-negatives (cell d). Cell b represents the false-positive findings in which the diagnostic test was found to be positive, yet the reference standard obtained a negative result. Cell c represents the false-negative findings, wherein the diagnostic test was found to be negative, yet the reference standard obtained a positive result.

The following is a fictitious example of how 2×2 contingency tables are used. A new test, the Palmer Pull test, has been purported to be effective in detecting anterior cruciate ligament (ACL) ruptures. This test has yet to be subjected to scientific scrutiny; therefore, its diagnostic accuracy is unknown. Diagnostic accuracy may be investigated with the use of a prospective, blind comparison of the Palmer Pull test and the reference standard—in this case, arthroscopic visualization. Recruited to participate in the study were 100 patients with knee pain and signs and symptoms that were possibly indicative of an ACL tear. Arthroscopic visualization identified 41 knees with ACL tears and 59 without. Data collected with the use of the Palmer Pull test are compared with those obtained through arthroscopic visualization *(Table 1–2)*.

At this stage, very little is known about the diagnostic accuracy of the Palmer Pull test, except that it accurately identified ACL tears (true-positives) in 29 cases and correctly ruled out an ACL tear in 49 cases (true-negative). In addition, the Palmer Pull test incorrectly clas-

	Reference Standard Positive	Reference Standard Negative
Clinical test positive	True-positive results a	False-positive results b
Clinical test negative	False-negative results c	True-negative results d

Table 1–1: *2×2 Contingency Table Used to Compare the Results of the Reference Standard With Those of the Test Under Investigation*

	Arthroscopic Visualizaton Positive (n = 41)		Arthroscopic Visualizaton Negative (n = 59)	
Palmer Pull test positive (n = 39)	29	a	b	10
Palmer Pull test negative (n = 61)	12	c	d	49

Table 1–2: *Comparison of Findings Obtained With Arthroscopic Visualization (the reference standard) and the Palmer Pull Test*

sified 10 patients as having an ACL tear (false-positives) and incorrectly identified 12 patients as not having an ACL tear (false-negatives). This preliminary information provides little indication of the clinical utility of the Palmer Pull test, and it does not assist the clinician in determining whether or not it should be incorporated into clinical practice.

Once a study undertaken to investigate the diagnostic utility of a clinical test has been completed and a comparison with the reference standard has been performed in the 2×2 contingency table, determination of clinical utility in terms of overall accuracy, PPVs and NPVs, sensitivity and specificity, and LRs can be calculated. These statistics will be useful to the clinician in determining if a diagnostic test is useful for ruling in or ruling out a disorder.

Overall Accuracy

The overall accuracy of a diagnostic test is determined by dividing the correct responses (true-positives and true-negatives) by the total number of patients.[9] Use of the 2×2 contingency table in determining overall accuracy includes the following equation:

$$\text{Overall accuracy} = 100\% \times (a + d)/(a + b + c + d)$$

When this principle is applied to the Palmer Pull test, the overall accuracy would be calculated as:

$$\text{Overall accuracy} = 100\% \times (29 + 49)/(29 + 10 + 12 + 49) = 78\%$$

A perfect test would exhibit an overall accuracy of 100%. This is most likely unattainable in that no clinical test is perfect, and each always exhibits at least a small degree of uncertainty. The accuracy of a diagnostic test should not be used to ascertain the clinical utility of that test because overall accuracy can be a bit misleading. The accuracy of a test can be significantly influenced by the prevalence, or total instances, of a disease in the population at a given time.[11, 12] Other statistics prove more useful in determining the usefulness of a clinical test or measure.

Positive and Negative Predictive Values

Positive predictive values estimate the likelihood that a patient with a positive test result actually has the disease.[11, 12, 23] PPVs, which are calculated horizontally in the 2×2 contingency table *(Table 1–3)*, indicate the percentage of patients accurately identified as having

	Reference Standard Positive	Reference Standard Negative	
Clinical test positive	True-positives a	False-positives b	PPV = a/a + b
Clinical test negative	False-negatives c	True-negatives d	NPV = d/c + d
	Sensitivity = a/a + c	Specificity = d/b + d	

Table 1–3: *2×2 Contingency Table Showing the Calculation of Positive and Negative Predictive Values Horizontally, and Sensitivity and Specificity Vertically*

the disorder (true-positive) divided by all the positive results of the test under investigation. A high PPV indicates that a positive result is a strong predictor that the patient has the disorder.[11, 12] The formula for calculating the PPV is:

$$PPV = 100\% \times a/(a + b)$$

NPVs estimate the likelihood that a patient with a negative test result does not have the disorder.[11, 12] NPVs are also calculated horizontally in the 2×2 contingency table (see *Table 1–3*) and indicate the percentage of patients accurately identified as not having the disorder (true-negative) divided by all the negative results of the test under investigation.[10] The formula for the NPV is as follows:

$$NPV = 100\% \times d/(c + d)$$

By applying these formulas to the Palmer Pull test, we determine the following:

$$PPV = 100\% \times 29/29 + 10 = 74\%$$

$$NPV = 100\% \times 49/12 + 49 = 80\%$$

We now know that when the Palmer Pull test is positive, we are 74% certain that the patient has an ACL tear, and when the Palmer Pull test is negative, we are 80% certain that the patient does not have an ACL tear.

Although the PPV and the NPV for the Palmer Pull test may appear useful in determining the presence or absence of an ACL tear, these values must be interpreted with caution.[24] Again, these data can be significantly altered according to the prevalence of the disorder.[1] Other statistics such as sensitivity and specificity may be of greater clinical value than the PPV and NPV values.

Sensitivity

The sensitivity of a diagnostic test indicates the test's ability to detect those patients who actually have the disorder, as indicated by the reference standard. This is also referred to as the true-positive rate.[1] Tests with high sensitivity are good for ruling out a particular disorder. The acronym SnNout can be used to remember that a test with high Sensitivity and a Negative result is good for ruling out the disorder.[1]

Consider, for example, a clinical test that, compared with the reference standard, exhibits a high sensitivity for detecting lumbar spinal stenosis. According to the rule above, if the test is negative, it reliably rules out lumbar spinal stenosis. If the test is positive, it is likely to accurately identify a high percentage of patients who present with stenosis. However, it also may identify as positive many of those without the disorder (false-positives). Thus, although a negative result can be relied on, a positive test result does not allow us to draw any conclusions *(Figure 1–1)*.

The sensitivity of a test also can be calculated from the 2×2 contingency table. However, it is calculated vertically (see *Table 1–3*). The formula for calculating a test's sensitivity is as follows:

$$\text{Sensitivity} = 100\% \times a/(a + c)$$

DIAGNOSTIC ACCURACY

Specificity

The specificity of a diagnostic test simply indicates the test's ability to detect those patients who actually do not have the disorder, as indicated by the reference standard. This is also

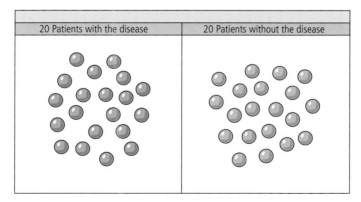

Figure 1–1: A. *20 patients with and 20 patients without the disorder.*

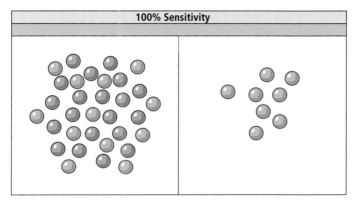

Figure 1–1: B. *100% sensitivity, inferring that if the test is positive, all those with the disease will be captured. However, note that although this test captured all those with the disease, it also captured many without. Yet, if the test is negative, we are confident that the disorder can be ruled out (SnNout).*

DIAGNOSTIC ACCURACY

referred to as the true-negative rate.[1] Tests with high specificity are good for ruling in a disorder. The acronym SpPin can be used to remember that a test with high Specificity and a Positive result is good for ruling in the disorder.[9, 25, 26]

Consider a test with high specificity. It would demonstrate a strong ability to accurately identify all patients who do not have the disorder. If a highly specific clinical test is negative, it is likely to identify a high percentage of those patients who do not have the disorder. However, it is also possible that the highly specific test with a negative result will identify as negative a number of patients who actually have the disease (false-negative). Therefore, we can be fairly confident that a highly specific test with a positive finding indicates that the disorder is present *(Figure 1–2)*.

The formula for calculating test specificity is as follows:

$$Specificity = 100\% \times d/(b + d)$$

By applying these principles to the Palmer Pull test, we calculate the sensitivity and specificity as follows *(Table 1–4)*:

$$Sensitivity = 100\% \times 29/(29 + 12) = 71\%$$

$$Specificity = 100\% \times 49/(10 + 49) = 83\%$$

We now see that the Palmer Pull test has a higher level of specificity than sensitivity, indicating greater diagnostic utility for ruling in an ACL tear (SpPin) than for ruling one out.

Sensitivity and specificity have been used for decades to determine a test's diagnostic utility; however, they are associated with a few clinical limitations.[10] Although sensitivity and specificity can be useful in assisting clinicians to select tests that are good for ruling in or out a particular disorder, few clinical tests demonstrate both high sensitivity and high specificity.[10] Also, sensitivity and specificity do not provide information regarding a change in the probability that a patient has a disorder if the test results are positive or negative.[17, 25] Instead, LRs have been advocated as the optimal statistics for determining a shift in the pretest probability that a patient has a specific disorder.

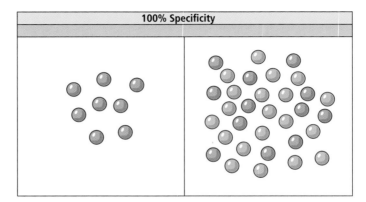

Figure 1–2: *100% specificity, inferring that if the test is negative, all those without the disease will be captured. However, note that although this test captured all those without the disease, it also captured many with. Yet, if the test is positive, we are confident that the patient has the disorder (SpPin).*

	Arthroscopic Visualizaton Positive (n = 41)	Arthroscopic Visualizaton Negative (n = 59)	
Palmer Pull test positive (n = 39)	True-positives = 29 a	False-positives = 10 b	PPV = 100 × 29/39 = 51%
Palmer Pull test negative (n = 61)	False-negatives = 12 c	True-negatives = 49 d	NPV = 100 × 49/61 = 80%
	Sensitivity = 100 × 29/41 = 71%	Specificity = 100 × 49/59 = 83%	

Table 1–4: *Calculation of Predictive Values and the Sensitivity and Specificity of the Palmer Pull Test*

Likelihood Ratios

A test's result is valuable only if it alters the pretest probability that a patient has a disorder.[27] LRs combine a test's sensitivity and specificity to indicate the shift of probability, given the specific test result; they are valuable in guiding clinical decision making.[17] LRs are a powerful measure that can significantly increase or reduce the probability that a patient has a disease.[28]

LRs can be positive or negative. A positive LR indicates a shift in probability that favors the existence of a disorder; a negative LR indicates a shift in probability that favors the absence of a disorder. Although LRs often are not reported in studies undertaken to investigate the diagnostic utility of the clinical examination, they can be calculated easily if a test's sensitivity and specificity are available. Throughout this text, for studies that did not report LRs but that did document a test's sensitivity and specificity, LRs that have been calculated by the author are provided.

The formula used to determine a positive LR is as follows:

$$\text{Positive LR} = \text{Sensitivity}/(1 - \text{Specificity})$$

The formula used to determine a negative LR is as follows:

$$\text{Negative LR} = (1 - \text{Sensitivity})/\text{Specificity}$$

A guide to interpreting test results can be found in Table 1–5. Positive LRs >1 increase the odds of a disorder given a positive test, and negative LRs <1 decrease the odds of a disorder given a negative test.[28] However, it is the magnitude of the shifts in probability that determines the usefulness of a clinical test. Positive LRs >10 and negative LRs close to zero often represent large and conclusive shifts in probability. An LR of 1 (either positive or negative), which does not alter the probability that the patient does or does not have the particular disorder, is of little clinical value.[28] Once the LRs have been calculated, they can be applied to the nomogram[29] *(Figure 1–3)*, or a mathematical equation[30] can be used to determine more precisely the shifts in probability given a specific test result. Both of these methods are described in further detail later in the chapter.

Positive Likelihood Ratio	Negative Likelihood Ratio	Interpretation Ratio
Greater than 10	Less than 0.1	Generate large and often conclusive shifts in probability
5–10	0.1–0.2	Generate moderate shifts in probability
2–5	0.2–0.5	Generate small but sometimes important shifts in probability
1–2	0.5–1	Alter probability to a small and rarely important degree

Table 1–5: *Interpretation of Likelihood Ratios*[28]

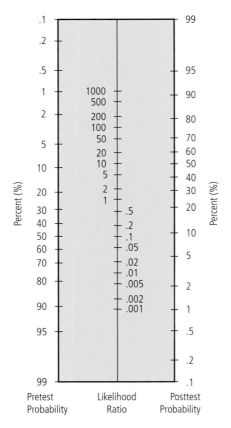

Figure 1–3: *Nomogram.*
Nomogram adapted with permission, Massachusetts Medical Society, Copyright 2005.

By applying the principles of LRs to the Palmer Pull test, we calculate the following:

$$\text{Positive LR} = .71/(1 - .83) = 4.2$$

$$\text{Negative LR} = (1 - .71)/.83 = .35$$

According to the established guidelines,[28] if the LR is found to be positive, the Palmer Pull test would generate small shifts in probability (4.1), and if it is found to be negative (.36), the Palmer Pull test would generate small, but perhaps clinically important, shifts in probability.

If a diagnostic test exhibits a specificity of 1, the positive LR cannot be calculated because the equation will result in a zero for the denominator. In these circumstances, it has been suggested that the 2×2 contingency table be modified by the addition of .5 to each cell in the table; this would allow for the calculation of LRs.[31]

Consider, for example, the diagnostic utility of the Crank test[11, 32] in detecting labral tears compared with arthroscopic examination, the reference standard. This is revealed in a 2×2 contingency table *(Table 1–6)*. The inability to calculate a positive LR becomes obvious when we set up the formula. In this circumstance, we have the following:

$$\text{Positive LR} = \text{Sensitivity}/(1 - \text{Specificity}) = 1/(1 - 1) = 1/0$$

We cannot have a fraction with zero as the denominator, so we will modify the 2×2 contingency table by adding .5 to each cell *(Table 1–7)*.

It should be recognized that addition of .5 to each cell could modify the results of many of the properties of diagnostic accuracy. For example, in this case, when .5 is added to each cell, the PPV changed from 100% to 95%. The NPV changed from 60% to 58%. The sensitivity was 83% before the 2×2 contingency table was modified, and afterward, it was 81%. Perhaps of greatest relevance is the significant change in specificity associated with this modification. The specificity was originally 100%, and it dropped to 87% with the addition of .5 to each cell.

	Arthroscopic Examination Positive (n = 12)	Arthroscopic Examination Negative (n = 3)	
Crank test positive	10 a	0 b	Positive predictive value = 100% × 10/10 = 100%
Crank test negative	2 c	3 d	Negative predictive value = 100% × 3/5 = 60%
	Sensitivity = 100% × 10/12 = 83%	Specificity = 100% × 3/3 = 100%	

Table 1–6: *Results of the Crank Test in Detecting Labral Tears When Compared With the Reference Standard of Arthroscopic Examination*[32]

	Arthroscopic Examination Positive (n = 12)	Arthroscopic Examination Negative (n = 3)	
Crank test positive	10.5 a	0.5 b	Positive predictive value = 100% × 10.5/11 = 95%
Crank test negative	2.5 c	3.5 d	Negative predictive value = 100% × 3.5/6 = 58%
	Sensitivity = 100% × 10.5/13 = 81%	Specificity = 100% × 3.5/4 = 87.5%	

Table 1–7: *Modification of the 2×2 Contingency Table to Allow for the Calculation of Positive Likelihood Ratio*

Although the addition of .5 to each cell is the only reported method of modifying the contingency table to prevent zero in the denominator of an LR calculation, when the changes that occur with the diagnostic properties of sensitivity, specificity, and predictive value are considered, this technique has not been used in this text. In circumstances in which the specificity is zero and the positive LR cannot be calculated, it will be documented as not available (NA). The reader should understand that, although we are not calculating the positive LR in this circumstance, the test will be indicative of a large shift in probability.

Hypothetically, let us use the 2×2 data before we modified them, from the study that investigated the diagnostic accuracy of the Crank test. The specificity was a perfect 100%, which did not allow us to calculate a positive LR. However, if we say that the specificity was not perfect (but close) at 99%, we can now calculate the positive LR as follows:

Positive LR = Sensitivity/(1 − Specificity) = .83/(1 − .99) = 83

Clearly, a positive LR of 83 is significant and would result in a major shift in the pretest probability that a patient has a disorder. However, this circumstance occurred in the presence of a high sensitivity as well. Consider the same circumstance with a lower sensitivity of 25%. We then would have the following formula:

Positive LR = Sensitivity/(1 − Specificity) = .25/(1 − .99) = 25

We still have a positive LR that would result in a considerable shift in pretest probability if the test were found to be positive. Therefore, although the positive LR cannot be mathematically calculated, we can assume that the shift in probability with a test that exhibits 100% specificity will be considerable.

Calculations of sensitivity, specificity, and LR are usually reported as point estimates, that is, they are single values that are representative of a sample of the population.[11] It is often more meaningful to have an interval estimate of the population that indicates the range in which all values of the population would fall.[11] One such estimate is known as the confidence interval (CI)—a range of scores around the standard error of measure that represents the boundaries within which all members of the population would be expected to fall.[33]

Since 1985, CIs have become a regular addition to research articles published in medical journals.[33] Although CIs were often reported in research articles, only recently have investigators begun to use them appropriately in the interpretation of data and the discussion of research results.[34] CIs are a measure of how precise an estimate is. Commonly, the 95% CI is calculated for studies undertaken to investigate the diagnostic utility of the clinical examination. A 95% CI indicates the spread of scores within which 95% of the population would be expected to fall.[11] The closer the boundaries are to the point estimate, the closer the data spread.[11] 95% CIs are reported in this text for all studies that provided this information.

The diagnostic utility of tests and measures is most commonly evaluated with the use of a 2×2 contingency table and the calculation of values for sensitivity, specificity, and LR. However, some studies investigate the correlation between a positive finding on a test or measure and the findings of the reference standard by subjecting the results to statistical tests to determine whether a relationship exists between the findings. A number of statistical procedures may be used, and a detailed description of these is beyond the scope of this text. With the use of correlational statistics, a significant relationship is considered to exist when probability (p) values are <0.05. A probability value <0.05 infers that there is a 95% probability that a true relationship exists between results of the outcome measures.[9]

As has previously been mentioned, LRs can assist the clinician in determining shifts in probability that would occur after a given test result has been obtained, according to the respective LR ratios of that given test. The quickest method of determining shifts in probability once an LR for a specific test is known is use of the nomogram[29] (see *Figure 1–3*). The nomogram is a diagram that illustrates pretest probability on the left and posttest probability on the right. In the middle are the LRs. When the shift in probability is determined, a mark is placed on the nomogram to represent pretest probability. Then, a mark is made on the nomogram at the level of the LR (either negative or positive). The two lines are connected with a straight edge, and the line is carried through the right of the diagram. The point at which the line crosses the posttest probability scale indicates the shift in probability.

For the Palmer Pull test, consider a pretest probability of 42%. We can apply the following results to the nomogram and investigate the posttest probability that a patient has the disorder, given a positive or a negative test result *(Figure 1–4)*.

A more precise determination of the shift in probability can be calculated algebraically with the use of the following formula[9]:

Step 1. Pretest odds = Pretest probability/1 − Pretest probability

Step 2. Pretest odds × LR = Posttest odds

Step 3. Posttest odds/Posttest odds + 1 = Posttest probability

When the calculation is applied to the Palmer Pull test, the following occurs:

Step 1. Pretest odds = .42/1 − .42 = .72

CALCULATING POSTTEST PROBABILITY

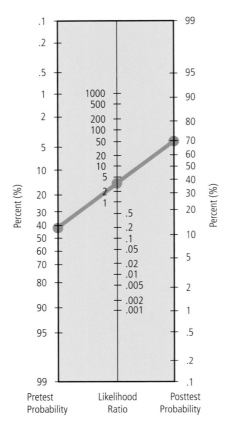

Figure 1–4: *Nomogram representing the change in pretest probability from 42% if the test was positive (positive likelihood ratio = 4.2) to a posttest probability of 71%.*

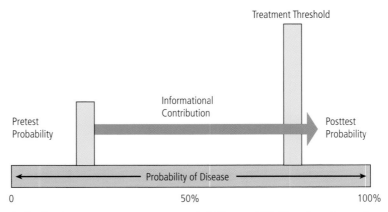

Figure 1–5: *Clinicians must use pretest probability and likelihood ratios to determine the treatment threshold, as indicated in this illustration.*

Step 2. $.72 \times 4.2 = 3.0$

Step 3. $3.0/(3.0 + 1) = .75$

The posttest probability that the patient will exhibit an ACL tear when the Palmer Pull test is positive is 75%.

The clinician must decide when the posttest probability is low enough to rule out the presence of a certain disease so that other alternatives should be investigated, or when the posttest probability is high enough that the presence of the disorder can be established with confidence. The level at which evaluation ceases and treatment begins is known as the treatment threshold *(Figure 1–5).*[9]

Often in clinical situations, test results do not stand alone, that is, the findings of multiple tests and measures are collected for determination of the probability that a patient has a specific disorder. A recent trend in the literature has shown an increase in the use of clinical prediction rules. Clinical prediction rules are tools used by clinicians to (1) determine the likelihood that a patient is presenting with a given disorder, based on a number of variables that have been shown to have predictive validity in revealing patients most likely to have specific disorders,[21, 35] or (2) identify those most likely to benefit from a specific treatment strategy.[36]

Clinical prediction rules may be used to enhance the clinician's accuracy in predicting a diagnosis or in determining appropriate management strategies. For example, a number of clinical prediction rules have been developed to improve the accuracy of clinicians in (1) identifying ankle or knee fractures after an injury,[37–40] (2) determining the need for cervical radiographs after neck trauma,[41–43] (3) assessing the likelihood of cervical radiculopathy presentation,[31] (4) considering the possible benefit a patient may gain from nonarthroplasty knee surgery,[44] and (5) determining the likelihood that a manipulation technique will reduce disability in a patient with low back pain.[36, 45] Clinical prediction rules are calculated through the use of the diagnostic properties previously mentioned, including sensitivity, specificity, and positive and negative LRs.

The development of clinical prediction rules that can be readily and accurately applied across a variety of settings by clinicians with varying experiences entails a multistep process. The first step in this process involves development of the rule. This requires the identification of variables that may be used to predict the probability that a disorder will occur, or that may predict an effective and efficient management strategy.[46] After these predictor variables have been identified, a prediction rule is developed.[21] Once the prediction rule has been established, the rule must then be validated.[21]

Validation entails investigating the accuracy of a clinical prediction rule in a different group of patients, with clinical tests performed by clinicians other than those who developed the rule.[21] Validation must occur in a variety of settings to enhance the rule's generalizability.[21] To further establish the usefulness of clinical prediction rules, an impact analysis must be performed to establish what impact the rule has had on changing clinical behaviors, and to assess whether or not economic benefits have resulted.

Clinical prediction rules can significantly enhance a clinician's abilities in detecting the presence of disease and in categorizing patients into classifications. Clinical prediction rules that are applicable to the orthopaedic population are included in this text.

CASE STUDY

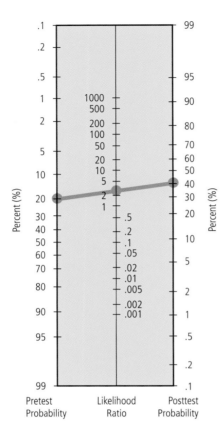

Figure 1–6: *If an investigator performs a test with a positive likelihood ratio of 2.33 on a patient with a pretest probability of 20% and receives a positive result, the probability is increased to only 37%.*

You are working in a sports medicine clinic at a local university, and most of your patients are athletes (both competitive and recreational). A 19-year-old baseball pitcher presents to your clinic with right shoulder pain of 3 months' duration. He notes that his symptoms are exacerbated during any overhand throwing motion, and he reports that he hears a "click" in his shoulder during the wind-up phase of pitching. Your experience is that approximately 20% of the baseball pitchers with shoulder pain that your clinic treats exhibit a labral tear. Therefore, your pretest probability is 20%.

You want to further investigate the likelihood that this particular patient is presenting with a labral tear. You must select from among a few special tests to further investigate your working hypothesis, and you first consider the O'Brien test, as described by Guanche and Jones[47] (see Chapter 10, page 394). When you investigate the diagnostic utility of the O'Brien test, as described by Guanche and Jones,[47] you realize that the test exhibits a positive LR of 2.33. Therefore, if you select the O'Brien test and determine the test to be positive, according to an LR of 2.33, the posttest probability that your patient presents with a labral tear would be 37% *(Figure 1–6)*. You realize that this test would not provide adequate clinical information, and you would continue to have significant uncertainty regarding the presence of a labral tear in your patient.

You decide to consider the use of another special test that, if the findings are determined to be positive, might reveal a greater probability that the patient is presenting with a labral

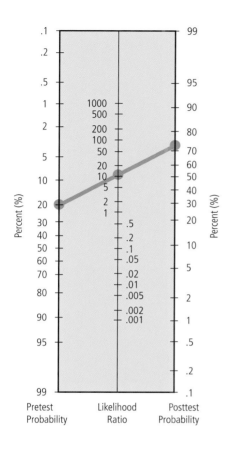

Pretest
Probability

Likelihood
Ratio

Posttest
Probability

Figure 1–7: *If an investigator performs a test with a positive likelihood ratio of 10.0 on a patient with a pretest probability of 20% and receives a positive result, the probability is increased to 71%.*

tear. This time, you investigate the diagnostic utility of the pain provocation test, as described by Mimori et al.[32] (see Chapter 10, page 396). You realize that Mimori et al.[32] investigated the diagnostic utility of this test in a group of athletes who reported pain with overhand throwing, which allows the results of their findings to be directly generalized to your patient. The positive LR for this test is 10.0. If you find the test to be positive, and the pretest probability of 20% is taken into consideration, the posttest probability would be 71% *(Figure 1–7)*. Bearing in mind the greater diagnostic utility of the pain provocation test, as described by Mimori et al.,[32] and the generalizability of their findings to your specific patient, you decide to use this test rather than the O'Brien.

SUMMARY

The reliability and diagnostic utility of tests and measures must be considered before they are included as components of the clinical examination. Tests and measures should demonstrate adequate reliability before they are used to guide clinical decision making. Throughout this text, data on the reliability of many tests and measures are reported. It is essential that clinicians consider these reported levels of reliability in the context of their own practice.

Before tests and measures are incorporated into the orthopaedic examination, the diagnostic utility of each test must be considered. Table 1–8 summarizes the statistics related to

	Reference Standard Positive	Reference Standard Negative
Diagnostic test positive	True-positive results a	False-positive results b
Diagnostic test negative	False-negative results c	True-negative results d

Statistic	Formula	Description
Overall accuracy	$(a + d)/(a + b + c + d)$	Percentage of patients who are correctly diagnosed
Sensitivity	$a/(a + c)$	Proportion of patients with the condition who have a positive test result
Specificity	$d/(b + d)$	Proportion of patients without the condition who have a negative test result
Positive predictive value	$a/(a + b)$	Proportion of patients with a positive test result who have the condition
Negative predictive value	$d/(c + d)$	Proportion of patients with a negative test result who do not have the condition
Positive likelihood ratio	Sensitivity/(1 − Specificity)	If the test is positive, the increase in odds favoring the condition
Negative likelihood ratio	(1 − Sensitivity)/Specificity	If the test is positive, the decrease in odds favoring the condition

Table 1–8: *2×2 Contingency Table and Statistics Used to Determine the Diagnostic Utility of a Test or Measure*

diagnostic accuracy, as well as the mathematical equations and operational definitions that pertain to each. The usefulness of a test or measure is most commonly considered in terms of the respective test's diagnostic properties. These can be described in terms of sensitivity, specificity, PPVs, and NPVs. However, perhaps the most useful diagnostic property is LRs, which can assist in altering the probability that a patient has a specific disorder.

No clinical test or measure provides absolute certainty as to the presence or absence of disease. However, clinicians can determine when enough data have been collected to alter the probability beyond the treatment threshold, at which point evaluation can cease and therapeutic management can begin.

1. Sackett DL, Straws SE, Richardson WS, Rosenberg W, Haynes RB. *Evidence-Based Medicine: How to Practice and Teach EBM*. 2nd ed. London: Harcourt Publishers Limited; 2000.

2. Kassirer JP. Our stubborn quest for diagnostic certainty: a cause of excessive testing. *N Eng J Med*. 1989;320:1489–1491.

3. Bossuyt P. The quality of reporting in diagnostic test research: getting better, still not optimal. *Clin Chem*. 2004;50:465–467.

4. Lijmer JG, Mol BW, Heisterkamp S, et al.. Empirical evidence of design-related bias in studies of diagnostic tests. *JAMA*. 1999;282:1061–1063.

5. Jette DU, Bacon K, Batty C, et al.. Evidence-based practice beliefs, attitudes, knowledge, and behaviors of physical therapists. *Phys Ther*. 2003;83:786–805.

6. Haynes B, Haines A. Barriers and bridges to evidence based clinical practice. *BMJ*. 1998;317:273–276.

7. Maher CG, Sherrington C, Elkins M, Herbert RD, Moseley AM. Challenges for evidence-based physical therapy: accessing and interpreting high-quality evidence on therapy. *Phys Ther*. 2004;84:644–654.

8. Schwartz JS. Evaluating diagnostic tests: what is done—what needs to be done. *J Gen Intern Med*. 1986;1:266–267.

9. Bernstein J. Decision analysis. *J Bone Joint Surg Am*. 1997;79:1404–1414.

10. Fritz JM, Wainner RS. Examining diagnostic tests: an evidence based perspective. *Phys Ther*. 2001;81:1546–1564.

11. Portney LG, Watkins MP. *Foundations of Clinical Research: Applications to Practice*. 2nd ed. Upper Saddle River, NJ: Prentice Hall Health; 2000.

12. Rothstein JM, Echternach JL. *Primer on Measurement: An Introductory Guide to Measurement Issues*. Alexandria, Va: American Physical Therapy Association; 1999.

13. Domholdt E. *Physical Therapy Research*. 2nd ed. Philadelphia, Pa: WB Saunders; 2000.

14. Gjorup T. Reliability of diagnostic tests. *Acta Obstet Gynecol Scand*. 1997;166:9–14.

15. Van Genderen F, De Bie R, Helders P, Van Meeteren N. Reliability research: towards a more clinically relevant approach. *Phys Ther Rev*. 2003;8.

16. Shrout PE, Fleiss JL. Intraclass correlations: uses in assessing rater reliability. *Psych Bull*. 1979;86:420–428.

17. Hayden SR, Brown MD. Likelihood ratio: a powerful tool for incorporating the results of a diagnostic test into clinical decision making. *Ann Emerg Med*. 1999;33:575–580.

18. Bossuyt PMM, Reitsma JB, Bruns DE, et al.. Towards complete and accurate reporting of studies of diagnostic accuracy: the STARD initiative. *Clin Chem*. 2003;49:1–6.

19. Jaeschke R, Guyatt GH, Sackett DL III. How to use an article about a diagnostic test. Are the results of the study valid? *JAMA*. 1994;271:389–391.

20. Bossuyt PMM, Reitsma JB, Bruns DE, et al.. The STARD statement for reporting studies of diagnostic accuracy: explanation and elaboration. *Clin Chem*. 2003;49:7–18.

21. McGinn T, Guyatt G, Wyer P, Naylor C, Stiell I, Richardson W. Users' guides to the medical literature XXII: how to use articles about clinical decision rules. *JAMA*. 2000;284:79–84.

22. Greenhalgh T. Papers that report diagnostic or screening tests. *BMJ*. 1997;315:540–543.

23. Potter NA, Rothstein JM. Intertester reliability for selected clinical tests of the sacroiliac joint. *Phys Ther*. 1985;65:1671–1675.

24. Hagen MD. Test characteristics: how good is that test? *Prim Care*. 1995;22:213–233.

REFERENCES

25. Boyko EJ. Ruling out or ruling in disease with the most sensitive or specific diagnostic test: short cut or wrong turn? *Med Decis Making.* 1994;14:175–180.

26. Riddle DL, Stratford PW. Interpreting validity indexes for diagnostic tests: an illustration using the Berg balance test. *Phys Ther.* 1999;79:939–948.

27. Simel DL, Samsa GP, Matchar DB. Likelihood ratios with confidence: sample size estimation for diagnostic test studies. *J Clin Epidemiol.* 1991;44:763–770.

28. Jaeschke R, Guyatt GH, Sackett DL III. How to use an article about a diagnostic test. B. What are the results and will they help me in caring for my patients? *JAMA.* 1994;271:703–707.

29. Fagan TJ. Nomogram for Bayes's theorem. *N Engl J Med.* 1975;293:257.

30. Sackett DL, Haynes RB, Guyatt GH, Tugwell P. *Clinical Epidemiology: A Basic Science for Clinical Medicine.* Boston: Little, Brown and Company; 1991.

31. Wainner RS, Fritz JM, Irrgang JJ, Boninger ML, Delitto A, Allison A. Reliability and diagnostic accuracy of the clinical examination and patient self-report measures for cervical radiculopathy. *Spine.* 2003;28:52–62.

32. Mimori K, Muneta T, Nakagawa T, Shinomiya K. A new pain provocation test for superior labral tears of the shoulder. *Am J Sports Med.* 1999;27:137–142.

33. Fidler F, Thomason N, Cumming G, Finch S, Leeman J. Editors can lead researchers to confidence intervals, but can't make them think. *Psychol Sci.* 2004;15:119–126.

34. Sackett DL. A primer on the precision and accuracy of the clinical examination. *JAMA.* 1992;267:2638–2644.

35. Laupacis A, Sekar N, Stiell IG. Clinical prediction rules: a review and suggested modifications of methodological standards. *JAMA.* 1997;277:488–494.

36. Flynn T, Fritz J, Whitman J, et al.. A clinical prediction rule for classifying patients with low back pain who demonstrate short term improvement with spinal manipulation. *Spine.* 2002;27:2835–2843.

37. Stiell IG, Greenberg GH, Wells GA, et al.. Prospective validation of a decision rule for the use of radiography in acute knee injuries. *JAMA.* 1996;275:611–615.

38. Stiell IG, McKnight DR, McDowell I, et al.. Implementation of the Ottawa Ankle Rules. *JAMA.* 1994;271:827–832.

39. Stiell I, Greenberg G, Wells G, et al.. Prospective validation of a decision rule for the use of radiography in acute injuries. *JAMA.* 1996;275:611–615.

40. Stiell I, Greenberg G, Wells G, et al.. Derivation of a decision rule for the use of radiography in acute knee injuries. *Ann Emerg Med.* 1995;26:405–413.

41. Stiell IG, Wells GA, Vandemheen KL, et al. The Canadian C-spine rule for radiography in alert and stable trauma patients. *JAMA.* 2001;286:1841–1848.

42. Stiell IG, Lesiuk H, Wells GA, et al. The Canadian CT Head Rule Study for patients with minor head injury: rationale, objectives, and methodology for phase I (derivation). *Ann Emerg Med.* 2001;38:160–169.

43. Stiell IG, Wells GA, Vandemheen K, et al. The Canadian CT Head Rule for patients with minor head injury. *Lancet.* 2001;357:1391–1396.

44. Solomon D, Avorn J, Warsi A, et al. Which patients with knee problems are likely to benefit from nonarthroplasty surgery? Development of a clinical prediction rule. *Arch Intern Med.* 2004;164:509–513.

45. Childs J, Fritz J, Flynn T, et al. Validation of a clinical prediction rule to identify patients with low back pain likely to benefit from spinal manipulation: a randomized controlled trial. *Ann Intern Med.* 2004;141:920–928.

46. Laupacis A, Sekar N, Stiell I. Clinical prediction rules: a review and suggested modifications of methodological standards. *JAMA.* 1997;277:488–494.

47. Guanche CA, Jones DC. Clinical testing for tears of the glenoid labrum. *Arthroscopy.* 2003;19:517–523.

Identification and Analysis of Articles Investigating the Diagnostic Utility of Clinical Tests and Measures

Chapter 2

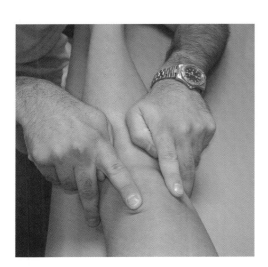

INTRODUCTION

Selecting the most appropriate tests and measures for incorporation into the clinical examination on the basis of available evidence can be daunting. New tests and measures are continually being developed and reported without consideration of their diagnostic utility. Too often, students and clinicians integrate new clinical examination techniques into clinical practice without regard for their ability to alter diagnostic probability. They may believe they do not have time for an evidence search, or they may be unable to access adequate search strategies. However, the diagnostic utility of a test always must be considered before it is incorporated into clinical practice.[1, 2]

This text has been written to describe the diagnostic properties of tests and measures that are currently used in clinical practice. This chapter focuses on efficient research strategies and methods for literature analysis so that clinicians can make accurate judgments regarding the diagnostic utility of new and established tests.

THE LITERATURE SEARCH

Development of accurate and efficient search strategies is crucial if the best available evidence is to be located in the literature. A few of the most commonly used search engines include Medline, Excerpta Medica (EMBASE), and the Cumulative Index of Nursing and Allied Health Literature (CINAHL).

Medline

Medline is the most widely used medical database. It contains more than 7 million references, lists more than 3500 journals, and is indexed by the US National Library of Medicine's Medical Subject Headings (MeSH) vocabulary.[3] MeSHs are biomedical terms that designate major concepts within the database.[4] Each new citation added to Medline is indexed with a number of MeSHs, which then distribute specific citations into smaller databases within Medline.

Medline queries can be performed with the use of pertinent MeSHs or keywords. Keyword searches involve the use of one or more words from the article's title or abstract. MeSHs are linked to both directly associated and closely associated articles within the database. Combining MeSHs and keywords in a search query yields the most sensitive search results (ie, ability to detect all citations in the database) in Medline, when compared with searching by either keywords or MeSHs.[3]

EMBASE

EMBASE is an electronic bibliographic database produced by Elsevier Science. EMBASE, which is considered one of the major biomedical databases, covers more than 3800 journals. One advantage of EMBASE over Medline is the higher prevalence of European journals.[5] Search strategies for EMBASE are similar to those recommended for Medline.[5]

Cumulative Index of Nursing and Allied Health Literature

The CINAHL database was developed in 1956 specifically for health care providers other than physicians.[6] CINAHL includes citations from 950 journals and publications, as well as from textbooks.[6] Keywords are used to search this database.[7]

Database searches do not retrieve only pertinent article citations related to keywords or MeSH headings. Search engines have various levels of recall and precision. Recall is the percentage of relevant citations identified through keyword searching compared with the number of relevant citations within the database.[4] The formula for calculating recall is as follows:

Recall = Number of relevant citations retrieved/Number of relevant citations in the database

Recall can be considered the sensitivity of a search, that is, recall describes how likely it is that a specific search strategy will be able to select key relevant articles from all the relevant articles available.[4] Recall is important to those who attempt to efficiently identify specific evidence without spending hours perusing study abstracts.[8]

The precision of a search refers to the percentage of relevant citations accurately identified compared with the total citations retrieved.[4] Precision can be likened to positive predictive value: of all those results identified as relevant (positive) by the search engine, what percentage actually are relevant (ie, actually discuss the disorder)?[3] Precision is often of greatest importance to persons who are performing an extensive review of the literature. It can be calculated with the following formula[4, 8]:

Precision = Number of relevant citations retrieved/Total number of citations retrieved

During a search in Medline for articles related to diagnostic utility, the most accurate searches entailed the keywords *sensitivity, specificity, false-negative,* and *accuracy*.[9] This search strategy exhibited a recall of 80% and a precision of 48%.[9]

The "numbers needed to read" (NNR) is an indicator of the number of citations that may need to be read before one citation satisfying the search strategy is identified.[10] This is calculated by dividing 1/precision. Clinicians might find it intimidating that well-developed searches in EMBASE have resulted in an NNR of 27, with the boundaries of a 95% confidence interval ranging from 21.0 to 34.8.[10] This means that, for any search in EMBASE, the clinician may need to read 27 citations to identify a single relevant citation. When the 95% confidence intervals are taken into consideration, this could increase to as many as 34 citations.

Once relevant articles have been retrieved, the next step is critical analysis of their content for adequate methodologic rigor. It has been reported that the methodologic quality of studies undertaken to investigate the diagnostic utility of the clinical examination is inferior to that of studies investigating the effectiveness of therapies.[11, 12] Unfortunately, studies with significant methodologic flaws that report on the usefulness of specific tests and measures can lead to premature incorporation of ineffective tests. This can result in inaccurate diagnoses and poor patient management. Alternatively, identification and use of rigorously appraised clinical tests can improve patient care and outcomes.[12]

A group of scientists from a variety of disciplines recently formed the Standards for Reporting of Diagnostic Accuracy (STARD) Steering Committee for the purpose of improving the methodologic quality of studies that report on diagnostic accuracy.[13] The STARD Committee refers to the test that is undergoing scientific scrutiny as the "index" test. Diagnostic accuracy is described in terms of agreement between the results of this index test and those of a reference standard.[13] The group has developed a 25-item checklist for use in evaluating the scientific rigor of studies *(Table 2–1)*. This checklist was created by narrowing the results from an extensive search of the literature that revealed the presence of 33 methodologic scoring lists with 75 individual items.[13, 14] This checklist is divided into the components of title, introduction, methods, results, and discussion.

Section and topic	Item no.	
TITLE/ABSTRACT/ KEYWORDS	1	Identify the article as a study of diagnostic accuracy (recommend MeSH heading "sensitivity and specificity")
INTRODUCTION	2	State the research questions or study aims, such as estimating diagnostic accuracy or comparing accuracy between tests or across participant groups
METHODS		
Participants	3	Describe the study population: the inclusion and exclusion criteria, setting and locations where the data were collected
	4	Describe participant recruitment: was recruitment based on presenting symptoms, results from previous tests or the fact that the participants had received the index tests or the reference standard?
	5	Describe participant sampling: was the study population a consecutive series of participants defined by the selection criteria in items 3 and 4? If not, specify how participants were further selected
	6	Describe data collection: was data collection planned before the index test and reference standard were performed (prospective study) or after (retrospective study)?
Test methods	7	Describe the reference standard and its rationale
	8	Describe technical specifications of material and methods involved including how and when measurements were taken, and/or cite references for index tests and reference standard
	9	Describe definition of and rationale for the units, cutoffs and/or categories of the results of the index tests and the reference standard

Table 2–1: *Checklist for Articles That Report Diagnostic Accuracy*

Section and topic	Item no.	
	10	Describe the number, training and expertise of the persons executing and reading the index tests and the reference standard
	11	Describe whether or not the readers of the index tests and reference standard were blind (masked) to the results of the other test and describe any other clinical information available to the readers
Statistical methods	12	Describe methods for calculating or comparing measures of diagnostic accuracy, and the statistical methods used to quantify uncertainty (e.g. 95% confidence intervals)
	13	Describe methods for calculating test reproducibility, if done
RESULTS		
Participants	14	Report when study was done, including beginning and ending dates of recruitment
	15	Report clinical and demographic characteristics of the study population (e.g. age, sex, spectrum of presenting symptoms, co-morbidity, current treatments, recruitment centres)
	16	Report the number of participants satisfying the criteria for inclusion that did or did not undergo the index tests and/or the reference standard; describe why participants failed to receive either test (a flow diagram is strongly recommended)
Test results	17	Report time interval from the index tests to the reference standard, and any treatment administered between
	18	Report distribution of severity of disease (define criteria) in those with the target condition; other diagnoses in participants without the target condition

Table 2–1: *Checklist for Articles That Report Diagnostic Accuracy (cont.)*

Section and topic	Item no.	
	19	Report a cross-tabulation of the results of the index tests (including indeterminate and missing results) by the results of the reference standard; for continuous results, the distribution of the test results by the results of the reference standard
	20	Report any adverse events from performing the index tests or the reference standard
Estimates	21	Report estimates of diagnostic accuracy and measures of statistical uncertainty (e.g. 95% confidence intervals)
	22	Report how indeterminate results, missing responses and outliers of the index tests were handled
	23	Report estimates of variability of diagnostic accuracy between subgroups of participants, readers or centres, if done
	24	Report estimates of test reproducibility, if done
DISCUSSION	25	Discuss the clinical applicability of the study findings

Table 2–1: *Checklist for Articles That Report Diagnostic Accuracy (cont.)*

Reprinted with permission from Bossuyt P, Reitsma JB, Bruns DE, et al. Towards complete and accurate reporting of studies of diagnostic accuracy: the STARD Initiative. *Clin Chem.* 2003;49:1–6.

Title/Abstract/Keywords

The STARD group has recommended that articles investigating the diagnostic utility of tests for clinical examination should use the words "sensitivity" and "specificity" in their titles, abstracts, and keywords.[13, 14] Search strategies that used both these terms identified only 51% of the relevant citations; searches that used either sensitivity or specificity identified 41% and 35% of relevant citations, respectively, indicating that studies have not used these terms sufficiently.[9] Consistent use of these terms in article titles may improve the efficiency of search strategies, making it easier for clinicians to locate evidence related to the diagnostic utility of specific tests and measures.

Introduction

Similar to studies investigating the effectiveness of therapies, the introduction of the article should support the need for the study under investigation.[13–15] In addition, the purpose of the study should be stated clearly.

Methods

Population

Several factors should be considered when it is determined whether a study's results will be applicable to a clinician's practice. Is the patient population similar—including age, severity of the disorder, and duration of symptoms?[16] An explicit description of the patient population's characteristics and demographics should be included so that readers can compare their patient population with that used in the study. Demographic features (eg, sex, age, ethnicity) can have an association with test performance, typically affecting test sensitivity rather than specificity.[17] If population characteristics, including demographics, do not resemble those of the clinician's population, the results of the study may be of limited use.

When reading an article for diagnostic accuracy, the clinician should be careful to ensure that bias was not introduced into the sample selection. One of the most common forms of bias is spectrum bias.[18–20] To prevent bias, an appropriate spectrum of patients should include a group of patients likely to undergo the test during clinical examination and those with cases of varying degrees of severity of the disorder.

The following example of spectrum bias came from a study that investigated the diagnostic utility of the Cyriax capsular pattern of the hip for detecting osteoarthritis.[21] This study excluded patients in severe stages of osteoarthritis as confirmed by radiographs, thereby creating a spectrum of patients that included only those with mild to moderate cases of osteoarthritis. Because of this, the results of the study confirm the validity of the Cyriax capsular pattern in detecting only mild to moderate cases of osteoarthritis of the hip; the findings do not apply to the population as a whole.

Another form of spectrum bias occurs when researchers use a group of asymptomatic persons and a group of patients with the disorder of interest.[18, 22] Appropriate subject selection includes patients with the target disorder and those with disorders that would commonly be confused with the condition of interest.[23] Clearly, clinical tests should be selected for their ability to differentiate between competing disorders rather than between asymptomatic persons and those with a disorder.

Consider the previously mentioned study undertaken to investigate the diagnostic utility of the Cyriax capsular pattern of the hip in detecting osteoarthritis. Subject selection for this study included 100 patients with symptom-free hips, creating a second spectrum bias that could affect the validity of the study results.[22, 23]

It is plausible for a new clinical test to be studied initially in a group of symptomatic and asymptomatic patients so it can be determined whether the test is capable of differentiating between persons with the disorder and those who are asymptomatic. If a test cannot make this differentiation, it is probably not worth investigating further. If it can make this differentiation, then it merits further investigation in a group of patients with the disorder and a group of patients with other disorders that could be confused clinically with the disorder of interest.[11]

It has been suggested that a possible solution to spectrum bias (and the need for optimal design of studies investigating diagnostic accuracy) is the use of a prospective, blinded comparison of the new test and the reference test in a consecutive series of patients from a relevant clinical population.[22, 24] The STARD committee[13, 14] has developed a prospective flow diagram for the inclusion of patients, consecutive patient selection, and progression through the study; it describes when the test under investigation and the reference test should be performed *(Figure 2–1)*.

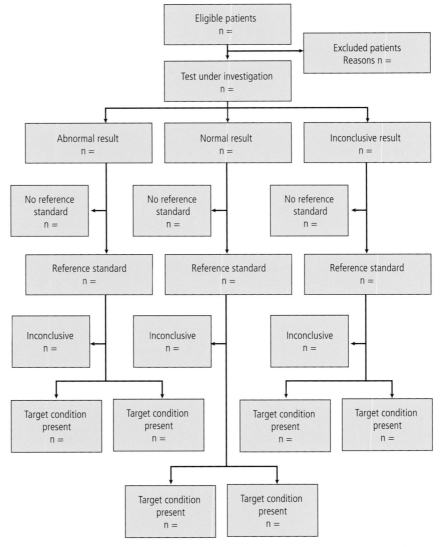

Figure 2–1: *Flow chart of a recommended sequence of carrying out a study of diagnostic accuracy. (Reprinted with permission from Bossuyt P, Reitsma JB, Bruns DE, et al. Towards complete and accurate reporting of studies of diagnostic accuracy: the STARD Initiative. Clin Chem. 2003;49:1–6.)*

Reference Standard

The reference standard, which is considered the "truth," is used to compare results of the test under investigation to determine its diagnostic accuracy.[16, 25] The reference standard should be clearly defined and should be the best method currently available for determining the presence of a disorder.[26] This does not mean that the reference standard is always completely accurate. Therefore, when the reference standard generates false-negatives or false-positives, this can alter the calculated diagnostic properties of the test under investigation. The validity of the reference standard should be discussed, or references should be provided to validate its ability to determine the "truth."

Studies also should note the order in which patients have been subjected to the test under investigation and the reference test.[23] The STARD group[13, 14] has suggested that patients should undergo examination with the use of the test under investigation before they are examined with the reference test, to prevent biasing of the test result caused by knowledge about the outcomes of the reference standard (see *Figure 2–1*).

Ethical issues can arise when the reference standard entails invasive procedures. In this circumstance, all subjects who warrant surgical intervention should be subjected to the reference standard (often arthroscopic visualization); those who do not warrant surgical intervention should not receive the reference standard. This has been referred to as verification bias or workup bias, and it occurs when only patients with positive findings on other tests undergo verification by the reference standard. This can significantly affect the evaluation of the diagnostic properties of the test under investigation.[12]

Consider the following investigation of a new pain provocation test for superior labral tears of the shoulder.[27] Researchers recruited 32 athletes who exhibited shoulder pain when throwing. The new pain provocation test was performed first; afterward, all athletes underwent magnetic resonance (MR) arthrography. MR arthrography results were compared with results of the pain provocation test, and the authors calculated the sensitivity and specificity of the pain provocation test based on the results of the MR arthrogram.

Although the authors reported that MR arthrography demonstrated greater diagnostic accuracy than did traditional MR imaging, the reference standard for identification of labral tears remains arthroscopic visualization.[28] The authors attempted to account for the possibility of false-negatives and false-positives diagnosed with the MR arthrogram by incorporating data from arthroscopic visualizations in 15 subjects who underwent surgical intervention after positive MR arthrogram findings were obtained. Results of the arthroscopic visualization were consistent with the MR arthrogram in all cases. However, this does not verify that the other 17 individuals (who did not undergo arthroscopy) had the same findings as the reference standard.

The possibility of false-negatives with the MR arthrogram had the potential to result in a workup bias that could lead to an underdiagnosis that may have resulted in escalated sensitivity.[29] However, in circumstances in which ethical issues prevent the use of the reference standard, such as with arthroscopic visualization, authors should use an alternative reference standard for comparison with the test under investigation, possibly creating a trade-off between ethics and the accuracy of results.[30] Authors investigating this new pain provocation test recognized this as a possible limitation to their study. In their defense, it may not be ethically possible to subject all persons undergoing the test under investigation to the reference standard when that standard entails an invasive procedure.

The Test Under Investigation

Studies investigating the diagnostic utility of a clinical test should describe the test procedure in explicit detail.[13, 14] They also should provide adequate descriptions of the intended use of the test, the exact physical performance of the test, and the scoring criteria.[22]

A test can be considered to produce results similar to those reported in a study only if it is performed under identical conditions and in the exact fashion outlined in the study.[22] If the test is performed differently than it was in the study, diagnostic properties could differ as well. For example, consider the diagnostic utility of the Neer test for identifying subacromial impingement. The Neer test, as described by one group of researchers, included elevation of the humerus.[31] The Neer test, as performed by a second group of researchers, entailed forced elevation in combination with internal rotation of the humerus.[32] These studies reported slightly different sensitivities and specificities. It is also essential that the scoring criteria for the test under investigation be clearly defined.[22] The article should include specific details as to what constitutes a positive and a negative score for the test under investigation.

As is shown in the STARD flow chart[13, 14] (see *Figure 2–1*), it is optimal for the test under investigation to be performed before the reference standard test is conducted because bias may be introduced when the results of a reference standard are known.[12] Knowledge of the results of the reference test has been reported to affect the outcome of the test under investigation, most often resulting in increased agreement between tests, which leads to artificially enhanced sensitivity and specificity for the test under investigation.[13, 14, 17]

One method for preventing this bias is the blinding of persons who are performing the test under investigation, as well as persons who are performing the reference test. Blinding of clinicians who are collecting data can considerably reduce the introduction of conscious or subconscious bias into test results.[15]

We must consider the fact that clinical examination techniques never stand alone. They are always affected by the patient's history, and their interpretation may vary on the basis of that history.[33] Therefore, it is possible that the diagnostic utility of a clinical examination reported alone might be underestimated when it is compared with the utility of the test in clinical circumstances in which other data can contribute to the overall clinical picture.

The reproducibility or reliability of a test under investigation can affect its diagnostic accuracy as well. It has been suggested that studies investigating diagnostic utility should subsequently investigate reliability.[13, 14] In addition, no clinical test stands alone, and perhaps we should consider the ability of a group of tests to alter the probability that a patient has a disorder.[33]

Consider the following study undertaken to investigate the reliability and diagnostic accuracy of the clinical examination in detecting cervical radiculopathy.[34] The authors investigated the reliability of the combined physical examination and historical questions while simultaneously investigating their diagnostic properties by comparing them with the reference standards of electromyography and nerve conduction studies. Results demonstrated that, when a combination of tests was used, the positive likelihood ratio was significantly greater than with any single test.

Generalizability should be considered when one is determining whether a clinical test is applicable to a particular patient population and setting. Each study should provide details about those who performed the clinical examination, including their background and previous training in performance of the test or measure. Was the study performed at one facility by highly trained clinicians? If so, this could result in a study's findings not being readily generalizable to all practice settings.[33] If this is the case, the diagnostic accuracy of the clinical test under investigation may require further validation in multiple settings with numerous examiners.[25]

Statistical Methods

Results of the clinical test under investigation should be compared with the reference standard in a 2×2 contingency table *(Table 2–2).*[19, 35] Once the 2×2 contingency table is complete, the diagnostic properties of positive and negative likelihood ratios, sensitivity, and specificity can be calculated. The likelihood ratio can be used to determine a shift in the probability that a patient has a particular disorder (see Chapter 1).

It is helpful for the study to report the 95% confidence intervals associated with the likelihood ratios.[18] The confidence interval provides an indication of the spread of scores likely to occur in 95% of the population, given the sample estimate of positive and negative likelihood ratios reported in the study. Articles with larger sample sizes typically present with smaller confidence intervals. Conversely, large 95% confidence intervals typically occur in studies with smaller sample sizes. In consideration of this, reports that indicate larger confidence intervals should be interpreted with caution.[18, 36]

Results

Studies undertaken to investigate the diagnostic accuracy of the clinical examination should discuss the number of patients who did not meet inclusion criteria or were determined to be ineligible for the study.[13, 14] Most often, this provides a representation of the percentage of the patient population that satisfied the study requirements.

The STARD committee[13, 14] has advocated that the time between performance of the test under investigation and performance of the reference standard should be reported. Concerns with these variables include the possibility that patient conditions may improve or

	Reference Standard Positive	Reference Standard Negative
Clinical test positive	True-positive results a	False-positive results b
Clinical test negative	False-negative results c	True-negative results d

Table 2–2: *2 × 2 Contingency Table*

worsen over time.[14, 37] Also of relevance is the disclosure of any adverse effects that may have resulted from testing procedures.[13, 14]

Discussion

In the discussion, as with any other research study, authors should speculate on the reasons for their results. Results should be compared with those of other studies, and the authors should suggest possible reasons for differing or similar findings. The practical and clinical implications of study results should be considered in the discussion. The authors should note limitations of their study, and areas for further research should be mentioned.

SUMMARY

It is difficult for busy clinicians and students to incorporate the best available evidence into clinical practice when selecting tests and measures; this text has been developed to help alleviate some commonly reported barriers to evidence-based practice, including the lack of access, resources, and time.[1, 2] Through the use of more efficient search strategies tailored to each of the major databases, clinicians should be better able to quickly locate literature pertinent to their practice. Careful analysis of the literature provides greater insight into the scientific rigor of each study and its performance, applicability, reliability, and reproducibility within a given clinical practice.

REFERENCES

1. Jette DU, Bacon K, Batty C, et al. Evidence-based practice beliefs, attitudes, knowledge, and behaviors of physical therapists. *Phys Ther.* 2003;83:786–805.
2. Maher CG, Sherrington C, Elkins M, Herbert RD, Moseley AM. Challenges for evidence-based physical therapy: accessing and interpreting high-quality evidence on therapy. *Phys Ther.* 2004;84:644–654.
3. van der Weijden T, IJzermans CJ, Dinant G, van Duijn N, de Vet R, Buntinx F. Identifying relevent diagnostic studies in *MEDLINE*. The diagnostic value of the erythrocyte sedimentation rate (ESR) and dipstick as an example. *Fam Pract.* 1997;14:204–208.
4. Lowe H, Barnett G. Understanding and using the medical subject headings (MeSH) vocabulary to perform literature searches. *JAMA.* 1994;271:1103–1108.
5. Avenell A, Handoll H, Grant AM. Lessons for search strategies from a systematic review, in The Cochrane Library, of nutritional supplementation trials in patients after a hip fracture. *Am J Clin Nutr.* 2001;73:505–510.
6. Domholdt E. *Physical Therapy Research.* 2nd ed. Philadelphia, Pa: WB Saunders; 2000.
7. Helewa A, Walker JM. *Critical Evaluation of Research in Physical Rehabilitation.* Philadelphia, Pa: WB Saunders; 2000.
8. Bachmann LM, Estermann P, Kronenberg C, Riet G. Identifying diagnostic accuracy studies in EMBASE. *J Med Libr Assoc.* 2003;91:341–346.
9. Deville WL, Bezemer PD, Bouter LM. Publications on diagnostic test evaluation in family medicine journals: an optimal search strategy. *J Clin Epidemiol.* 2000;53:65–69.
10. Bachmann LM, Coray R, Estermann P, ter Riet G. Identifying diagnostic studies in MEDLINE: reducing the number needed to read. *J Am Med Inform Assoc.* 2002;9:653–658.

11. Moons KG, Biesheuvel CJ, Grobbee DE. Test research versus diagnostic research. *Clin Chem*. 2004;50:473–476.

12. Reid MC, Lachs MS, Feinstein AR. Use of methodological standards in diagnostic test research. *JAMA*. 1995;274:645–651.

13. Bossuyt PM, Reitsma JB, Bruns DE, et al. Towards complete and accurate reporting of studies of diagnostic accuracy: the STARD initiative. *Clin Chem*. 2003;49:1–6.

14. Bossuyt PM, Reitsma JB, Bruns DE, et al. The STARD statement for reporting studies of diagnostic accuracy: explanation and elaboration. *Clin Chem*. 2003;49:7–18.

15. Portney LG, Watkins MP. *Foundations of Clinical Research: Applications to Practice*. 2nd ed. Upper Saddle River, NJ: Prentice Hall Health; 2000.

16. Jaeschke R, Guyatt GH, Sackett DL. Users' guides to medical literature. III. How to use an article about a diagnostic test. B. What are the results and will they help me in caring for my patients? *JAMA*. 1994;271:703–707.

17. Whiting P, Rutjes AW, Reitsma JB, Glas AS, Bossuyt PM, Kleijnen J. Sources of variation and bias in studies of diagnostic accuracy: a systematic review. *Ann Intern Med*. 2004;140:189–202.

18. Greenhalgh T. How to read a paper: papers that report diagnostic or screening tests. *BMJ*. 1997;315:540–543.

19. Sackett DL, Haynes RB, Guyatt GH, Tugwell P. *Clinical Epidemiology: A Basic Science for Clinical Medicine*. Boston, Mass: Little, Brown and Company; 1991.

20. Mulherin SA, Miller WC. Spectrum bias or spectrum effect? Subgroup variation in diagnostic test evaluation. *Ann Intern Med*. 2002;137:598–603.

21. Klassabo M, Harms-Ringdahl K, Larsson G. Examination of passive ROM and capsular patterns in the hip. *Physiother Res Int*. 2003;8:1–12.

22. Fritz JM, Wainner RS. Examining diagnostic tests: an evidence based perspective. *Phys Ther*. 2001;81:1546–1564.

23. Sackett DL. A primer on the precision and accuracy of the clinical examination. *JAMA*. 1992;267:2638–2644.

24. Lijmer JG, Mol BW, Heisterkamp S, et al. Empirical evidence of design-related bias in studies of diagnostic tests. *JAMA*. 1999;282:1061–1066.

25. McGinn T, Guyatt G, Wyer P, Naylor C, Stiell I, Richardson W. Users' guides to the medical literature: XXII: How to use articles about clinical decision rules. *JAMA*. 2000;284:79–84.

26. Irwig L, Tosteson AN, Gatsonis C, et al. Guidelines for meta-analyses evaluating diagnostic tests. *Ann Intern Med*. 1994;120:667–676.

27. Mimori K, Muneta T, Nakagawa T, Shinomiya K. A new pain provocation test for superior labral tears of the shoulder. *Am J Sports Med*. 1999;27:137–142.

28. Liu SH, Henry MH, Nuccion SL. A prospective evaluation of a new physical examination in predicting glenoid labral tears. *Am J Sports Med*. 1996;24:721–725.

29. Ransohoff DF, Feinstein AR. Problems of spectrum bias in evaluating the efficacy of diagnostic tests. *N Engl J Med*. 1978;299:926–930.

30. Begg CB. Biases in the assessment of diagnostic tests. *Stat Med*. 1987;6:411–423.

31. Calis M, Akgun K, Birtane M, Karacan I, Calis H, Tuzun F. Diagnostic values of clinical diagnostic tests in subacromial impingement syndrome. *Ann Rheum Dis*. 2000;59:44–47.

32. MacDonald P, Clark P, Sutherland K. An analysis of the diagnostic accuracy of the Hawkins and Neer subacromial impingement signs. *J Shoulder Elbow Surg*. 2000;9:299–301.

REFERENCES

REFERENCES

33. Begg CB. Methodologic standards for diagnostic test assessment studies. *J Gen Intern Med*. 1988;3:518–520.

34. Wainner RS, Fritz JM, Irrgang JJ, Boninger ML, Delitto A, Allison A. Reliability and diagnostic accuracy of the clinical examination and patient self-report measures for cervical radiculopathy. *Spine*. 2003;28:52–62.

35. Sackett DL, Straws SE, Richardson WS, Rosenberg W, Haynes RB. *Evidence-Based Medicine: How to Practice and Teach EBM*. 2nd ed. London: Harcourt Publishers Limited; 2000.

36. Simel DL, Samsa GP, Matchar DB. Likelihood ratios with confidence: sample size estimation for diagnostic test studies. *J Clin Epidemiol*. 1991;44:763–770.

37. Glas AS, Pijnenburg B, Lijmer JG, et al. Comparison of diagnostic decision rules and structured data collection in assessment of acute ankle injury. *CMAJ*. 2002;166:727–733.

Temporomandibular Joint

Chapter 3

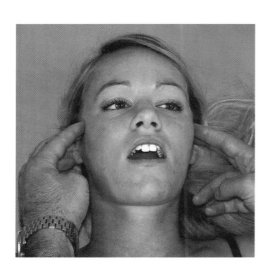

OSTEOLOGY   Bony Framework of Head and Neck

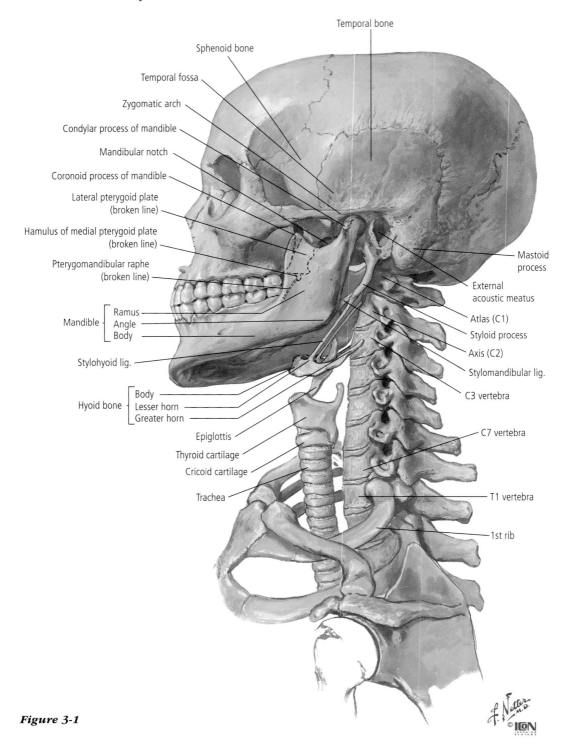

Figure 3-1

Mandible

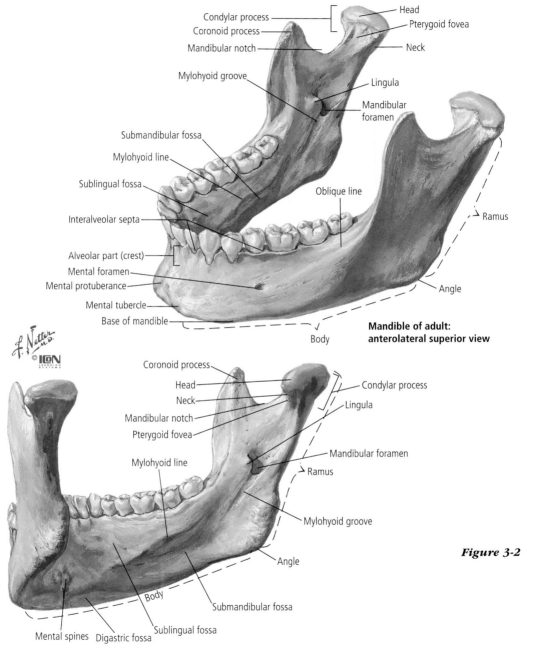

Mandible of adult:
anterolateral superior view

Figure 3-2

Mandible of adult:
left posterior view

OSTEOLOGY   Lateral Skull

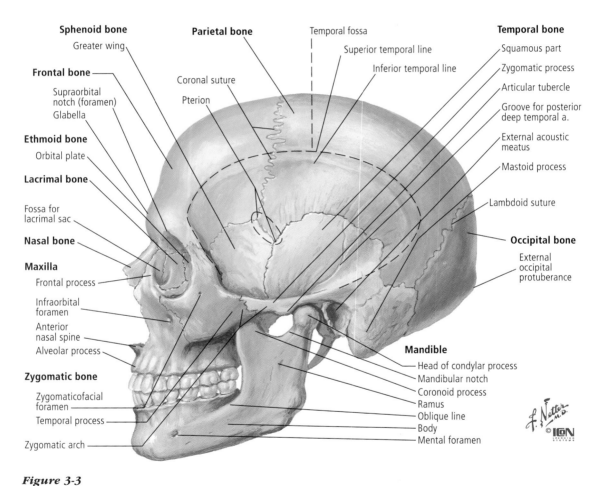

Sphenoid bone
Greater wing

Frontal bone
Supraorbital notch (foramen)
Glabella

Ethmoid bone
Orbital plate

Lacrimal bone
Fossa for lacrimal sac

Nasal bone

Maxilla
Frontal process
Infraorbital foramen
Anterior nasal spine
Alveolar process

Zygomatic bone
Zygomaticofacial foramen
Temporal process
Zygomatic arch

Parietal bone
Coronal suture
Pterion

Temporal fossa
Superior temporal line
Inferior temporal line

Temporal bone
Squamous part
Zygomatic process
Articular tubercle
Groove for posterior deep temporal a.
External acoustic meatus
Mastoid process
Lambdoid suture

Occipital bone
External occipital protuberance

Mandible
Head of condylar process
Mandibular notch
Coronoid process
Ramus
Oblique line
Body
Mental foramen

Figure 3-3

Temporomandibular Joint

The temporomandibular joint (TMJ) is divided by an intra-articular biconcave disc that separates the joint cavity into two distinct functional components. The upper joint is a plane-gliding joint that permits translation of the mandibular condyles. The lower joint is a hinge joint that permits rotation of the condyles.[1] The closed pack position of the TMJ is full occlusion. A unilateral restriction pattern primarily limits contralateral excursion, but also affects mouth opening and protrusion.

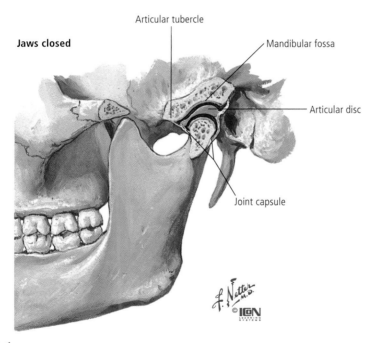

Figure 3-4

ARTHROLOGY   Temporomandibular Joint Mechanics

During mandibular depression from a closed mouth position, initial movement occurs at the lower joint as the condyles pivot on the intra-articular disc. This motion continues to approximately 11 mm of depression. With further mandibular depression, motion begins to occur at the upper joint and causes anterior translation of the disc on the articular eminence. Normal mandibular depression is between 40 and 50 mm.

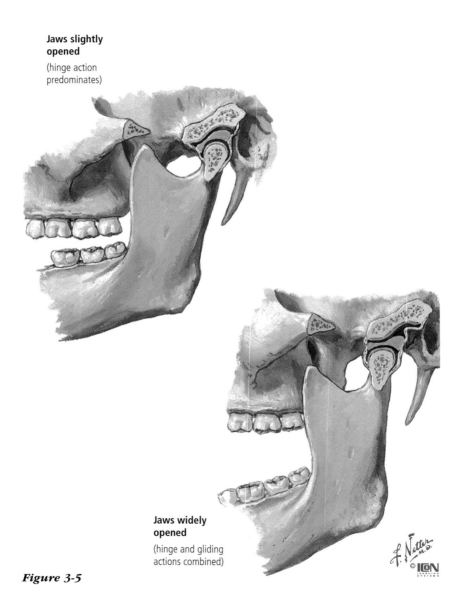

Jaws slightly opened

(hinge action predominates)

Jaws widely opened

(hinge and gliding actions combined)

Figure 3-5

Temporomandibular Joint Ligaments   **LIGAMENTS**

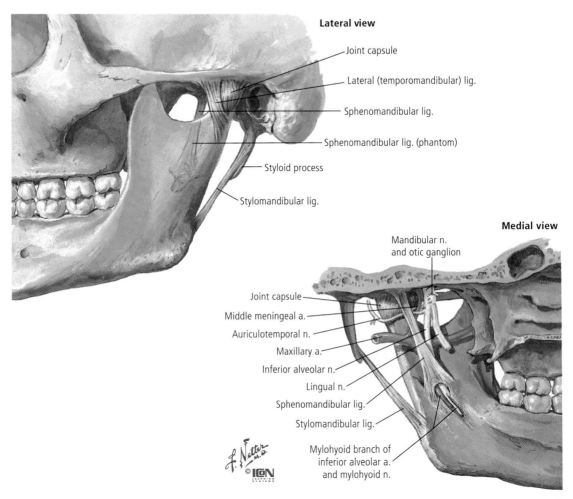

Lateral view

- Joint capsule
- Lateral (temporomandibular) lig.
- Sphenomandibular lig.
- Sphenomandibular lig. (phantom)
- Styloid process
- Stylomandibular lig.

Medial view

- Mandibular n. and otic ganglion
- Joint capsule
- Middle meningeal a.
- Auriculotemporal n.
- Maxillary a.
- Inferior alveolar n.
- Lingual n.
- Sphenomandibular lig.
- Stylomandibular lig.
- Mylohyoid branch of inferior alveolar a. and mylohyoid n.

Figure 3-6

Ligaments	Attachments	Function
Temporomandibular	Thickening of anterior joint capsule extending from neck of mandible to zygomatic arch	Strengthen the TMJ laterally
Sphenomandibular	Sphenoid bone to mandible	Serve as a fulcrum and reinforcement to TMJ motion
Stylomandibular	Styloid process to angle of the mandible	Provide minimal support to the joint

MUSCLES   Muscles Involved in Mastication

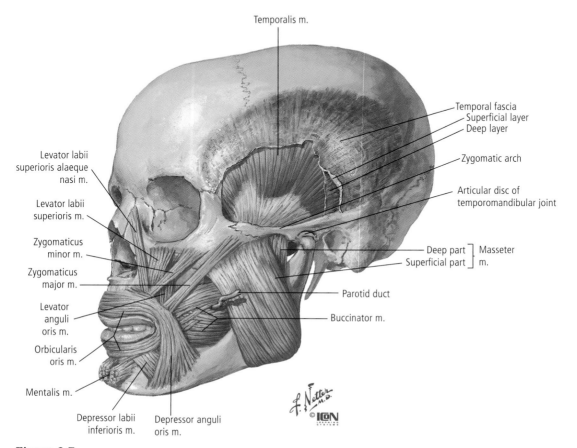

Figure 3-7

Muscle	Proximal Attachment	Distal Attachment	Nerve and Segmental Level	Action
Temporalis	Temporal fossa	Coronoid process and anterior ramus of mandible	Deep temporal branches of mandibular nerve	Elevate mandible
Masseter	Inferior and medial aspects of zygomatic arch	Coronoid process and lateral ramus of mandible	Mandibular nerve via masseteric nerve	Elevate and protrude mandible

Muscles Involved in Mastication (cont.)   **MUSCLES**

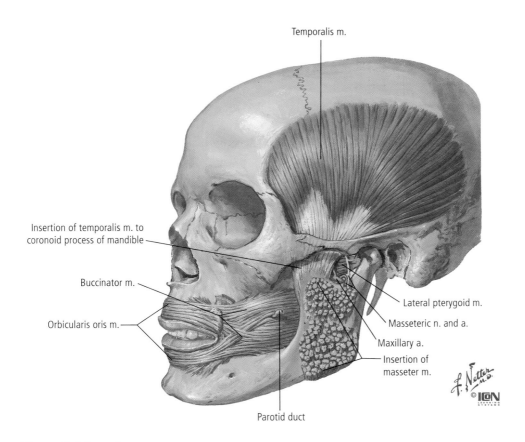

Temporalis m.

Insertion of temporalis m. to
coronoid process of mandible

Buccinator m.

Orbicularis oris m.

Lateral pterygoid m.

Masseteric n. and a.

Maxillary a.

Insertion of
masseter m.

Parotid duct

Figure 3-7 (cont.)

MUSCLES   Posterior and Lateral Muscles Involved in Mastication

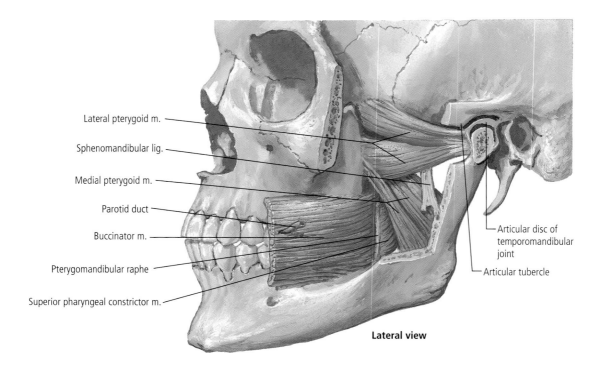

Lateral pterygoid m.

Sphenomandibular lig.

Medial pterygoid m.

Parotid duct

Buccinator m.

Pterygomandibular raphe

Superior pharyngeal constrictor m.

Articular disc of temporomandibular joint

Articular tubercle

Lateral view

Figure 3-8

Muscle		Proximal Attachment	Distal Attachment	Nerve and Segmental Level	Action
Medial pterygoid		Medial surface of lateral pterygoid plate, pyramidal process of palatine bone, and tuberosity of maxilla	Medial aspect of mandibular ramus	Mandibular nerve via medial pterygoid nerve	Elevate and protrude mandible
Lateral pterygoid	Superior head	Lateral surface of greater wing of sphenoid bone	Neck of mandible, articular disc, and TMJ capsule	Mandibular nerve via lateral pterygoid nerve	Acting bilaterally: protrude and depress mandible Acting unilaterally: laterally deviate mandible
	Inferior head	Lateral surface of lateral pterygoid plate			

Posterior and Lateral Muscles Involved in Mastication (cont.)   **MUSCLES**

Posterior view

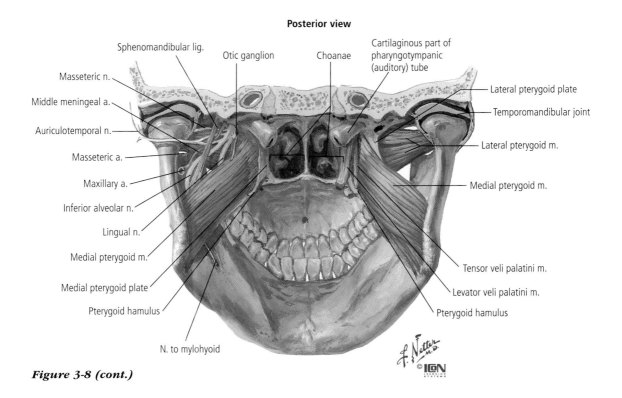

Sphenomandibular lig.

Otic ganglion

Choanae

Cartilaginous part of pharyngotympanic (auditory) tube

Masseteric n.

Middle meningeal a.

Auriculotemporal n.

Masseteric a.

Maxillary a.

Inferior alveolar n.

Lingual n.

Medial pterygoid m.

Medial pterygoid plate

Pterygoid hamulus

N. to mylohyoid

Lateral pterygoid plate

Temporomandibular joint

Lateral pterygoid m.

Medial pterygoid m.

Tensor veli palatini m.

Levator veli palatini m.

Pterygoid hamulus

Figure 3-8 (cont.)

MUSCLES   Floor of Mouth

Lateral, slightly inferior view

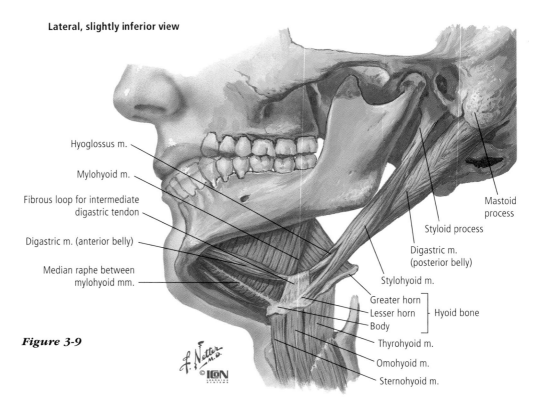

Hyoglossus m.

Mylohyoid m.

Fibrous loop for intermediate
digastric tendon

Digastric m. (anterior belly)

Median raphe between
mylohyoid mm.

Figure 3-9

Mastoid
process

Styloid process

Digastric m.
(posterior belly)

Stylohyoid m.

Greater horn
Lesser horn   Hyoid bone
Body

Thyrohyoid m.

Omohyoid m.

Sternohyoid m.

Muscle		Proximal Attachment	Distal Attachment	Nerve and Segmental Level	Action
Mylohyoid		Mylohyoid line of mandible	Hyoid bone	Mylohyoid nerve (branch of cranial nerve [CN] V₃)	Elevates hyoid bone
Stylohyoid		Styloid process of temporal bone	Hyoid bone	Cervical branch of facial nerve	Elevates and retracts hyoid bone
Geniohyoid		Inferior mental spine of mandible	Hyoid bone	C1 via the hypoglossal nerve	Elevates hyoid bone anterosuperiorly
Digastric	Anterior belly	Digastric fossa of mandible	Intermediate tendon to hyoid bone	Mylohyoid nerve	Depresses mandible, raises and stabilizes hyoid bone
	Posterior belly	Mastoid notch of temporal bone		Facial nerve	

Floor of Mouth (cont.)

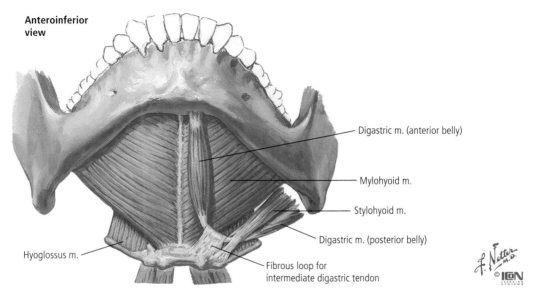

Anteroinferior view

- Digastric m. (anterior belly)
- Mylohyoid m.
- Stylohyoid m.
- Digastric m. (posterior belly)
- Fibrous loop for intermediate digastric tendon
- Hyoglossus m.

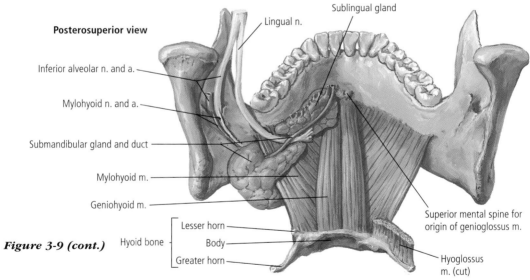

Posterosuperior view

- Lingual n.
- Sublingual gland
- Inferior alveolar n. and a.
- Mylohyoid n. and a.
- Submandibular gland and duct
- Mylohyoid m.
- Geniohyoid m.
- Superior mental spine for origin of genioglossus m.
- Hyoid bone
  - Lesser horn
  - Body
  - Greater horn
- Hyoglossus m. (cut)

Figure 3-9 (cont.)

NERVES

Mandibular Nerve

Medial view

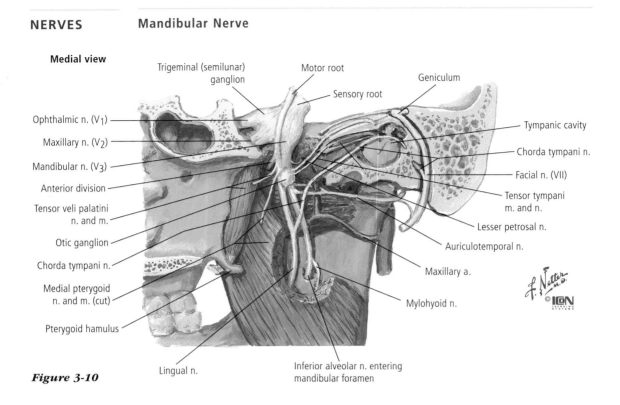

Trigeminal (semilunar) ganglion
Motor root
Geniculum
Sensory root
Ophthalmic n. (V₁)
Maxillary n. (V₂)
Mandibular n. (V₃)
Anterior division
Tensor veli palatini n. and m.
Otic ganglion
Chorda tympani n.
Medial pterygoid n. and m. (cut)
Pterygoid hamulus
Lingual n.
Tympanic cavity
Chorda tympani n.
Facial n. (VII)
Tensor tympani m. and n.
Lesser petrosal n.
Auriculotemporal n.
Maxillary a.
Mylohyoid n.
Inferior alveolar n. entering mandibular foramen

Figure 3-10

Nerves	Segmental Levels	Sensory	Motor
Mandibular	CN V₃	Skin of inferior third of face	Temporalis, masseter, lateral pterygoid, medial pterygoid, digastric, mylohyoid
Nerve to mylohyoid	CN V₃	No sensory	Mylohyoid
Buccal	CN V₃	Cheek lining and gingiva	No motor
Lingual	CN V₃	Anterior tongue and floor of mouth	No motor
Maxillary	CN V₂	Skin of middle third of face	No motor
Ophthalmic	CN V₁	Skin of superior third of face	No motor

CN V = Trigeminal Nerve

Mandibular Nerve (cont.)

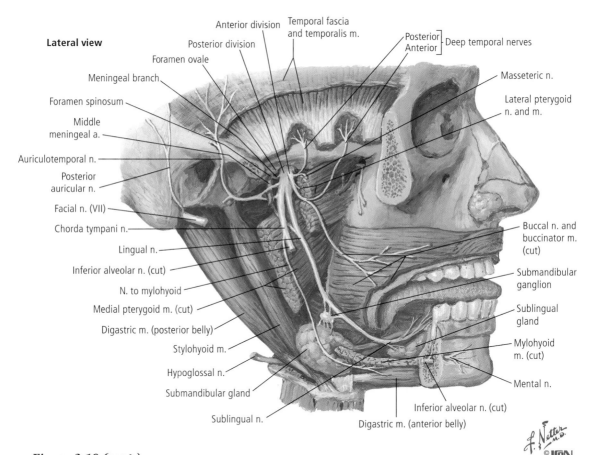

Lateral view

Anterior division

Temporal fascia
and temporalis m.

Posterior division

Posterior
Anterior ⎤ Deep temporal nerves

Foramen ovale

Meningeal branch

Masseteric n.

Foramen spinosum

Lateral pterygoid
n. and m.

Middle
meningeal a.

Auriculotemporal n.

Posterior
auricular n.

Facial n. (VII)

Chorda tympani n.

Buccal n. and
buccinator m.
(cut)

Lingual n.

Inferior alveolar n. (cut)

Submandibular
ganglion

N. to mylohyoid

Sublingual
gland

Medial pterygoid m. (cut)

Digastric m. (posterior belly)

Mylohyoid
m. (cut)

Stylohyoid m.

Hypoglossal n.

Mental n.

Submandibular gland

Inferior alveolar n. (cut)

Sublingual n.

Digastric m. (anterior belly)

Figure 3-10 (cont.)

EXAMINATION: HISTORY

Initial Hypotheses Based on Historical Findings

History	Initial Hypothesis
Patient reports jaw crepitus and pain during mouth opening and closing. Might also report limited opening with translation of the jaw to the affected side at the end range of opening	Osteoarthrosis[2] Capsulitis Internal derangement consisting of an anterior disc displacement without reduction[3-5]
Patient reports jaw clicking during opening and closing of the mouth and pain	Internal derangement consisting of anterior disc displacement with reduction[3, 6-8]
Patient reports limited motion to about 20 mm with no joint sounds	Capsulitis Internal derangement consisting of an anterior disc displacement without reduction[3, 6]

Range-of-Motion Measurements of the Temporomandibular Joint

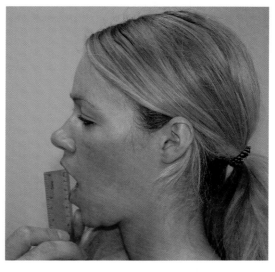

Figure 3-11: *Measurement of active range of motion in mouth opening.*

Test and Measure		Test Procedure	Population	Inter-examiner Reliability ICC	Intra-examiner Reliability ICC
Opening	Without TMJ disorder	Patient is instructed to open mouth as much as possible without causing pain. Intercisal distance is measured to the nearest millimeter with a plastic ruler		.98	.77–.89
	With TMJ disorder			.99	.94
Overbite	Without TMJ disorder	A horizontal line is made on the lower incisor at the level of the upper incisor with the TMJ closed. The vertical distance between the line and the superior aspect of the lower incisor is measured		.98	.90–.96
	With TMJ disorder			.95	.90–.97
Excursion left	Without TMJ disorder	Vertical marks are made in the median plane on the anterior surface of the lower central incisors in relationship to the upper central incisors. The patient is instructed to move the jaw as far laterally as possible, and a measurement is recorded	15 subjects with and 15 subjects without a TMJ disorder	.95	.91–.92
	With TMJ disorder			.94	.85–.92
Excursion right	Without TMJ disorder			.90	.70–.87
	With TMJ disorder			.96	.75–.82
Protrusion	Without TMJ disorder	Two vertical lines are made on the first upper and lower canine incisors. The subject is instructed to move the jaw as far forward as possible, and a measurement is taken between the two marks		.95	.85–.93
	With TMJ disorder			.98	.89–.93
Overjet	Without TMJ disorder	The horizontal distance between the upper and lower incisors is measured when the mouth is closed		1.0	.98
Walker et al.[9]	With TMJ disorder			.99	.98–.99

RELIABILITY OF THE CLINICAL EXAMINATION

Measuring Mandibular Opening With Different Head Positions

Test and Measure	Test Procedure	Population	Inter-examiner Reliability ICC	Intra-examiner Reliability ICC
Forward head position	Patient slides the jaw as far forward as possible, and vertical mandibular opening is measured	40 healthy subjects	.92	.97
Neutral head position	Patient is placed in a position where a plumb line bisects the ear, and vertical mandibular opening is measured		.93	.93
Retracted head position *Higbie et al.[10]*	Patient slides the jaw as far backward as possible, and vertical mandibular opening is measured		.92	.92

Patient Reports of Pain in Temporomandibular Joint Disorders

Test and Measure	Test Procedure	Population	Reliability Kappa Values
Visual analog scale	100-mm line with the ends defined as no pain and worst pain imaginable	38 consecutive patients referred with TMJ disorders	κ = .38
Numeric scale	10-point scale with 0 indicating no pain and 10 representing worst pain		κ = .36
Behavior rating scale	6-point scale ranging from minor discomfort to very strong discomfort		κ = .68
Verbal scale *Magnusson et al.[11]*	5-point scale ranging from no pain to very severe pain		κ = .44

Detecting the Presence of Bruxism

Test and Measure	Test Procedure	Population	Inter-examiner Reliability Kappa Value	Intra-examiner Reliability Kappa Value
Visual determination of bruxism *Marbach et al.[12]*	20 examiners rate the casts for severity of bruxism on a 4-point scale from none to severe	29 augmented sets of dental models	κ = .32–.33	κ = .46

RELIABILITY OF THE CLINICAL EXAMINATION

Determining the Presence of Pain During Palpation

Test and Measure	Test Procedure	Population	Reliability Kappa Values
Intra-examiner			
Lateral palpation	Examiner palpates anterior to the ear over TMJ	61 patients with TMJ pain	κ = .53
Posterior palpation *Manfredini et al.*[13]	Examiner palpates TMJ through external meatus		κ = .48
Inter-examiner			
Extraoral	Examiner palpates temporalis, masseter, posterior cervical, and sternocleidomastoid muscles	64 healthy volunteers	κ = .91
Intraoral *Dworkin et al.*[14]	Examiner palpates tendon of the temporalis, lateral pterygoid, masseter, and body of tongue		κ = .90
Masseter muscle	Examiner palpates mid belly of masseter muscle	79 randomly selected patients referred to a craniomandibular disorder department	κ = .33
Temporalis muscle	Examiner palpates mid belly of temporalis muscle		κ = .42
Medial pterygoid	Examiner palpates insertion of the medial pterygoid		κ = .23
Palpation of TMJ *Lobbezoo-Scholte et al.*[15]	Examiner palpates lateral and dorsal aspects of the condyle		κ = .33
Masseter	Examiner palpates superficial and deep portions of masseter muscle	79 patients referred to a TMJ disorder and orofacial pain department	κ = .33
Temporalis	Examiner palpates anterior and posterior aspects of temporalis muscle		κ = .42
Medial pterygoid attachment	Examiner palpates medial pterygoid muscles extraorally		κ = .23
Palpation of TMJ *de Wijer et al.*[16]	Examiner palpates lateral pole of condyle in open and closed mouth positions. The dorsal pole is palpated posteriorly through the external auditory meatus		κ = .33

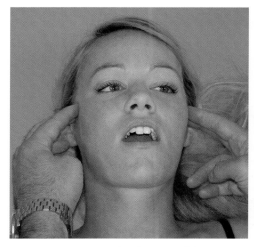

Figure 3-12: *Lateral palpation of the temporomandibular joint.*

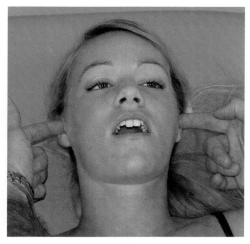

Figure 3-13: *Posterior palpation of the temporomandibular joint through external auditory meatus.*

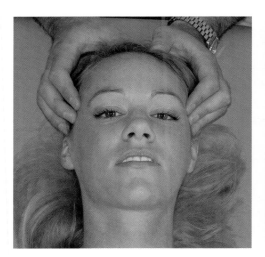

Figure 3-14: *Palpation of the temporalis.*

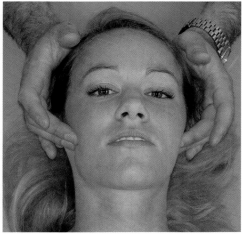

Figure 3-15: *Palpation of the masseter.*

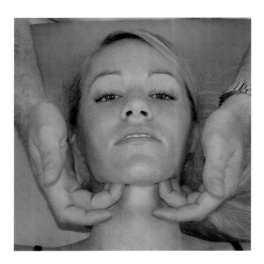

Figure 3-16: *Palpation of the medial pterygoid.*

RELIABILITY OF THE CLINICAL EXAMINATION

Determining the Presence of Pain During Dynamic Movements

Test and Measure	Test Procedure	Population	Reliability Kappa Values
Intra-examiner			
Mandibular movements	Patient is asked if pain is felt during opening, closing, lateral excursion, protrusion, and retrusion	61 patients with TMJ pain	κ = .43
Maximum assisted opening Manfredini et al.[13]	Examiner applies overpressure to the end range of mandibular depression		κ= −.05
Inter-examiner			
Pain on opening	Patient opens mouth maximally	79 patients referred to a TMJ disorder and orofacial pain department	κ = .28
Pain on lateral excursion right	Patient moves the mandible in a lateral direction as far as possible		κ = .28
Pain on lateral excursion left			κ = .28
Pain on protrusion de Wijer et al.[16]	Patient actively protrudes the jaw		κ = .36
Passive opening	At the end of active opening, the examiner applies a passive stretch to increase mouth opening	79 randomly selected patients referred to a craniomandibular disorder department	κ = .34
Active opening Lobbezoo-Scholte et al.[15]	Patient opens mouth as wide as possible		κ = .32

Determining the Presence of Pain During Dynamic Movements (cont.)

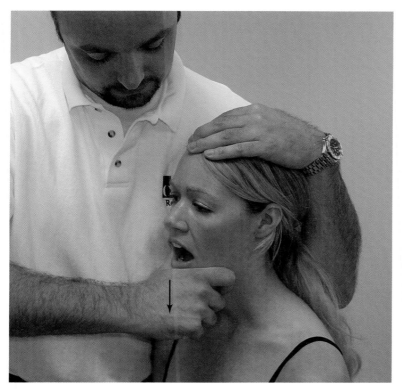

Figure 3-17: *Assessment of pain during passive opening.*

RELIABILITY OF THE CLINICAL EXAMINATION

Determining the Presence of Pain During Joint Play

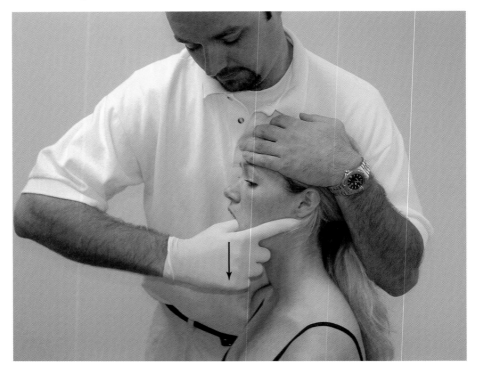

Figure 3-18: *Temporomandibular traction.*

Test and Measure	Test Procedure	Population	Reliability Kappa Values
Intra-examiner			
Joint play Manfredini et al.[13]	Examiner performs passive traction and translation movements	61 patients with TMJ pain	κ = .20
Inter-examiner			
Joint play test Lobbezoo-Scholte et al.[15]	Examiner applies a traction and a translation (medial/lateral) force through the TMJ	79 randomly selected patients referred to a craniomandibular disorder department	κ = .46
Traction right	Examiner moves the mandibular condyle in an inferior direction for traction and a mediolateral direction for translation. Presence of pain is recorded.	79 patients referred to a TMJ disorder and orofacial pain department	κ = −.08
Traction left			κ = .25
Translation right			κ = .50
Translation left de Wijer et al.[16]			κ = .28

Detecting Joint Sounds During Active Motion in Patients With Temporomandibular Disorders

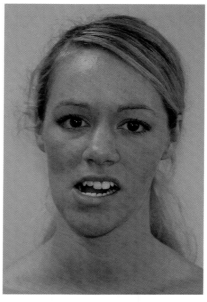

Figure 3-19: *Lateral excursion right.*

Test and Measure		Test Procedure	Population	Reliability Kappa Values
Intra-examiner				
Click sounds during mouth opening		During mouth opening, examiner records presence of a click sound	61 patients with TMJ pain	κ = .12
Crepitus sounds during mouth opening *Manfredini et al.*[13]		During mouth opening, examiner records presence of a grating or grinding sound		κ = .15
Inter-examiner				
Active maximal mouth opening	Clicking	Intensity of clicking and crepitation is graded on a 0 to 2 scale from none to clearly audible	79 randomly selected patients referred to a craniomandibular disorder department	κ = .70
	Crepitation			κ = .29
Joint sounds *Lobbezoo-Scholte et al.*[15]		Examiner records presence of joint sounds		κ = .24
Opening		Examiner records the presence of joint sounds during mandibular opening, lateral excursion right and left, and protrusion	79 patients referred to a TMJ disorder and orofacial pain department	κ = .59
Lateral excursion right				κ = .57
Lateral excursion left				κ = .50
Protrusion *de Wijer et al.*[16]				κ = .47

**Detecting Joint Sounds During Joint Play in Patients With
Temporomandibular Disorders**

Test and Measure	Test Procedure	Population	Inter-examiner Reliability Kappa Values
Joint sounds during joint play *Lobbezoo-Scholte et al.*[15]	Examiner records presence of joint sounds during traction and translation	79 randomly selected patients referred to a craniomandibular disorder department	$\kappa = -.01$
Traction right	Examiner moves mandibular condyle in an inferior direction for traction and a medial-lateral direction for translation. Examiner records presence of joint sounds during translation and traction	79 patients referred to a TMJ disorder and orofacial pain department	$\kappa = -.02$
Traction left			$\kappa = .66$
Translation right			$\kappa = .07$
Translation left *de Wijer et al.*[16]			$\kappa = -.02$

Joint Play and End-Feel Assessment of the TMJ

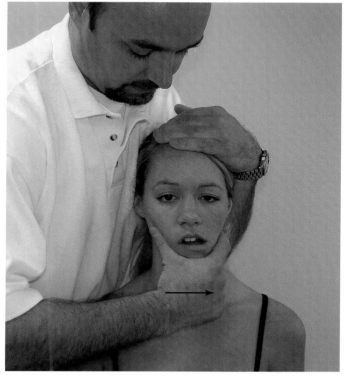

Figure 3-20: *Translation of mandible left.*

Test and Measure	Test Procedure	Population	Inter-examiner Reliability Kappa Values	
			Joint Play	End-Feel
Traction and translation *Lobbezoo-Scholte et al.*[15]	Examiner records presence of restriction of movement at end-feel during traction and translation of the TMJ	79 randomly selected patients referred to a craniomandibular disorder department	Restriction of movement κ = .08	End-feel κ = .07
Traction right	Examiner moves mandibular condyle in an inferior direction for traction and a medial-lateral direction for translation, and grades of joint play and end-feel are recorded as normal or abnormal	79 patients referred to a TMJ disorder and orofacial pain department	κ = −.03	κ = −.05
Traction left			κ = .08	κ = .20
Translation right			κ = −.05	κ = −.05
Translation left *de Wijer et al.*[16]			κ = −.1	κ = .13

Detecting Pain During Resistance Tests

Test and Measure	Test Procedure	Population	Reliability Kappa Values
Intra-examiner			
Dynamic tests *Manfredini et al.*[13]	Patient performs opening, closing, lateral excursion, protrusion, and retrusion movements while examiner applies resistance	61 patients with TMJ pain	κ = .20
Inter-examiner			
Opening	Examiner applies isometric resistance during opening, closing, and lateral excursions right and left of the TMJ and records presence of pain	79 patients referred to a TMJ disorder and orofacial pain department	κ = .24
Closing			κ = .30
Lateral excursion right			κ = .28
Lateral excursion left *de Wijer et al.*[16]			κ = .26
Static pain test *Lobbezoo-Scholte et al.*[15]	Examiner applies resistance against patient's mandible in upward, downward, and lateral directions	79 randomly selected patients referred to a craniomandibular disorder department	κ = .15

Compression Test

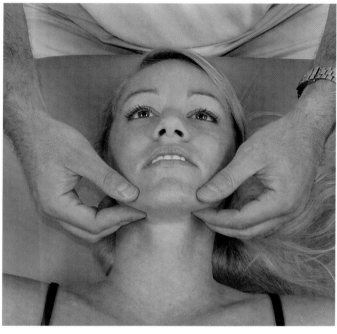

Figure 3-21: *Bilateral temporomandibular compression.*

Test and Measure		Test Procedure	Population	Inter-examiner Reliability Kappa Values
Compression right	Pain	Examiner loads the intra-articular structures by moving the mandible in a dorsocranial direction and records presence of pain and joint sounds	79 patients referred to a TMJ disorder and orofacial pain department	κ = .19
	Sounds			NR
Compression left de Wijer et al.[16]	Pain			κ = .47
	Sounds			κ = 1.0
Compression	Pain		79 randomly selected patients referred to a craniomandibular disorder department	κ = .40
Lobbezoo-Scholte et al.[15]	Joint sounds			κ = .66

NR, not recorded.

DIAGNOSTIC UTILITY OF THE CLINICAL EXAMINATION

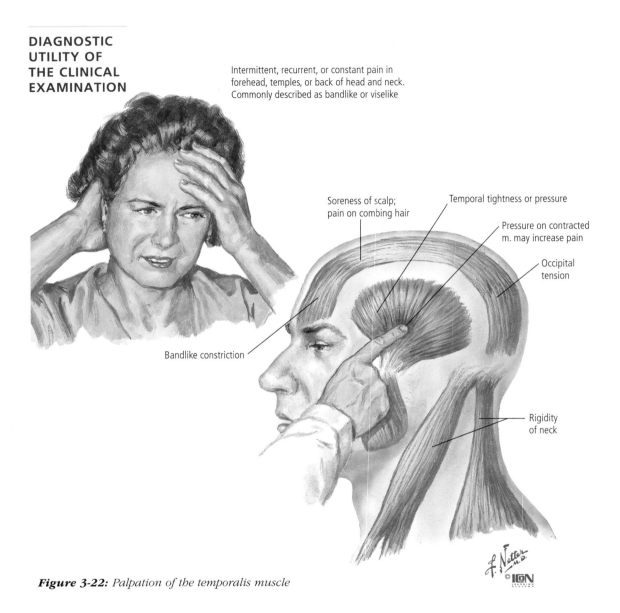

Intermittent, recurrent, or constant pain in forehead, temples, or back of head and neck. Commonly described as bandlike or viselike

Soreness of scalp; pain on combing hair

Temporal tightness or pressure

Pressure on contracted m. may increase pain

Occipital tension

Bandlike constriction

Rigidity of neck

Figure 3-22: *Palpation of the temporalis muscle*

Historical Examination

History	Population	Sens	Spec	+LR	−LR
Patient reports of headaches *Cacchiotti et al.[17]*	41 patients with TMJ disorders and 40 controls	.63	.67	1.91	.55

Sens, sensitivity; Spec, specificity; LR, likelihood ratio.

Accuracy of the Patient History for Detecting Anterior Disc Displacement

History	Population	Sens		Spec		+LR		−LR	
		DR	DDR	DR	DDR	DR	DDR	DR	DDR
Clicking		.82	.86	.19	.24	1.01	1.13	.95	.58
Locking		.53	.86	.22	.52	.68	1.79	2.14	.27
Restriction after clicking		.26	.66	.40	.74	.43	2.54	1.85	.46
Periodic restriction		.6	.12	.9	.95	6.0	2.4	.44	.93
Continuous restriction	90 patients with TMJ disorders	.35	.78	.26	.62	.47	2.05	2.5	.35
Function related to joint pain		.82	.96	.10	.24	.91	1.26	1.80	.17
Complaint of clicking		.28	.82	.24	.69	.37	2.65	3.0	.26
Complaint of movement-related pain		.71	.74	.31	.36	1.03	1.16	.94	.72
Complaint of severe restriction *Stegenga et al.*[18]		.6	.38	.65	.93	1.71	5.43	.62	.67

Sens, sensitivity; Spec, specificity; LR, likelihood ratio; DR, disc reduces; DDR, disc does not reduce

The Association of Oral Habits With Temporomandibular Disorders

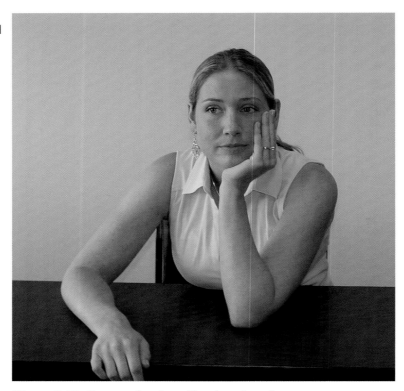

Figure 3-23: *Frequent leaning of head on the palm*

Gavish and colleagues[19] investigated the association of oral habits with signs and symptoms of TMJ disorders in 248 randomly selected high school females. Results demonstrated that chewing of gum, jaw play (nonfunctional jaw movements), chewing of ice, and frequent leaning of the head on the palm were associated with the presence of TMJ disorders.

Accuracy of the Historical Examination in Detecting Temporomandibular Joint Disorders in Children

History	Population	Sens	Spec	+LR	−LR
Any pain complaints		.31	.82	1.72	.84
Presence of joint sounds		.29	.85	1.93	.84
Reports of grinding	1342 patients aged 6 to 19 years reporting TMJ symptoms	.19	.81	1.00	1.0
Headache		.28	.81	1.47	.89
Pain during opening Riolo et al.[20]		.33	.80	1.65	.84

Differentiating Between Patients With and Without Temporomandibular Joint Disorders

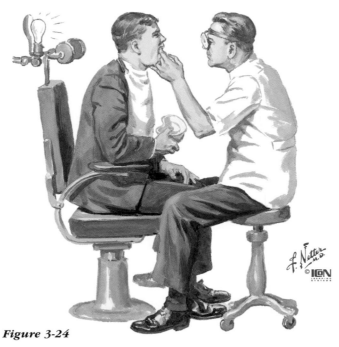

Figure 3-24

Test and Measure	Test Procedure	Determination of Findings	Population	Reference Standard	Sens	Spec	+LR	−LR
Palpation of masticatory muscles	Examiner performs routine muscle palpation of the muscles of mastication	Examiner grades response to palpation on a 0 to 3 scale, with 0 indicating no response and 3 indicating that patient pulls the head away in anticipation of palpation, along with significant pain	41 persons seeking treatment for TMJ disorders and 40 not seeking treatment	Subject report of TMJ pain	.76	.90	7.6	.27
Palpation of cervical musculature	Examiner performs routine muscle palpation of the cervical musculature				.40	.97	13.33	.62
Restrictions of maximal mouth opening *Cacchiotti et al.*[17]	ROM measurements taken to the nearest .5 mm	>6 mm of restriction			.26	.97	8.67	.76

ROM, range of motion.

DIAGNOSTIC UTILITY OF THE CLINICAL EXAMINATION

Detecting Osteoarthrosis

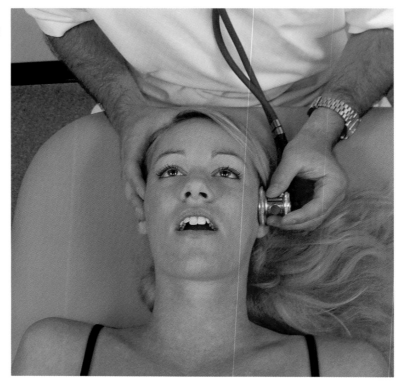

Figure 3-25: *Auscultation performed with a stethoscope*

Test and Measure	Test Procedure and Determination of Positive Findings	Population	Reference Standard	Sens	Spec	+LR	−LR
Presence of crepitus Israel et al.[21]	OA based on the presence of crepitus during auscultation. Positive if crepitus present	84 patients with symptoms of TMJ pain	Arthroscopic visualization	.70	.43	1.23	.70
Presence of crepitus Holmlund and Axelsson[22]	Auscultation performed with stethoscope. Positive if crepitus present	200 consecutive patients with TMJ disease	Arthroscopic visualization	OA1 = .45 OA2 = .67	OA1 =.84 OA2 = .86	OA1 = 2.81 OA2 = 4.79	OA1 = .65 OA2 = .38

OA1 = smooth, glossy white surfaces of the disc and fibrocartilage.
OA2 = 1 or more of the following features: pronounced fibrillation of the articular cartilage and disc; exposure of subchondral bone; disc perforation.
OA, osteoarthritis

Identifying Temporomandibular Joint Synovitis

Test and Measure	Test Procedure	Determination of Findings	Population	Reference Standard	Sens	Spec	+LR	−LR
Palpation Israel et al.[21]	Palpation of lateral and posterior aspects of the TMJ and assessment of pain response with active movement	Positive if patient reports pain with palpation or active movement	84 patients with TMJ pain	Arthroscopic visualization	.92	.21	1.16	.38
Palpation Holmlund and Axelsson[22]	Joint palpation	Examiner palpates the lateral and posterior aspects of the joint with one finger and determines the presence of tenderness	200 consecutive patients with TMJ disorder	Arthroscopic visualization	.88	.36	1.38	.33

Detecting the Presence of Temporomandibular Joint Effusion

Test and Measure	Test Procedure	Determination of Findings	Population	Reference Standard	Sens	Spec	+LR	−LR
Pain with lateral palpation	Examiner palpates the lateral pole of the condyle with the index finger	Positive if pain is present	61 patients with TMJ pain	MRI	.83	.69	2.68	.25
Pain with posterior palpation	Examiner palpates the posterior portion of the condyle with the little finger in the patient's ear				.85	.62	2.24	.24
Pain during mandibular movement	Patient opens, closes, protrudes, retrudes, and performs lateral excursion of the mandible				.82	.61	2.10	.30
Pain during maximum opening and overpressure	Patient performs the movements above while examiner applies resistance				.93	.016	.95	4.38
Pain during dynamic tests	Patient opens the mouth as wide as possible, and examiner applies overpressure				.74	.44	1.32	.59
Pain during joint play	Examiner passively performs translation and traction of the TMJ				.80	.39	1.31	.51
Presence of click sounds	Examiner auscultates for sounds during joint movement	Positive if click sound is heard			.69	.51	1.41	.61
Presence of crepitus sounds *Manfredini et al.*[13]	Examiner auscultates for sounds during joint movement	Positive if grating or grinding sounds are heard			.85	.30	1.21	.50

MRI, magnetic resonance imaging

Detecting Anterior Disc Displacement of the Temporomandibular Joint

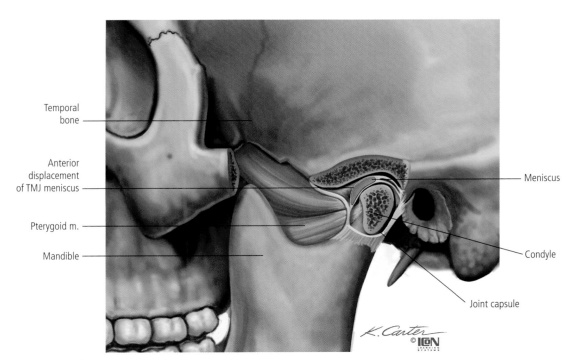

Temporal bone

Anterior displacement of TMJ meniscus

Pterygoid m.

Mandible

Meniscus

Condyle

Joint capsule

Figure 3-26: *Anterior disc displacement*

DIAGNOSTIC UTILITY OF THE CLINICAL EXAMINATION

Detecting Anterior Disc Displacement of the Temporomandibular Joint (cont.)

Test and Measure	Test Procedure	Determination of Findings	Population	Reference Standard	Sens DR	Sens DDR	Spec DR	Spec DDR	+LR DR	+LR DDR	–LR DR	–LR DDR
Detection of disc displacement without reduction Emshoff et al.[24]	Examiner performs evaluation of mandibular ROM and joint pain, and auscultation of joint sounds	Mandibular ROM is measured for maximum opening and lateral excursion. TMJ is auscultated with a stethoscope during the above movements	69 patients referred with TMJ disorders	MRI	.75		.83		4.41		.3	
Reproducible clicking	Auscultation with a stethoscope	Positive if observed at least 4 times during 5 repetitions of mouth opening	70 patients (90 TMJs) referred with complaints of craniomandibular pain	MRI	.10	.71	.40	.90	.17	7.10	2.25	.32
Reciprocal clicking		Positive if a click on opening is followed by a click on closing			.4	.76	.52	.95	.83	15.2	1.51	.25
Deviation with correction	Examiner observes active mouth opening	Positive if a deviation occurs and the mandible returns to midline			.14	.44	.57	.83	.33	2.59	1.51	.67
Deviation without correction		Positive if the mandible does not return to midline after deviation			.18	.66	.41	.83	.31	3.88	2.0	.41
Restriction range functional		Measurement is taken at the end range of active mouth opening			.38	.86	.21	.62	.48	2.26	2.95	.23

Detecting Anterior Disc Displacement of the Temporomandibular Joint (cont.)

Test and Measure	Test Procedure	Determination of Findings	Population	Reference Standard	Sens DR	Sens DDR	Spec DR	Spec DDR	+LR DR	+LR DDR	−LR DR	−LR DDR
Restriction range passive opening	Measurement is taken at the end range of passive mouth opening after 15 sec	Not reported	70 patients (90 TMJs) referred with complaints of craniomandibular pain	MRI	.29	.76	.29	.69	.41	2.45	2.45	.35
Restricted translation	Not reported	Patient demonstrates inability to obtain full movement			.15	.66	.38	.81	.24	3.47	2.24	.42
Restricted protrusion	Measurement is taken at the end range of active mandibular protrusion	Patient demonstrates inability to obtain full movement			.29	.62	.38	.64	.47	1.72	1.87	.59
Restricted contralateral movement	Measurement is taken at the end of contralateral movement from the midline	Patient demonstrates inability to obtain full movement			.15	.66	.34	.76	.23	2.75	2.50	.45
Joint pain on opening	Patient opens mouth as wide as possible	Positive if patient reports pain			.44	.74	.31	.57	.64	1.72	1.81	.46
Tender joint on palpation	Examiner palpates the lateral and posterior aspects of the joint	Positive if patient reports tenderness or pain			.38	.66	.41	.67	.64	2.0	1.51	.51
Pain contralateral motion *Stegenga et al.*[18]	Patient performs lateral excursion contralateral to the side of joint involvement	Positive if patient reports pain			.6	.34	.69	.93	1.94	4.86	.58	.71

DIAGNOSTIC UTILITY OF THE CLINICAL EXAMINATION

DIAGNOSTIC UTILITY OF THE CLINICAL EXAMINATION

Detecting Anterior Disc Displacement of the Temporomandibular Joint

Test and Measure	Test Procedure	Determination of Findings	Population	Reference Standard	Sens	Spec	+LR	−LR
With Reduction								
No deviation of the mandible on maximal opening	Patient opens mouth maximally while examiner views the mandibular position at end range	Horizontal difference between the upper and lower central incisors is considered a deviation	146 patients attending a TMJ and craniofacial pain clinic	Magnetic resonance imaging (MRI)	.84	.20	1.05	.80
No TMJ pain during assisted opening	At the end of maximal mouth opening, the examiner applies 2 to 3 lb of overpressure	The presence or absence of pain is recorded			.83	.21	1.05	.81
No limitation of maximal mouth opening	Patient opens mouth maximally, and examiner measures the distance in millimeters	<40 mm is considered a restriction			.81	.21	1.03	.90
No restriction of condylar translation	Patient opens mouth maximally while examiner palpates condylar movement	Examiner records any limitation of condylar translation			.76	.33	1.13	.73
Clicking	Examiner palpates the lateral aspect of the TMJ during opening and closing	Audible palpable clicking is recorded by the examiner			.51	.83	3.0	.59

Detecting Anterior Disc Displacement of the Temporomandibular Joint (cont.)

Test and Measure	Test Procedure	Determination of Findings	Population	Reference Standard	Sens	Spec	+LR	–LR
Without Reduction								
Restriction of condylar translation	Patient opens mouth maximally while examiner palpates condylar movement	Examiner records any limitation of condylar translation	146 patients attending a TMJ and craniofacial pain clinic	MRI	.69	.81	3.63	.38
TMJ pain during assisted opening	At the end of maximal mouth opening, the examiner applies 2 to 3 lb of overpressure	The presence or absence of pain is recorded			.55	.91	6.11	.49
Deviation of the mandible	Patient opens the mouth maximally	Positive if the midline of the upper and lower incisors does not line up			.32	.87	2.46	.78
Limitation of maximal mouth opening	Patient opens the mouth maximally and examiner measures the distance in millimeters	<40 mm is considered a restriction			.32	.83	1.88	.82
No clicking *Orsini et al.*[5]	Examiner palpates the lateral aspect of the TMJ during opening and closing	Audible palpable clicking is recorded by the examiner			.77	.24	1.01	.96

Accuracy of Combined Tests for Detecting Anterior Disc Displacement With Reduction

Test and Measure	Population	Reference Standard	Sens	Spec	+LR	−LR
No deviation of the mandible No pain during assisted opening			.76	.30	1.09	.80
No deviation of the mandible No limitation of opening			.76	.27	1.04	.89
No deviation of the mandible No restriction of condylar translation			.75	.37	1.19	.68
No deviation of the mandible Clicking	146 patients attending a TMJ and craniofacial pain clinic	MRI	.51	.85	3.40	.58
No deviation of the mandible No pain during opening No limitation of opening			.71	.35	1.09	.83
No deviation of the mandible No pain during opening No limitation of opening No restriction of condylar translation			.68	.37	1.08	.86
No deviation of the mandible No pain during opening No limitation of opening No restriction of condylar translation Clicking *Orsini et al.*[5]			.44	.86	3.14	.65

Accuracy of Combined Tests for Detecting Anterior Disc Displacement With Reduction (cont.)

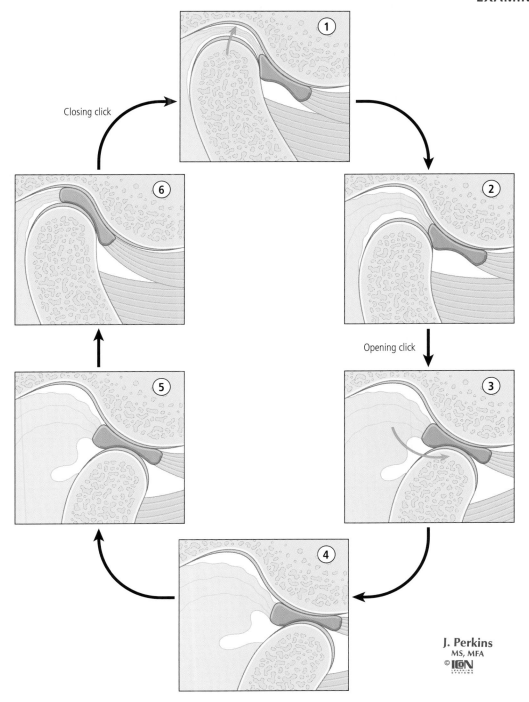

Figure 3-27: *Anterior disc displacement with reduction*

Combined Tests for Detecting Anterior Disc Displacement Without Reduction

Test and Measure	Population	Reference Standard	Sens	Spec	+LR	−LR
Motion restriction No clicking			.61	.82	3.39	.48
Motion restriction Pain during assisted opening			.54	.93	7.71	.49
Motion restriction Limitation of maximal mouth opening			.31	.87	2.38	.79
Motion restriction Deviation of the mandible			.30	.90	3.0	.78
Motion restriction No clicking TMJ pain with assistive opening	146 patients attending a TMJ and craniofacial pain clinic	MRI	.46	.94	7.67	.59
Motion restriction No clicking TMJ pain with assistive opening Limitation of maximum mouth opening			.22	.96	5.50	.81
Motion restriction No clicking TMJ pain with assistive opening Limitation of maximum mouth opening Deviation of the mandible *Orsini et al.*[5]			.11	.98	5.5	.91

Combined Tests for Detecting Anterior Disc Displacement Without Reduction (cont.)

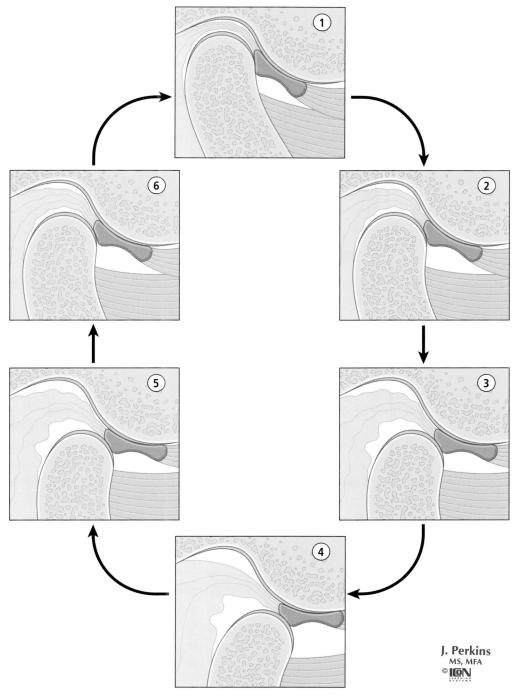

J. Perkins
MS, MFA
©IGN

Figure 3-28: *Anterior disc displacement without reduction*

Diagnostic Criteria for Detecting Intra-articular Temporomandibular Disorders

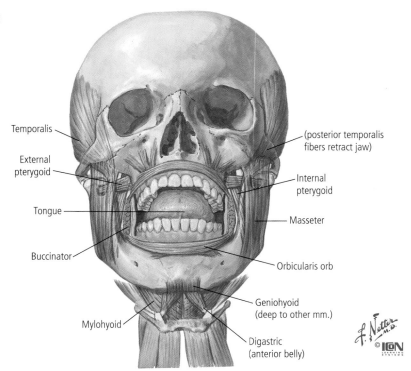

Figure 3-29: *Musculature of the temporomandibular joint*

History and Examination	Normal	Internal Derangement With Reduction	Internal Derangement Without Reduction/ Acute	Internal Derangement Without Reduction/ Chronic
History	None	None	Positive history of mandibular limitation	Positive history of TMJ sounds
Examination *Schiffman et al.*[24]	1. No reciprocal click 2. No coarse crepitus 3. Passive stretch ≥40 mm 4. Lateral movements ≥7 mm 5. If S-curve deviation is present, then joint must be silent	1. No reciprocal click 2. No coarse crepitus 3. Passive stretch ≥40 mm	1. No reciprocal click 2. No coarse crepitus 3. Maximal mouth opening ≥35 mm 4. Passive stretch ≥40 mm 5. Contralateral movement ≥7 mm 6. No S-curve deviation	1. No reciprocal click 2. Coarse crepitus or joint sound other than #1

Schiffman et al.[24] investigated the overall sensitivity and specificity of the following criteria for classifying intra-articular TMJ disorders compared with arthrotomography. The sensitivity is determined to be .85, specificity .81, +LR 4.47, and –LR .19.

Accuracy of Clinical Criteria for Classifying Internal Derangement and Arthrosis

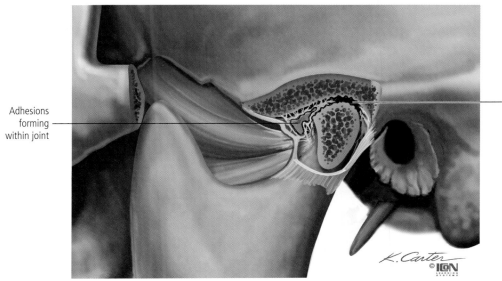

Adhesions forming within joint

Rupture of meniscus causing bony surfaces to rub

Figure 3-30: *Temporomandibular arthrosis*

Normal Superior Disc Position and Normal Function	Disc Displacement With Reduction	Disc Displacement Without Reduction	Disc Displacement Without Reduction Associated With Arthrosis
Maximal mouth opening >40 mm, movement to opposite side >8. No palpable or audible joint sound. No joint pain	Reciprocal clicking that could be eliminated by starting the opening movements from a protruded position	A history of sudden onset of restricted mouth opening and impaired lateral movement toward the opposite side, usually associated with disappearance of clicking or transient locking	Same as disc displacement without reduction but associated with audible or palpable crepitations

Paesani et al.[25] investigated the accuracy of the above clinical criteria for detecting the presence of internal derangement or arthrosis of the TMJ. Compared with MRI on 220 joints, clinical criteria demonstrated a sensitivity of .78, specificity of .52, +LR of 1.63, and –LR of .42 in the identification of internal derangement, with a sensitivity of .42, specificity of .90, +LR of 4.2, and –LR of .64 for the identification of joint arthrosis.

DIAGNOSTIC UTILITY OF THE CLINICAL EXAMINATION

Identifying Patients with Craniomandibular Pain

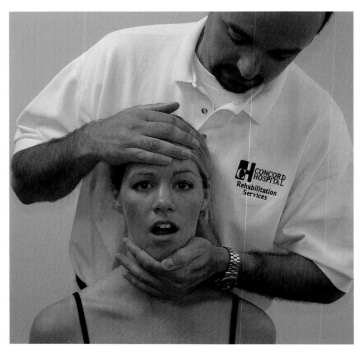

Figure 3-31A: *Manual resistance applied during mouth opening*

Test and Measure	Test Procedure	Determination of Findings	Population	Reference Standard	Sens	Spec	+LR	−LR
Palpation	Examiner palpates the TMJ laterally and posteriorly, the temporalis muscle, and the masseter muscle				.75	.67	2.27	.37
Dynamic/ static	Examiner applies manual resistance during mouth opening, closing, protrusion, and lateral deviation	Examiner records the presence of pain on a verbal scale and a visual analog scale	147 patients referred for craniomandibular complaints and 103 asymptomatic individuals	Patient report of tenderness in the masticatory muscles, the preauricular area, or the temporomandibular area in the past month	.63	.93	.90	.40
Active movement	Patient maximally depresses, protrudes, and deviates mandible right and left				.87	.67	2.64	.19
Passive movement *Visscher et al.*[26]	Examiner gently applies overpressure at the end of maximal mouth opening				.80	.64	2.22	.31

Identifying Patients with Craniomandibular Pain (cont.)

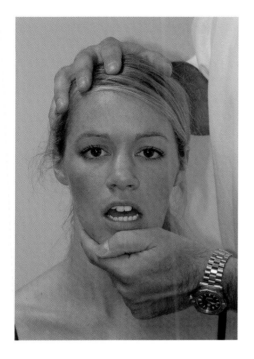

Figure 3-31B: *Manual resistance applied during mouth closing*

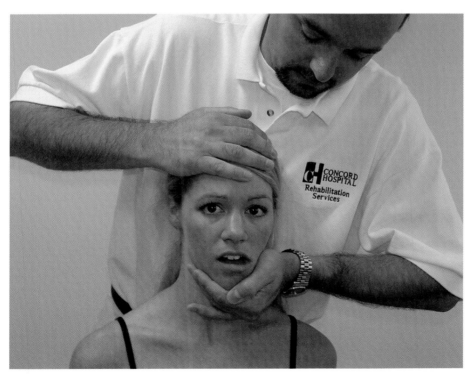

Figure 3-31C: *Manual resistance applied during lateral deviation*

REFERENCES

1. Bennett AC. Temporomandibular disorder and orofacial pain. In: *Physical Therapy for the Cervical Spine and Temporomandibular Joint*. La Crosse: Orthopaedic Section, American Physical Therapy Association; 2003.

2. Widmer CG. Evaluation of temporomandibular disorders. In: Kraus SL, ed. *TMJ Disorders: Management of the Craniomandibular Complex*. New York: Churchill Livingstone; 1988:79-112.

3. Barclay P, Hollender L, Maravilla K, Truelove E. Comparison of clinical and magnetic resonance imaging diagnoses in patients with disc displacement in the temporomandibular joint. *Oral Surg Oral Med Oral Pathol*. 1999;88:37-43.

4. Cholitgul W, Nishiyama H, Sasai T, Uchiyama Y, Fuchihata H, Rohlin M. Clinical and magnetic resonance imaging findings in temporomandibular joint disc displacement. *Dentomaxillofac Radiol*. 1997;26:183-188.

5. Orsini MG, Kuboki T, Terada S, Matsuka Y, Yatani H, Yamashita A. Clinical predictability of temporomandibular joint disc displacement. *J Dent Res*. 1999;78:650-660.

6. Hertling DL. The temporomandibular joint. In: Hall CM, ed. *Therapeutic Exercise: Moving Toward Function*. Philadelphia: Lippincott Williams & Wilkins; 1999:499-520.

7. Gross A, Haines T, Thomson M, Goldsmith C, McIntosh J. Diagnostic tests for temporomandibular disorders: an assessment of the methodological quality of research reviews. *Man Ther*. 1996;1:250-257.

8. Haley D, Schiffman E, Lindgren B, Anderson Q, Andreason K. The relationship between clinical and MRI findings in patients with unilateral temporomandibular joint pain. *J Am Dent Assoc*. 2001;132:476-481.

9. Walker N, Bohannon RW, Cameron D. Discriminant validity of temporomandibular joint range of motion measurements obtained with a ruler. *J Orthop Sports Phys Ther*. 2000;30:484-492.

10. Higbie EJ, Seidel-Cobb D, Taylor LF, Cummings GS. Effect of head position on vertical mandibular opening. *J Orthop Sports Phys Ther*. 1999;29:127-130.

11. Magnusson T, List T, Helkimo M. Self-assessment of pain and discomfort in patients with temporomandibular disorders: a comparison of five different scales with respect to their precision and sensitivity as well as their capacity to register memory of pain and discomfort. *J Oral Rehabil*. 1995;22:549-556.

12. Marbach JJ, Raphael KG, Janal MN, Hirschkorn-Roth R. Reliability of clinician judgements of bruxism. *J Oral Rehabil*. 2003;30:113-118.

13. Manfredini D, Tognini F, Zampa V, Bosco M. Predictive value of clinical findings for temporomandibular joint effusion. *Oral Surg Oral Med Oral Pathol*. 2003;96:521-526.

14. Dworkin SF, LeResche L, DeRouen T, Von Korff M. Assessing clinical signs of temporomandibular disorders: reliability of clinical examiners. *J Prosthet Dent*. 1990;63:574-579.

15. Lobbezoo-Scholte AM, de Wijer A, Steenks MH, Bosman F. Interexaminer reliability of six orthopaedic tests in diagnostic subgroups of craniomandibular disorders. *J Oral Rehabil*. 1994;21:273-285.

16. de Wijer A, Lobbezoo-Scholte AM, Steenks MH, Bosman F. Reliability of clinical findings in temporomandibular disorders. *J Orofac Pain*. 1995;9:181-191.

17. Cacchiotti DA, Plesh O, Bianchi P, McNeill C. Signs and symptoms in samples with and without temporomandibular disorders. *J Craniomandib Disord.* 1991;5:167-172.

18. Stegenga B, de Bont L, van der Kuijl B, Boering G. Classification of temporomandibular joint osteoarthrosis and internal derangement. Part 1: Diagnostic significance of clinical and radiographic symptoms and signs. *J Craniomandib Pract.* 1992;10:96-117.

19. Gavish A, Halachmi M, Winocur E, Gazit E. Oral habits and their association with signs and symptoms of temporomandibular disorders in adolescent girls. *J Oral Rehabil.* 2000;27:22-32.

20. Riolo ML, TenHave TR, Brandt D. Clinical validity of the relationship between TMJ signs and symptoms in children and youth. *ASDC J Dent Child.* 1988;55:110-113.

21. Israel H, Diamond B, Saed-Nejad F, Ratcliffe A. Osteoarthritis and synovitis as major pathoses of the temporomandibular joint: comparison of the clinical diagnosis with arthroscopic morphology. *J Oral Maxillofac Surg.* 1998;56:1023-1028.

22. Holmlund AB, Axelsson S. Temporomandibular arthropathy: correlation between clinical signs and symptoms and arthroscopic findings. *Int J Oral Maxillofac Surg.* 1996;25:178-181.

23. Emshoff R, Innerhofer K, Rudisch A, Bertram S. Clinical versus magnetic resonance imaging findings with internal derangement of the temporomandibular joint: an evaluation of anterior disc displacement without reduction. *J Oral Maxillofac Surg.* 2002;60:36-41.

24. Schiffman E, Anderson G, Fricton J, Burton K, Schellhas K. Diagnostic criteria for intraarticular TM disorders. *Community Dent Oral Epidemiol.* 1989;17:257.

25. Paesani D, Westesson PL, Hatala M, Tallents RH, Brooks S. Accuracy of clinical diagnosis for TMJ internal derangement and arthrosis. *Oral Surg Oral Med Oral Pathol.* 1992;73:360-363.

26. Visscher CM, Lobbezoo F, de Boer W, van der ZJ, Verheij JG, Naeije M. Clinical tests in distinguishing between persons with or without craniomandibular or cervical spinal pain complaints. *Eur J Oral Sci.* 2000;108:475-483.

REFERENCES

Cervical Spine

Chapter 4

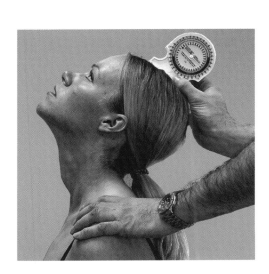

OSTEOLOGY   Bony Framework of the Head and Neck

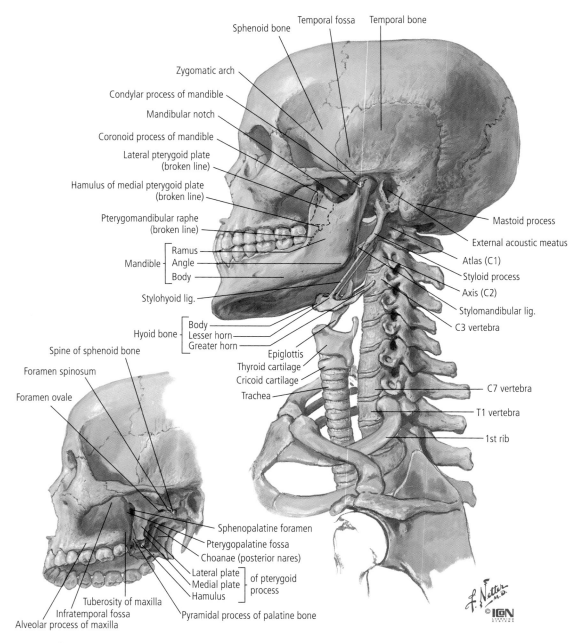

Sphenoid bone
Temporal fossa
Temporal bone
Zygomatic arch
Condylar process of mandible
Mandibular notch
Coronoid process of mandible
Lateral pterygoid plate (broken line)
Hamulus of medial pterygoid plate (broken line)
Pterygomandibular raphe (broken line)
Ramus
Mandible - Angle
Body
Stylohyoid lig.
Body
Hyoid bone - Lesser horn
Greater horn
Spine of sphenoid bone
Foramen spinosum
Foramen ovale

Mastoid process
External acoustic meatus
Atlas (C1)
Styloid process
Axis (C2)
Stylomandibular lig.
C3 vertebra
Epiglottis
Thyroid cartilage
Cricoid cartilage
Trachea
C7 vertebra
T1 vertebra
1st rib

Sphenopalatine foramen
Pterygopalatine fossa
Choanae (posterior nares)
Lateral plate
Medial plate   of pterygoid
Hamulus   process
Tuberosity of maxilla
Infratemporal fossa
Alveolar process of maxilla
Pyramidal process of palatine bone

Figure 4-1

Cervical Vertebrae

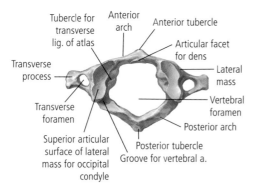

Atlas (C1): superior view

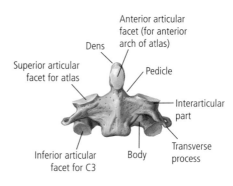

Axis (C2): anterior view

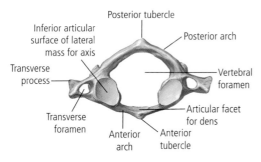

Atlas (C1): inferior view

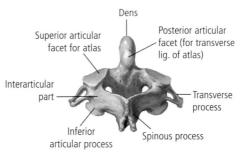

Axis (C2): posterosuperior view

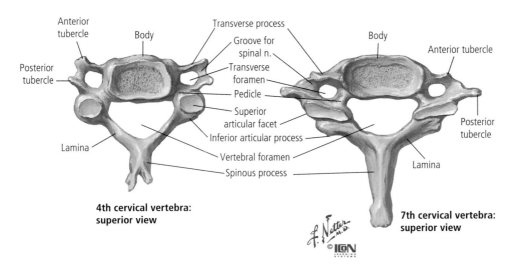

4th cervical vertebra: superior view

7th cervical vertebra: superior view

Figure 4-2

ARTHROLOGY   Joints of the Cervical Spine

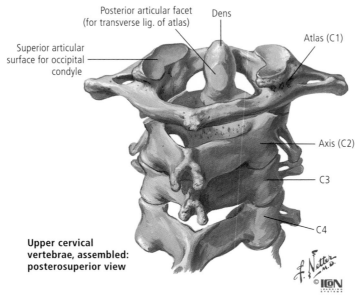

Figure 4-3: *Upper cervical vertebrae*

Joint	Type and Classification	Closed Packed Position	Capsular Pattern
Atlanto-occipital	Synovial: plane	NR	NR
Atlanto-odontoid/ dens	Synovial: trochoid	Extension	NR
Atlantoaxial apophyseal	Synovial: plane	Extension	NR
C3-C7 apophyseal	Synovial: plane	Full extension	Limitation in side bending = rotation = extension
C3-C7 intervertebral	Amphiarthrodial	Not applicable	Not applicable

NR, not reported

Joints of the Cervical Spine (cont.)

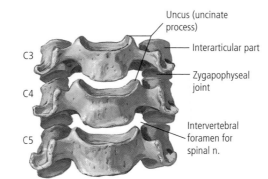

Uncus (uncinate process)

Interarticular part

C3

Zygapophyseal joint

C4

Intervertebral foramen for spinal n.

C5

3rd, 4th and 5th cervical vertebrae: anterior view

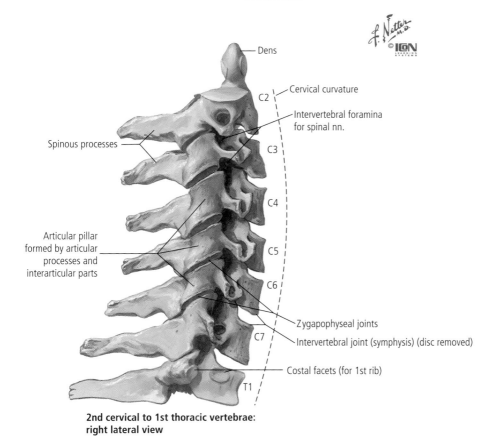

Dens

Cervical curvature

C2

Intervertebral foramina for spinal nn.

Spinous processes

C3

C4

Articular pillar formed by articular processes and interarticular parts

C5

C6

Zygapophyseal joints

Intervertebral joint (symphysis) (disc removed)

C7

Costal facets (for 1st rib)

T1

2nd cervical to 1st thoracic vertebrae: right lateral view

Figure 4-4: *Joints of the cervical vertebrae*

LIGAMENTS   Ligaments of the Atlanto-occipital Joint

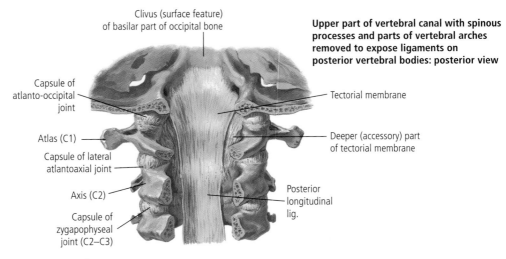

Clivus (surface feature) of basilar part of occipital bone

Upper part of vertebral canal with spinous processes and parts of vertebral arches removed to expose ligaments on posterior vertebral bodies: posterior view

Capsule of atlanto-occipital joint

Tectorial membrane

Atlas (C1)

Deeper (accessory) part of tectorial membrane

Capsule of lateral atlantoaxial joint

Axis (C2)

Posterior longitudinal lig.

Capsule of zygapophyseal joint (C2–C3)

Figure 4-5

Ligaments		Attachments	Function
Alar		Sides of dens to lateral aspects of foramen magnum	Limits ipsilateral head rotation and contralateral side bending
Apical		Dens to posterior aspect of foramen magnum	Limits separation of dens from occiput
Tectorial membrane		Body of C2 to occiput	Limits forward flexion
Cruciform ligament	Superior longitudinal	Transverse ligament to occiput	Maintains contact between dens and anterior arch of atlas
	Transverse	Extends between lateral tubercles of C1	
	Inferior	Transverse ligament Longitudinal to body of C2	

Ligaments of the Atlanto-occipital Joint (cont.)

LIGAMENTS

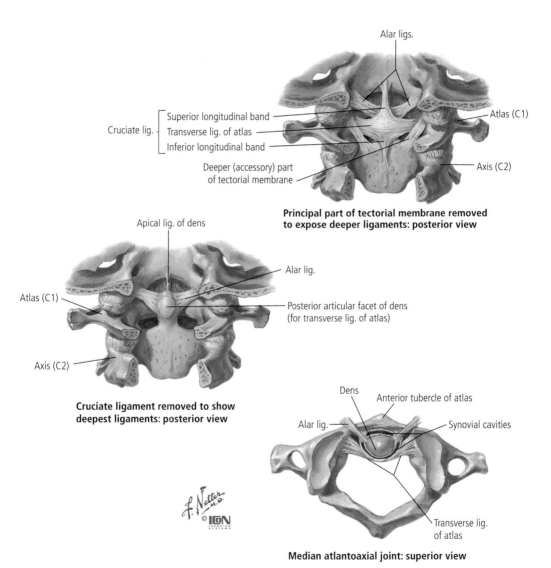

Alar ligs.

Superior longitudinal band
Cruciate lig. — Transverse lig. of atlas
Inferior longitudinal band

Atlas (C1)

Deeper (accessory) part
of tectorial membrane

Axis (C2)

**Principal part of tectorial membrane removed
to expose deeper ligaments: posterior view**

Apical lig. of dens

Alar lig.

Atlas (C1)

Posterior articular facet of dens
(for transverse lig. of atlas)

Axis (C2)

**Cruciate ligament removed to show
deepest ligaments: posterior view**

Dens   Anterior tubercle of atlas

Alar lig.

Synovial cavities

Transverse lig.
of atlas

Median atlantoaxial joint: superior view

Figure 4-5 (cont.)

LIGAMENTS   Spinal Ligaments

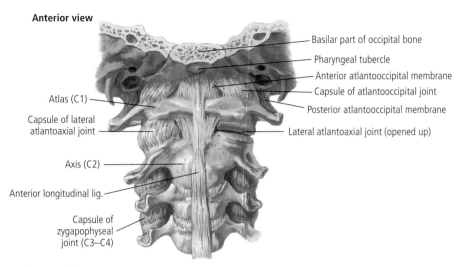

Anterior view

- Basilar part of occipital bone
- Pharyngeal tubercle
- Anterior atlantooccipital membrane
- Capsule of atlantooccipital joint
- Posterior atlantooccipital membrane
- Lateral atlantoaxial joint (opened up)

Atlas (C1)

Capsule of lateral
atlantoaxial joint

Axis (C2)

Anterior longitudinal lig.

Capsule of
zygapophyseal
joint (C3–C4)

Figure 4-6

Ligament	Attachments	Function
Anterior longitudinal	Extends from anterior sacrum to anterior tubercle of C1. Connects anterolateral vertebral bodies and disks	Maintains stability of vertebral body joints and prevents hyperextension of vertebral column
Posterior longitudinal	Extends from sacrum to C2. Runs within vertebral canal, attaching posterior vertebral bodies	Prevents hyperflexion of vertebral column and posterior disk protrusion
Ligamentum nuchae	Extension of supraspinous ligament (occipital protuberance to C7)	Prevents cervical hyperflexion
Ligamenta flava	Attach lamina above each vertebra to lamina below	Prevent separation of vertebral laminae
Supraspinous	Connect apices of spinous processes C7-S1	Limit separation of spinous processes
Interspinous	Connect adjoining spinous processes C1-S1	Limit separation of spinous processes
Intertransverse	Connect adjacent transverse processes of vertebrae	Limit separation of transverse processes

Spinal Ligaments (cont.)   **LIGAMENTS**

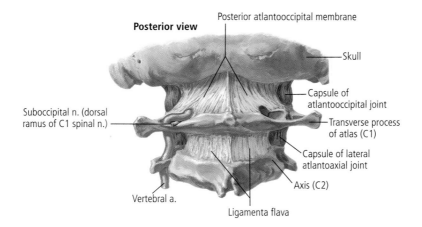

Posterior view

Posterior atlantooccipital membrane

Skull

Capsule of atlantooccipital joint

Suboccipital n. (dorsal ramus of C1 spinal n.)

Transverse process of atlas (C1)

Capsule of lateral atlantoaxial joint

Axis (C2)

Vertebral a.

Ligamenta flava

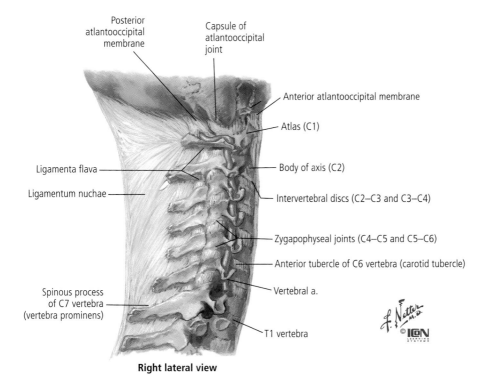

Posterior atlantooccipital membrane

Capsule of atlantooccipital joint

Anterior atlantooccipital membrane

Atlas (C1)

Ligamenta flava

Body of axis (C2)

Ligamentum nuchae

Intervertebral discs (C2–C3 and C3–C4)

Zygapophyseal joints (C4–C5 and C5–C6)

Anterior tubercle of C6 vertebra (carotid tubercle)

Vertebral a.

Spinous process of C7 vertebra (vertebra prominens)

T1 vertebra

Right lateral view

Figure 4-6 (cont.)

MUSCLES   **Anterior Muscles of the Neck**

Muscle		Proximal Attachment	Distal Attachment	Nerve and Segmental Level	Action
Sternocleidomastoid		Mastoid process and lateral superior nuchal line	Sternal head: anterior manubrium Clavicular head: superior medial clavicle	Spinal root of accessory nerve	Neck flexion, ipsilateral side bending, and contralateral rotation
Scalenes	Anterior	Transverse processes of vertebrae C4-C6	1st rib	C4, C5, C6	Elevates 1st rib, ipsilateral side bending, and contralateral rotation
	Middle	Transverse processes of vertebrae C1-C4	Superior aspect of 1st rib	Ventral rami of cervical spinal nerves	Elevates 1st rib, ipsilateral side bending, and contralateral rotation
	Posterior		External aspect of 2nd rib	Ventral rami of cervical spinal nerves C3, C4	Elevates 2nd rib, ipsilateral side bending, and contralateral rotation
Platysma		Inferior mandible	Fascia of pectoralis major and deltoid	Cervical branch of facial nerve	Draws skin of neck superiorly with clenched jaw, draws corners of mouth inferiorly

Anterior Muscles of the Neck (cont.)   **MUSCLES**

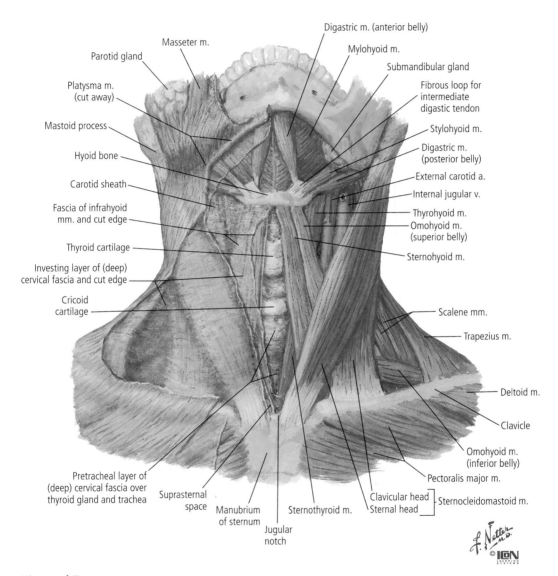

Figure 4-7

MUSCLES   Suprahyoids/Infrahyoids

Muscle		Proximal Attachment	Distal Attachment	Nerve and Segmental Level	Action
Suprahyoids	Mylohyoid	Mandibular mylohyoid line	Hyoid bone	Mylohyoid nerve	Elevates hyoid bone, floor of mouth, and tongue
	Geniohyoid	Mental spine of mandible	Body of hyoid bone	Hypoglossal nerve	Elevates hyoid bone anterosuperiorly, widens pharynx
	Stylohyoid	Styloid process of temporal bone	Body of hyoid bone	Cervical branch of facial nerve	Elevates and retracts hyoid bone
	Digastric	Anterior belly: digastric fossa of mandible Posterior belly: mastoid notch of temporal bone	Greater horn of hyoid bone	Anterior belly: mylohyoid nerve Posterior belly: facial nerve	Depresses mandible and raises hyoid
Infrahyoids	Sternohyoid	Manubrium and medial clavicle	Body of hyoid bone	Branch of ansa cervicalis (C1, C2, C3)	Depresses hyoid bone after it has been elevated
	Omohyoid	Superior border of scapula	Inferior aspect of hyoid bone	Branch of ansa cervicalis (C1, C2, C3)	Depresses and retracts hyoid bone
	Sternothyroid	Posterior aspect of manubrium	Thyroid cartilage	Branch of ansa cervicalis (C2, C3)	Depresses hyoid bone and larynx
	Thyrohyoid	Thyroid cartilage	Body and greater horn of hyoid bone	Hypoglossal nerve (C1)	Depresses hyoid bone, elevates larynx

Suprahyoids/Infrahyoids (cont.)   **MUSCLES**

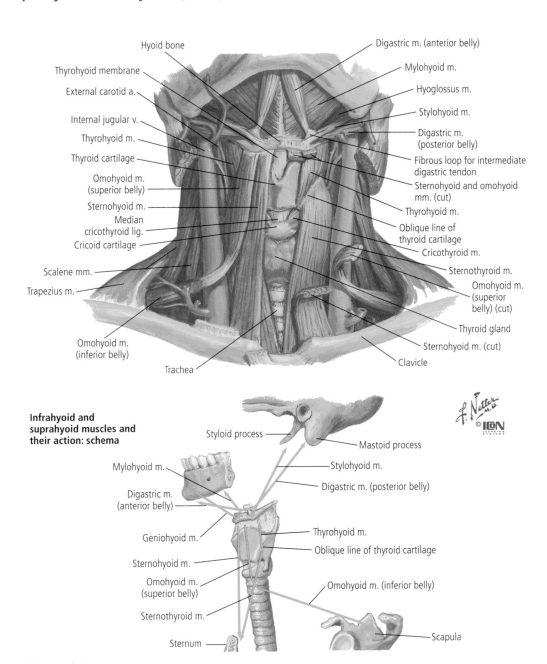

Hyoid bone

Thyrohyoid membrane

External carotid a.

Internal jugular v.

Thyrohyoid m.

Thyroid cartilage

Omohyoid m. (superior belly)

Sternohyoid m.

Median cricothyroid lig.

Cricoid cartilage

Scalene mm.

Trapezius m.

Omohyoid m. (inferior belly)

Trachea

Digastric m. (anterior belly)

Mylohyoid m.

Hyoglossus m.

Stylohyoid m.

Digastric m. (posterior belly)

Fibrous loop for intermediate digastric tendon

Sternohyoid and omohyoid mm. (cut)

Thyrohyoid m.

Oblique line of thyroid cartilage

Cricothyroid m.

Sternothyroid m.

Omohyoid m. (superior belly) (cut)

Thyroid gland

Sternohyoid m. (cut)

Clavicle

Infrahyoid and suprahyoid muscles and their action: schema

Styloid process

Mastoid process

Mylohyoid m.

Stylohyoid m.

Digastric m. (anterior belly)

Digastric m. (posterior belly)

Geniohyoid m.

Thyrohyoid m.

Oblique line of thyroid cartilage

Sternohyoid m.

Omohyoid m. (superior belly)

Omohyoid m. (inferior belly)

Sternothyroid m.

Sternum

Scapula

Figure 4-8

MUSCLES   **Scalene and Prevertebral Muscles**

Muscle	Proximal Attachment	Distal Attachment	Nerve and Segmental Level	Action
Longus capitis	Basilar aspect of occipital bone	Anterior tubercles of transverse processes C3-C6	Ventral rami of C1-C3 spinal nerves	Flexes head on neck
Longus colli	Anterior tubercle of C1, bodies of C1-C3, and transverse processes of C3-C6	Bodies of C3-T3 and transverse processes of C3-C5	Ventral rami of C2-C6 spinal nerves	Neck flexion, ipsilateral side bending and rotation
Rectus capitis anterior	Base of skull anterior to occipital condyle	Anterior aspect of lateral mass of C1	Branches from loop between C1 and C2 spinal nerves	Flexes head on neck
Rectus capitis lateralis	Jugular process of occipital bone	Transverse process of C1		Flexes head and assists in stabilizing head on neck

Scalene and Prevertebral Muscles (cont.) MUSCLES

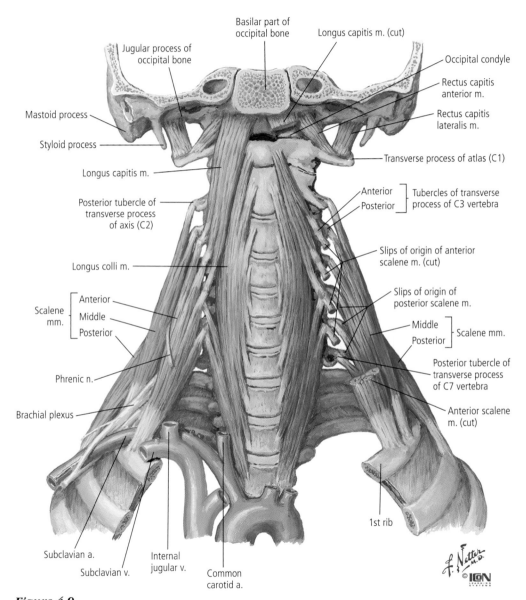

Figure 4-9

MUSCLES   Posterior Muscles of the Neck

Muscle Attachment		Proximal Attachment	Distal Segmental Level	Nerve and	Action
Upper trapezius		Superior nuchal line, occipital protuberance, nuchal ligament, spinous processes of C7-C12	Lateral clavicle, acromion, and spine of scapula	Spinal root of accessory nerve	Elevation of scapula
Levator scapulae		Transverse processes of C1-C4	Superomedial border of scapula	Dorsal scapular nerve (C3, C4, C5)	Elevaion of scapula and inferior rotation of glenoid fossa
Semispinalis capitis and cervicis		Cervical and thoracic spinous processes	Superior spinous processes and occipital bone	Dorsal rami of spinal nerves	Bilaterally: extension of the neck Unilaterally: ipsilateral side bending
Splenius capitis and cervicis		Spinous processes of T1-T6 and ligamentum nuchae	Mastoid process and lateral superior nuchal line	Dorsal rami of middle cervical spinal nerves	Bilaterally: head and neck extension Unilaterally: ipsilateral rotation
Longissimus capitis and cervicis		Superior thoracic tranverse processes and cervical transverse processes	Mastoid process of temporal bone and cervical transverse processes	Dorsal rami of cervical spinal nerves	Head extension, ipsilateral side bending, and rotation of head and neck
Spinalis cervicis		Lower cervical spinous processes of vertebrae	Upper cervical spinous processes of vertebrae	Dorsal rami of spinal nerves	Bilaterally: extension of the neck Unilaterally: ipsilateral side bending of neck
Posterior occipitals	Rectus capitis posterior major	Spinous process of C2	Lateral inferior nuchal line of occipital bone	Suboccipital nerve (C1)	Head extension and ipsilateral rotation
	Rectus capitis posterior minor	Posterior arch of C1	Medial inferior nuchal line	Suboccipital nerve (C1)	Head extension and ipsilateral rotation
	Obliquus capitis superior	Transverse process of C1	Occipital bone	Suboccipital nerve (C1)	Head extension and side bending
	Obliquus capitis inferior	Spinous process of C2	Transverse process of C1	Suboccipital nerve (C1)	Ipsilateral neck rotation

Posterior Muscles of the Neck (cont.)   **MUSCLES**

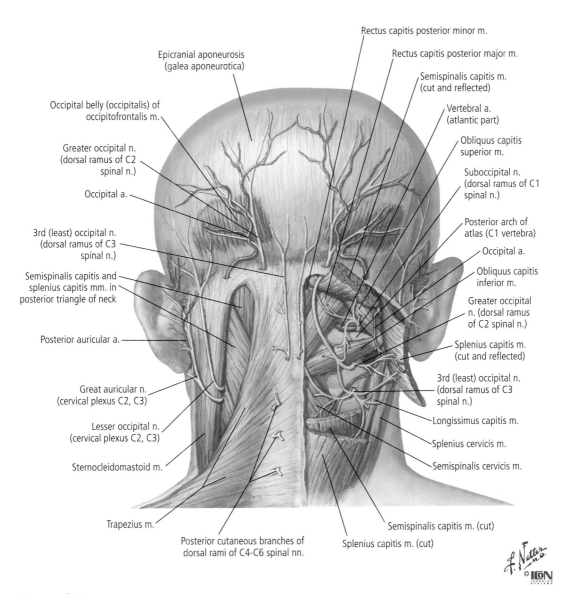

Rectus capitis posterior minor m.

Epicranial aponeurosis
(galea aponeurotica)

Rectus capitis posterior major m.

Semispinalis capitis m.
(cut and reflected)

Occipital belly (occipitalis) of
occipitofrontalis m.

Vertebral a.
(atlantic part)

Greater occipital n.
(dorsal ramus of C2
spinal n.)

Obliquus capitis
superior m.

Suboccipital n.
(dorsal ramus of C1
spinal n.)

Occipital a.

3rd (least) occipital n.
(dorsal ramus of C3
spinal n.)

Posterior arch of
atlas (C1 vertebra)

Occipital a.

Semispinalis capitis and
splenius capitis mm. in
posterior triangle of neck

Obliquus capitis
inferior m.

Greater occipital
n. (dorsal ramus
of C2 spinal n.)

Posterior auricular a.

Splenius capitis m.
(cut and reflected)

3rd (least) occipital n.
(dorsal ramus of C3
spinal n.)

Great auricular n.
(cervical plexus C2, C3)

Longissimus capitis m.

Lesser occipital n.
(cervical plexus C2, C3)

Splenius cervicis m.

Semispinalis cervicis m.

Sternocleidomastoid m.

Trapezius m.

Semispinalis capitis m. (cut)

Posterior cutaneous branches of
dorsal rami of C4-C6 spinal nn.

Splenius capitis m. (cut)

Figure 4-10

NERVES

Nerves of the Neck

Nerves	Segmental Levels	Sensory	Motor
Dorsal scapular	C4, C5	No sensory	Rhomboids, levator scapulae
Suprascapular	C4, C5, C6	No sensory	Supraspinatus, infraspinatus
Nerve to subclavius	C5, C6	No sensory	Subclavius
Lateral pectoral	C5, C6, C7	No sensory	Pectoralis major
Medial pectoral	C8, T1	No sensory	Pectoralis major Pectoralis minor
Long thoracic	C5, C6, C7	No sensory	Serratus anterior
Medial cutaneous of arm	C8, T1	Medial aspect of arm	No motor
Medial cutaneous of forearm	C8, T1	Medial aspect of forearm	No motor
Upper subscapular	C5, C6	No sensory	Subscapularis
Lower subscapular	C5, C6, C7	No sensory	Subscapularis, teres major
Thoracodorsal	C6, C7, C8	No sensory	Latissimus dorsi
Axillary	C5, C6	Lateral shoulder	Deltoid, teres minor
Radial	C5, C6, C7, C8, T1	Dorsal lateral aspect of hand, including the thumb and up to the base of digits 2 and 3	Triceps brachii, brachioradialis, anconeus, extensor carpi radialis longus, extensor carpi radialis brevis
Median	C5, C6, C7, C8, T1	Palmar aspect of lateral hand, including lateral half of 4th digit and dorsal distal half of digits 1 to 3 and lateral border of 4	Pronator teres, flexor carpi radialis, palmaris longus, flexor digitorum superficialis, flexor pollicis longus, flexor digitorum profundus (lateral half), pronator quadratus, lumbricals to digits 2 and 3, thenar muscles
Ulnar	C8, T1	Medial border of both palmar and dorsal hand, including medial half of 4th digit	Flexor carpi ulnaris, flexor digitorum profundus (medial half), palmar interossei, adductor pollicis, palmaris brevis, dorsal interossei, lumbricals to digits 4 and 5, hypothenar muscles
Musculocutaneous	C5, C6, C7	Lateral forearm	Coracobrachialis, biceps brachii, brachialis

Nerves of the Neck (cont.)

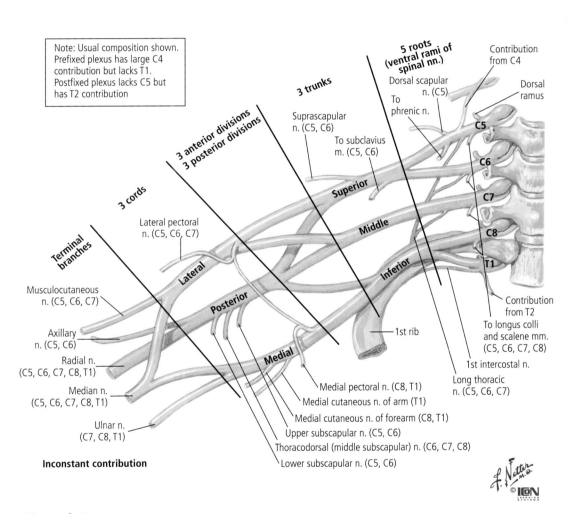

Note: Usual composition shown. Prefixed plexus has large C4 contribution but lacks T1. Postfixed plexus lacks C5 but has T2 contribution

5 roots (ventral rami of spinal nn.)

3 trunks

3 anterior divisions
3 posterior divisions

3 cords

Terminal branches

Dorsal scapular n. (C5)

To phrenic n.

Contribution from C4

Dorsal ramus

Suprascapular n. (C5, C6)

To subclavius m. (C5, C6)

Superior

Middle

Inferior

C5

C6

C7

C8

T1

Lateral pectoral n. (C5, C6, C7)

Lateral

Posterior

Medial

Musculocutaneous n. (C5, C6, C7)

Axillary n. (C5, C6)

Radial n. (C5, C6, C7, C8, T1)

Median n. (C5, C6, C7, C8, T1)

Ulnar n. (C7, C8, T1)

Inconstant contribution

1st rib

Medial pectoral n. (C8, T1)

Medial cutaneous n. of arm (T1)

Medial cutaneous n. of forearm (C8, T1)

Upper subscapular n. (C5, C6)

Thoracodorsal (middle subscapular) n. (C6, C7, C8)

Lower subscapular n. (C5, C6)

Contribution from T2

To longus colli and scalene mm. (C5, C6, C7, C8)

1st intercostal n.

Long thoracic n. (C5, C6, C7)

Figure 4-11

EXAMINATION: HISTORY

Initial Hypotheses Based on Historical Findings

History	Initial Hypothesis
Patient reports diffuse nonspecific neck pain that is exacerbated by neck movements	Mechanical neck pain[1] Cervical facet syndrome[2] Cervical muscle strain or sprain
Patient reports pain in certain postures that is alleviated by positional changes	Upper crossed postural syndrome[3, 4]
Traumatic mechanism of injury with complaint of nonspecific cervical symptoms that are exacerbated in the vertical position and relieved with the head supported in supine position	Cervical instability, especially if patient reports that dysesthesias of the face occur with neck movement[5]
Reports of nonspecific neck pain with numbness and tingling into one upper extremity	Cervical radiculopathy
Reports of neck pain with bilateral upper extremity symptoms and occasional reports of loss of balance or lack of coordination of the lower extremities	Cervical myelopathy

Reliability of the Cervical Spine Historical Examination

Historical Question	Population	Reliability Kappa Value (95% confidence interval [CI])
Which of the following symptoms is most bothersome for you? 1. Pain 2. Numbness 3. Tingling 4. Loss of feeling *Wainner et al.*[6]	50 patients with suspected cervical radiculopathy or carpal tunnel syndrome	κ = .74 (.55, .93)
Where are your symptoms most bothersome? 1. Neck 2. Shoulder or shoulder blade 3. Arm above elbow 4. Arm below elbow 5. Hands and/or fingers *Wainner et al.*[6]		κ = .83 (.68, .96)
Which of the following best describes the behavior of your symptoms? 1. Constant 2. Intermittent 3. Variable *Wainner et al.*[6]		κ = .57 (.35, .79)
Does your entire affected limb and/or hand feel numb? *Wainner et al.*[6]		κ = .53 (.26, .81)
Do your symptoms keep you from falling asleep? *Wainner et al.*[6]		κ = .70 (.48, .92)
Do your symptoms improve with movement of your neck? *Wainner et al.*[6]		κ = .67 (.44, .90)

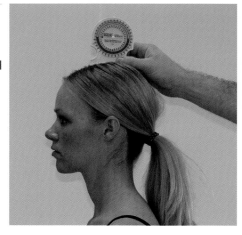

Figure 4-12: Positioning of inclinometer to measure flexion and extension

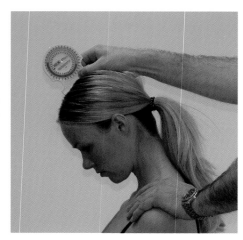

Figure 4-13: Measurement of flexion

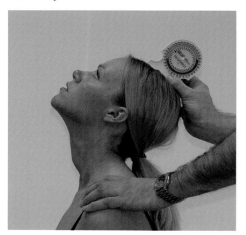

Figure 4-14: Measurements of extension

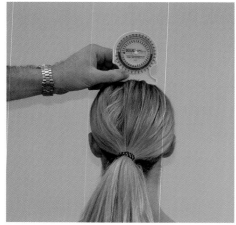

Figure 4-15: Positioning of inclinometer to measure side bending

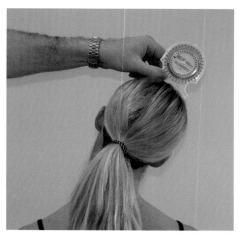

Figure 4-16: Measurement of side bending to the right

Range of Motion

Test and Measure	Instrumentation	Population	Inter-examiner Reliability ICC (95% CI)
Flexion	Inclinometer	50 patients with suspected cervical radiculopathy or carpal tunnel syndrome	.79 (.65, .88)
Extension	Inclinometer		.84 (.70, .95)
Left rotation	Goniometer		.75 (.59, .85)
Right rotation	Goniometer		.63 (.22, .82)
Left side bending	Inclinometer		.63 (.40, .78)
Right side bending *Wainner et al.[6]*	Inclinometer		.68 (.62, .87)
Flexion	CROM	60 patients with neck pain	(CI not reported) .58
Extension			.97
Right side bending			.96
Left side bending			.94
Right rotation			.96
Left rotation			.98
Protraction			.49
Retraction *Olson et al.[7]*			.35
Flexion/extension	Inclinometer CROM	30 asymptomatic subjects	Inclinometer = .84 CROM = .88
Side bending			Inclinometer = .82 CROM = .84
Rotation *Hole et al.[8]*			Inclinometer = .81 CROM = .92
Flexion	CROM UG VE	60 patients in whom the assessment of cervical ROM testing would be appropriate during the PT evaluation	CROM = .86 UG = .57 VE = .42
Extension			CROM = .86 UG = .79 VE = .42
Left side bending			CROM = .73 UG = .79 VE = .63
Right side bending			CROM = .73 UG = .79 VE = .63
Left rotation			CROM = .82 UG = .54 VE = .70
Right rotation *Youdas et al.[9]*			CROM = .92 UG = .62 VE = .82

CROM, cervical range of motion device; UG, Universal goniometer; VE, Visual estimate; PT, physical therapy.

Passive Intervertebral Motion

Test and Measure	Test Procedure and Determination of Positive Findings	Population	Inter-examiner Reliability Kappa Values
Rotation of C1-C2 *Smedmark et al.*[10]	Patient seated. C2 is stabilized while C1 is rotated on C2 until the end of passive ROM. Positive if decreased rotation on one side compared with contralateral side	61 patients with nonspecific neck problems	κ = .28
Lateral flexion of C2-C3 *Smedmark et al.*[10]	Patient supine. Examiner's left hand stabilizes the head while the right hand performs side-bending flexion of C2-C3 until the end of passive ROM. This is repeated in the contralateral direction. Positive if reduced lateral flexion on one side compared with contralateral side		κ = .43
Flexion and extension *Smedmark et al.*[10]	Patient sidelying. Examiner stabilizes the neck with one hand while palpating the movement at C7-T1 with the other hand. Positive if flexion and extension are "stiff" compared with the vertebrae superior and inferior		κ = .36
1st rib *Smedmark et al.*[10]	Patient supine. The cervical spine is rotated toward the side being tested. The 1st rib is pressed in a ventral and caudal direction. Positive if the rib is more "stiff" than the contralateral side		κ = .35

ROM, range of motion.

Passive Intervertebral Motion (cont.)

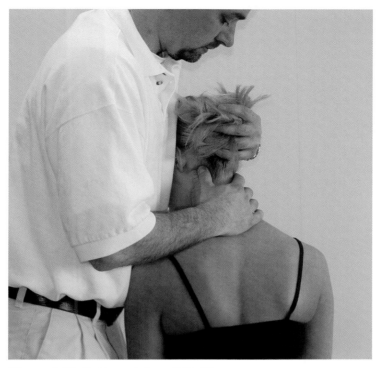

Figure 4-17: *Testing rotation of C1-C2*

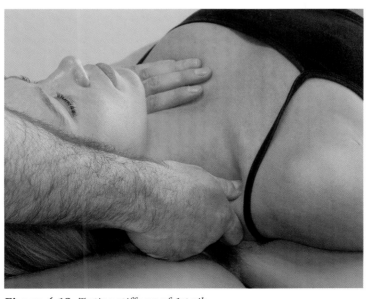

Figure 4-18: *Testing stiffness of 1st rib*

RELIABILITY OF THE CLINICAL EXAMINATION

Testing Side Bending

Test and Measure	Test Procedure and Determination of Positive Findings	Population	Inter-examiner Reliability Values			
			Limited Movements		Pain	
			Right	Left	Right	Left
C0-C1 *Pool et al.*[11]	Patient supine. Passive flexion is performed. Motion classified as limited or not limited, and patient pain response assessed on 11-point numeric pain rating (NPR) scale		κ = .29*		ICC = .73*	
C1-C2 *Pool et al.*[11]	Patient supine. Rotation is performed and classified as limited or not limited, and patient pain response assessed on 11-point NPR scale	32 patients with neck pain	κ = .20	κ = .37	ICC = .56	ICC = .35
C2-C3			κ = .34	κ = .63	ICC = .50	ICC = .78
C3-C4			κ = .20	κ = .26	ICC = .62	ICC = .75
C4-C5	Patient supine. Fixation of lower segment with side bending to the right and left. Motion classified as limited or not limited, and patient pain response assessed on 11-point NPR scale		κ = .16	κ = -.09	ICC = .62	ICC = .55
C5-C6			κ = .17	κ = .09	ICC = .66	ICC = .65
C6-C7			κ = .34	κ = .03	ICC = .59	ICC = .22
C7-T1			κ = .08	κ = .14	ICC = .45	ICC = .34
T1-T2 *Pool et al.*[11]			κ = .33	κ = .46	ICC = .80	ICC = .54

*Kappa and ICC values were calculated only for flexion of C0-C1.

Testing Side Bending (cont.)

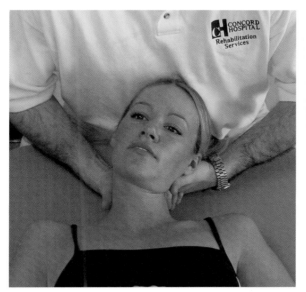

Figure 4-19: *Testing side bending of C5-C6*

RELIABILITY OF THE CLINICAL EXAMINATION

Assessment of Pain Responses During Active Physiologic Motion

Test and Measure	Test Procedure and Determination of Positive Findings	Population	Inter-examiner Reliability Kappa Values (95% CI)
Flexion	Patient seated with back supported. Patient is asked to perform full flexion, and pressure is applied by the examiner. Pain responses are recorded on 11-point NPR scale		$\kappa = .63$
Extension			$\kappa = .71$
Rotation right			$\kappa = .70$
Rotation left			$\kappa = .66$
Side bending right		32 patients with neck pain	$\kappa = .65$
Side bending left *Pool et al.[11]*			$\kappa = .45$
Flexion C0-C1	Patient is asked to perform high cervical flexion/extension by nodding. Pain responses are recorded on 11-point NPR scale		$\kappa = .36$
Extension C0-C1 *Pool et al.[11]*			$\kappa = .56$
Flexion	Patient performs AROM and pain is determined to be either present or not present	24 patients with headaches	$\kappa = .53 (.17, .89)$
Extension			$\kappa = .67 (.34, .99)$
Rotation right			$\kappa = .65 (.31, .99)$
Rotation left *van Suijlekom et al.[12]*			$\kappa = .46 (.10, .79)$

AROM, active range of motion.

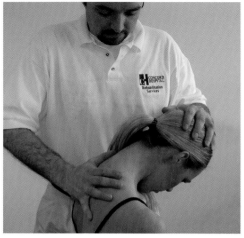

Figure 4-20A: *Testing flexion with overpressure*

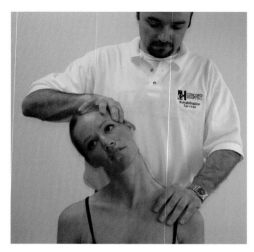

Figure 4-20B: *Testing side bending with overpressure*

Pain With Palpation

Test and Measure	Population	Inter-examiner Reliability Kappa Values (95% CI)	
Upper cervical spinous process	52 patients with cervical spondylosis (32); neurologic tumor (6); disseminated sclerosis (2); peripheral upper limb paresis (2); brachial plexus involvement (2); miscellaneous (5); unknown (3)	κ = .47	
Lower cervical spinous process		κ = .52	
Right suprascapular area		κ = .53	
Left suprascapular area *Viikari-Juntura[13]*		κ = .60	
Zygapophyseal joint pressure	24 patients with headache		
High cervical		κ = .14 (−.12, .39)	
Middle cervical		κ = .37 (.12, .85)	
Low cervical		κ = .31 (.28, .90)	
(Method of classification for high, middle, and low not described) *van Suijlekom et al.[12]*			
		With Knowledge of History	**Without Knowledge of History**
Spinous process C1-C3	100 patients with neck and/or shoulder problems with or without radiating pain	.60	.49
Spinous process C4-C7		.42	.50
Spinous process T1-T3 *Bertilson et al.[14]*		.55	.79

RELIABILITY OF THE CLINICAL EXAMINATION

Neck and Radicular Upper Extremity Pain

Test and Measure	Test Procedure and Determination of Positive Findings	Population	Inter-examiner Reliability Kappa Values (95% CI)
Straight compression *Bertilison et al.*[14]	Patient seated with examiner standing behind patient. Examiner exerts pressure on head. Positive if pain is provoked	100 patients with neck and/or shoulder problems with or without radiating pain	$\kappa = .34$ without knowledge of patient history $\kappa = .44$ with knowledge of patient history
Neck compression with: Right shoulder/arm pain	Cervical compression performed in sitting. Examiner passively rotates and side bends the head to the right and/or left. A compression force of 7 kg is applied. Presence and location of pain, paresthesias, or numbness is recorded	52 patients with varying disorders: cervical spondylosis (32); neurologic tumor (6); disseminated sclerosis (2); peripheral upper limb paresis (2); brachial plexus involvement (2); miscellaneous (5); unknown (3)	Right: $\kappa = .61$ Left: not available
Left shoulder/arm pain			Right: not available Left: $\kappa = .40$
Right forearm/ hand pain			Right: $\kappa = .77$ Left: $\kappa = .54$
Right forearm/ hand pain *Viikari-Juntura*[13]			Right: not available Left: $\kappa = .62$
Spurling A *Wainner et al.*[6]	Patient seated with neck side bent toward ipsilateral side. 7 kg of overpressure is applied	50 patients with suspected cervical radiculopathy or carpal tunnel syndrome	$\kappa = .60$ (.32, .87)
Spurling B *Wainner et al.*[6]	Patient seated with extension and side bending/rotation to ipsilateral side. 7 kg of overpressure is applied		$\kappa = .62$ (.25, .99)
Spurling to the right	Cervical compression performed in sitting. Examiner passively rotates and side bends head to right or left and applies compression force of 7 kg. Presence and location of pain, paresthesias, or numbness are recorded	100 patients with neck and/or shoulder problems with or without radiating pain	$\kappa = .37$ without knowledge of patient history $\kappa = .28$ with knowledge of patient history
Spurling to the left *Bertilison et al.*[14]			$\kappa = .37$ without knowledge of patient history $\kappa = .46$ with knowledge of patient history

Neck and Radicular Upper Extremity Pain (cont.)

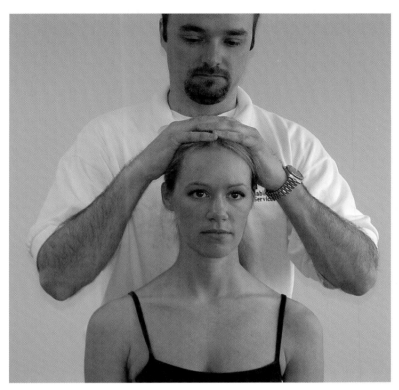

Figure 4-21: *Cervical compression test*

RELIABILITY OF THE CLINICAL EXAMINATION

Neck Distraction and Traction Tests

Test and Measure	Test Procedure and Determination of Positive Findings	Population	Inter-examiner Reliability Kappa Values (95% CI)
Axial manual traction *Viikari-Juntura*[13]	Patient supine. Examiner applies axial distraction force of 10 to15 kg. Positive if radicular symptoms decrease	52 patients with: cervical spondylosis (32); neurologic tumot (6); disseminated sclerosis (2); peripheral upper limb paresis (2); brachial plexus involvement (2); miscellaneous (5); unknown (3)	κ = .50
Neck distraction test *Wainner et al.*[6]	Patient supine. Examiner grasps under chin and occiput while slightly flexing patient's neck and applies distraction force of 14 lb. Positive if symptoms are reduced	50 patients with suspected cervical radiculopathy or carpal tunnel syndrome	κ = .88 (.64, 1.0)
Traction *Bertilson et al.*[14]	Patient seated. Examiner stands behind patient with hands underneath each maxilla and thumbs on the back of the head. Positive if symptoms are reduced during traction	100 patients with neck and/or shoulder problems with or without radiating pain	κ = .56 without knowledge of history κ = .41 with knowledge of history

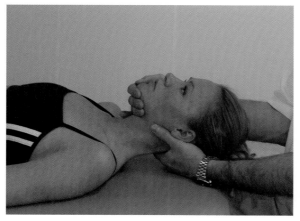

Figure 4-22: *Neck distraction test*

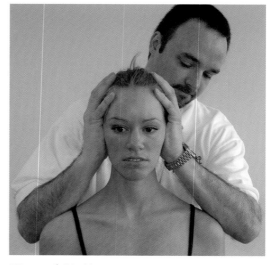

Figure 4-23: *Traction test*

Shoulder Abduction Test

Test and Measure	Test Procedure and Determination of Positive Findings	Population	Inter-examiner Reliability Kappa Values (95% CI)
Shoulder abduction test Wainner et al.[6]	Patient is seated and is asked to place the symptomatic extremity on the head. Positive if symptoms are reduced	50 patients with suspected cervical radiculopathy or carpal tunnel syndrome	$\kappa = .20$ (.00, .59)
Shoulder abduction test Viikari-Juntura[13]	Patient is seated and is asked to raise the symptomatic extremity above the head. Positive if symptoms are reduced	52 patients with: cervical spondylosis (32); neurologic tumor (6); disseminated sclerosis (2); peripheral upper limb paresis (2); brachial plexus involvement (2); miscellaneous (5); unknown (3)	Right side $\kappa = .21$ Left side $\kappa = .40$

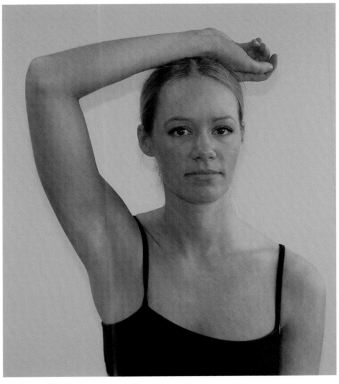

Figure 4-24

Upper Limb Tests

Test and Measure	Test Procedure and Determination of Positive Findings	Population	Inter-examiner Reliability Kappa Values (95% CI)
Upper limb tension test A *Wainner et al.*[6]	With patient supine, examiner performs the following movements: 1. Scapular depression 2. Shoulder abduction 3. Forearm supination, wrist and finger extension 4. Shoulder lateral rotation 5. Elbow extension 6. Contralateral/ipsilateral cervical side bending	50 patients with suspected cervical radiculopathy or carpal tunnel syndrome	$\kappa = .76$ (.51, 1.0)
Upper limb tension test B *Wainner et al.*[6]	With patient supine and shoulder abducted 30°, examiner performs the following movements: 1. Scapular depression 2. Shoulder medial rotation 3. Full elbow extension 4. Wrist and finger flexion 5. Contralateral/ipsilateral cervical side bending		$\kappa = .83$ (.65, 1.0)
Brachial plexus test *Viikari-Juntura*[13]	With patient supine, examiner abducts the humerus to the limit of pain-free motion, then adds lateral rotation of the arm and elbow flexion. If no limitation of motion is noted, the humerus is abducted to 90°. The appearance of symptoms is recorded	52 patients with: cervical spondylosis (32); neurologic tumor (6); disseminated sclerosis (2); peripheral upper limb paresis (2); brachial plexus involvement (2); miscellaneous (5); unknown (3)	Right $\kappa = .35$ Left not calculated because prevalence of positive findings was <10%

Nonspecific Neck Pain

Test and Measure	Test Procedure and Determination of Positive Findings	Population	Reference Standard	Sens	Spec	+LR	−LR
Active flexion and extension of the neck *Sandmark and Nisell*[15]	Active flexion and extension performed to the extremes of the range. Positive if subject reported pain with procedure			.27	.90	2.70	.81
Spurling test *Sandmark and Nisell*[15]	Extension of the neck with rotation and side bending to the same side. Positive if subject reported pain with procedure			.77	.92	9.63	.25
Upper limb tension test *Sandmark and Nisell*[15]	Patient seated, arm in extension, abduction and ER of the glenohumeral joint, extension of the elbow, the forearm in supination, and the wrist and fingers in extension. Contralateral flexion of the neck is added. Positive if subject reported pain with procedure	75 males (22 with neck pain)	Patient reports of neck pain	.77	.94	12.83	.25
Palpation over the facet joints in the cervical spine *Sandmark and Nisell*[15]	Articulations were palpated 2 cm lateral to the spinous process. Positive if patient reported pain with procedure			.82	.79	3.90	.23

ER, external rotation.

DIAGNOSTIC UTILITY OF THE CLINICAL EXAMINATION

Cervical Zygapophyseal Pain Syndromes

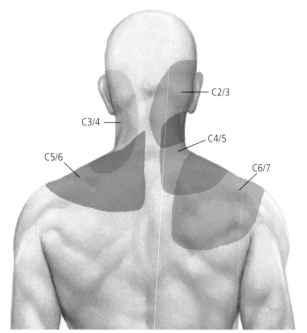

C2/3

C3/4

C4/5

C5/6

C6/7

Figure 4-25A: Distribution of zygapophyseal pain referral patterns as described by Dwyer et al.[16]

Test and Measure	Test Procedure	Determination of Positive Findings	Population	Reference Standard	Sens	Spec	+LR	−LR
Manual examination *Jull et al.*[18]	Subjective examination followed by central posteroanterior glides, followed by passive physiologic iintervertebral movements of flexion, extension, side bending, and rotation	Joint dysfunction was diagnosed if the examiner concluded that the joint demonstrated an abnormal end-feel, abnormal quality of resistance to motion, and the reproduction of pain	20 patients with cervical pain	Radiologically controlled diagnostic nerve block	1.0	1.0	Not available	Not available

Cervical Zygapophyseal Pain Syndromes (cont.)

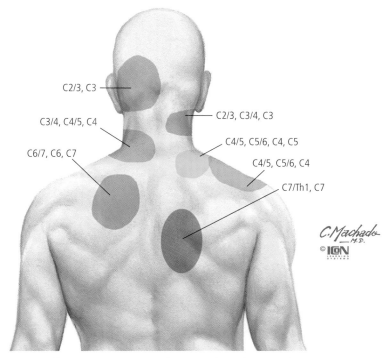

C2/3, C3

C3/4, C4/5, C4

C6/7, C6, C7

C2/3, C3/4, C3

C4/5, C5/6, C4, C5

C4/5, C5/6, C4

C7/Th1, C7

Figure 4-25B: Distribution of zygapophyseal pain referral patterns as described by Fukui et al.[17]

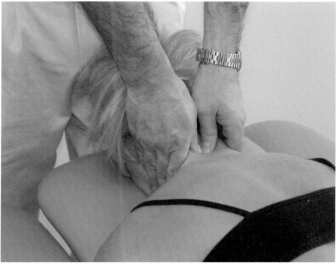

Figure 4-26: Posteroanterior central glides to the mid cervical spine

DIAGNOSTIC UTILITY OF THE CLINICAL EXAMINATION

Cervical Radiculopathy

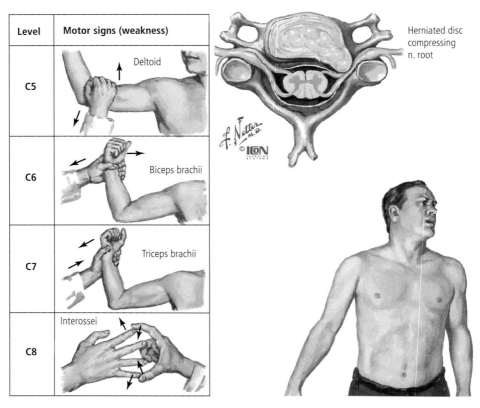

Level	Motor signs (weakness)
C5	Deltoid
C6	Biceps brachii
C7	Triceps brachii
C8	Interossei

Herniated disc compressing n. root

Figure 4-27

History

Patient Reports	Population	Reference Standard	Sensitivity	Specificity	+LR	−LR
Weakness			.65	.39	1.07	.90
Numbness	183 patients referred to electrodiagnostic laboratories	Electrodiagnostics	.79	.25	1.05	.84
Arm pain			.65	.26	.88	1.35
Neck pain			.62	.35	.95	1.09
Tingling			.72	.25	.96	1.92
Burning Lauder et al.[19]			.33	.63	.89	1.06

Cervical Radiculopathy (cont.)

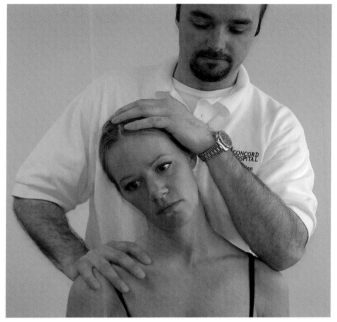

Figure 4-28: *Spurling A test*

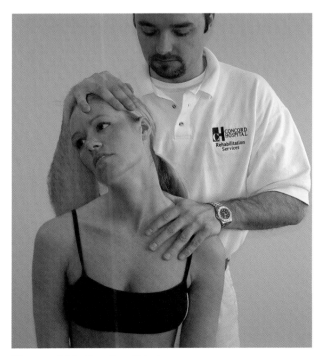

Figure 4-29: *Spurling B test*

Physical Examination

Test and Measure	Test Procedure and Determination of Positive Findings	Population	Reference Standard	Sens	Spec	+LR	−LR
Spurling test *Tong et al.*[20]	Patient side bends and extends the neck, and examiner applies compression. Positive if pain or tingling starts in the shoulder and radiates distally to the elbow	255 consecutive patients referred to a physiatrist with upper extremity nerve disorders	Electrodiagnostic testing	.30	.93	4.29	.75
Spurling A *Wainner et al.*[6]	Patient is seated, the neck is side bent toward the ipsilateral side, and 7 kg of overpressure is applied (Figure 4-32). Positive is symptoms are reproduced	82 consecutive patients referred to an electrophysiologic laboratory with suspected diagnosis of cervical radiculopathy or carpal tunnel syndrome	Needle electromyography and nerve conduction studies	0.50	0.88	.58 (.36, .94)	3.5 (1.6, 7.5)
Spurling B *Wainner et al.*[6]	Patient seated. Extension and side bending/rotation to the ipsilateral side, then 7 kg of overpressure is applied (Figure 4-33). Positive if symptoms are reproduced			0.50	0.74	.67 (.42, 1.1)	1.9 (1.0, 3.6)
Neck compression test *Viikari-Juntura et al.*[21]	Patient seated. Examiner side bends and slightly rotates patient's head. A compression force of 7 kg is exerted. Positive if test aggravates radicular pain, numbness, or paresthesias			.28 right .33 left	.92 right 1.0 left	1.05 right Left not available	.78 right .67 left
Axial manual traction *Viikari-Juntura et al.*[22]	With patient supine, examiner provides axial distraction force between 10 and 15 kg. Positive if symptoms are reduced or disappear	69 consecutive patients of a neurosurgery department	Cervical myelography	.26	1.0	Not available	.74
Shoulder abduction test *Viikari-Juntura et al.*[21]	The patient lifts the hand above the head. Positive if symptoms are reduced or disappear			.31 right .42 left	1.05 right 1.0 left	Not available	.69 right .58 left

Cervical Radiculopathy: Pin-Prick Sensation Testing

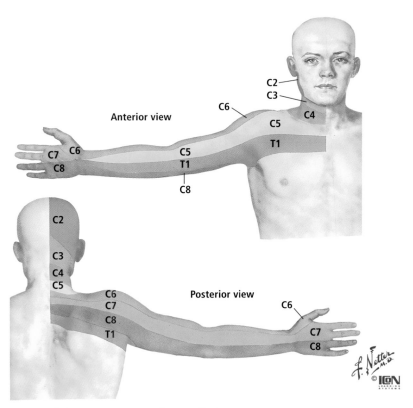

Figure 4.30: *Dermatomes of upper limb*

Test and Measure	Test Procedure and Determination of Positive Findings	Population	Reference Standard	Sens	Spec	+LR	−LR
C5				.29	.86	.82 (.60, 1.1)	2.1 (.79, 5.3)
C6	Pin-prick sensation testing. Graded as reduced, normal, or increased	82 consecutive patients referred to an electrophysiologic laboratory with suspected diagnosis of cervical radiculopathy or carpal tunnel syndrome	Needle electromyography and nerve conduction studies	.24	.66	1.16 (.84, 1.6)	.69 (.28, 1.8)
C7				.18	.77	1.07 (.83, 1.4)	.76 (.25, 2.3)
C8				.12	.81	1.09 (.88, 1.4)	.61 (.15, 2.5)
T1 *Wainner et al.[6]*				.28	.79	1.05 (.81, 1.4)	.83 (.27, .6)
Decreased vibration of pin prick *Lauder et al.[19]*	Not specifically described	183 patients referred to electrodiagnostic laboratories	Electrodiagnostics	.49	.64	1.36	.80

DIAGNOSTIC UTILITY OF THE CLINICAL EXAMINATION

Cervical Radiculopathy: Muscle Stretch Reflexes

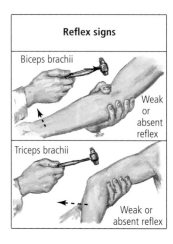

Figure 4.31: *Reflex testing*

Muscle Stretch Reflexes	Determination of Findings	Population	Reference Standard	Sens	Spec	+LR	−LR
Biceps brachii *Wainner et al.*[6]	Graded as absent/ reduced, normal, or increased	82 consecutive patients referred to an electrophysiologic laboratory with suspected diagnosis of cervical radiculopathy or carpal tunnel syndrome	Needle electromyography and nerve conduction studies	.24	.95	.80 (.61, 1.1)	4.9 (1.2, 20.0)
Brachioradialis *Wainner et al.*[6]				.06	.95	.99 (.87, 1.1)	1.2 (.14, 11.1)
Triceps *Wainner et al.*[6]				.03	.93	1.05 (.94, 1.2)	40 (.02, 7.0)
Biceps *Lauder et al.*[19]	Not specifically described	183 patients referred to electrodiagnostic laboratories	Electrodiagnostics	.10	.99	10.0	.91
Triceps *Lauder et al.*[19]				.10	.95	2.0	.95
Brachioradialis *Lauder et al.*[19]				.08	.99	8.0	.93

Cervical Radiculopathy: Test Item Cluster (TIC)

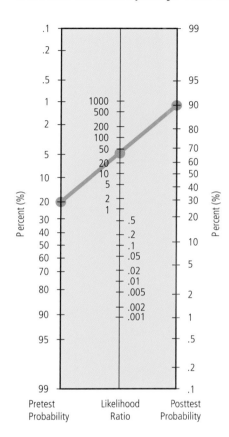

Figure 4-34: *Considering the 20%
prevalence or pretest probability of cervical
radiculopathy in the Wainner et al.[6] study,
the nomogram demonstrates the major shifts
in probability that occur when all 4 tests
from the TIC are positive.*
(Reprinted with permission from Fagan TJ. Nomogram
for Baye's theorem. N Engl Med. 1975;293:257.
Copyright © 2005 Massachusetts Medical Society. All
rights reserved.)

Wainner et al.[6] identified a test item cluster (TIC), or the optimal clinical examination tests, to determine the likelihood that the patient will present with cervical radiculopathy. The four predictor variables most likely to identify patients who present with cervical radiculopathy are the upper limb tension test A, the Spurling A test, the distraction test, and cervical rotation less than 60° to the ipsilateral side. This table demonstrates how positive tests increase the posttest probability that a patient will present with cervical radiculopathy.

Number of Positive TICs	Sens	Spec	+LR	Posttest Probability
Two positive tests from the TIC	.39	.56	.88 (1.5, 2.5)	21%
Three positive tests from the TIC	.39	.94	6.1 (2.0, 18.6)	65%
Four positive tests from the TIC	.24	.99	30.3 (1.7, 38.2)	90%

Cervical Radiculopathy: Upper Limb Tension Tests

Test and Measure	Test Procedure	Determination of Findings	Population	Reference Standard	Sens	Spec	+LR	−LR
Upper limb tension test A *Wainner et al.*[6]	With patient supine, examiner performs the following movements: 1. Scapular depression 2. Shoulder abduction 3. Forearm supination, wrist and finger extension 4. Shoulder lateral rotation 5. Elbow extension 6. Contralateral/ ipsilateral cervical side bending	1. Patient symptoms reproduced 2. Side-to-side differences in elbow extension >10 3. Contralateral cervical side bending increases symptoms, or ipsilateral side bending decreases symptoms	82 consecutive patients referred to an electrophysiologic laboratory with suspected diagnosis of cervical radiculopathy or carpal tunnel syndrome	Needle electromyography and nerve conduction studies	.44	.22	.12 (.40, .90)	.85 (.37, 1.9)
Upper limb tension test B *Wainner et al.*[6]	With patient supine and shoulder abducted 30°, examiner performs the following movements: 1. Scapular depression 2. Shoulder medial rotation 3. Full elbow extension 4. Wrist and finger flexion 5. Contralateral/ ipsilateral cervical side bending				.97	.33	.85 (.37, 1.9)	1.1 (.77, 1.5)

Cervical Radiculopathy: Upper Limb Tension Tests (cont.)

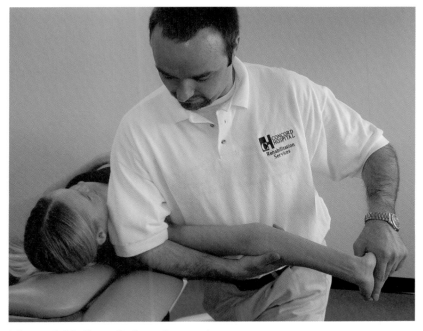

Figure 4.32: Upper limb tension test A

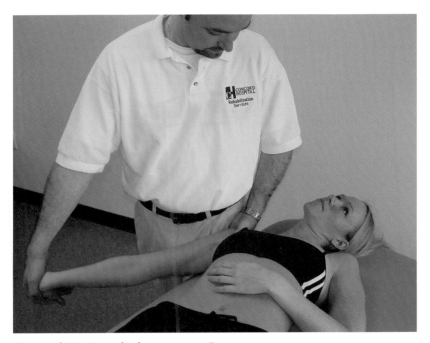

Figure 4.33: Upper limb tension test B

DIAGNOSTIC UTILITY OF THE CLINICAL EXAMINATION

Cervical Instability

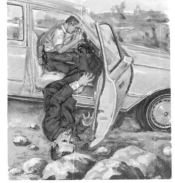

Compression–rotation injury may occur when person is thrown from car or upended in football or other sports accident

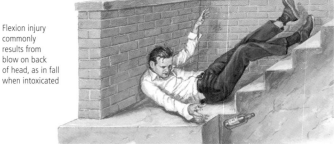

Flexion injury commonly results from blow on back of head, as in fall when intoxicated

Figure 4-35: *Cervical trauma*

Test and Measure	Test Procedure	Determination of Findings	Population	Reference Standard	Sens	Spec	+LR	−LR
Sharp-Purser test *Uitvlugt and Indenbaum*[23]	Patient sits with neck in a semiflexed position. Examiner places palm of one hand on patient's forehead and index finger of the other hand on the spinous process of the axis	When posterior pressure is applied through the forehead, a sliding motion of the head posteriorly in relation to the axis indicates a positive test for atlantoaxial instability	123 consecutive outpatients with rheumatoid arthritis	Full flexion and extension lateral radiographs. Atlanto-dens interval greater than 3 mm was considered abnormal	.69	.96	17.25	.32

Cervical Instability (cont.)

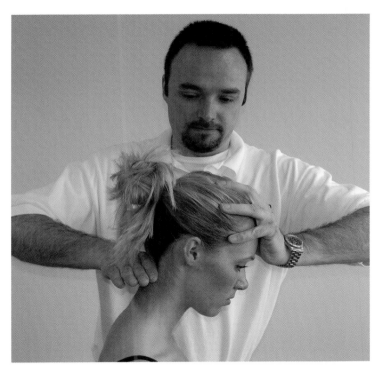

Figure 4-36: *Sharp-Purser test*

DIAGNOSTIC UTILITY OF THE CLINICAL EXAMINATION

Cervical Cord Compression

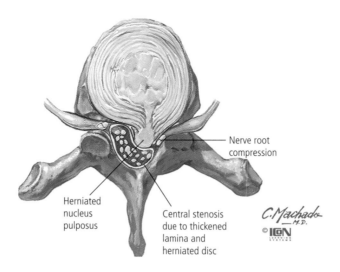

Figure 4-37

Test and Measure	Test Procedure	Determination of Findings	Population	Reference Standard	Sens	Spec	+LR	−LR
Compression of brachial plexus *Uchihara et al.*[24]	Firm compression and squeezing of the brachial plexus with the thumb	Positive only when pain radiates to the shoulder or upper extremity	65 patients who had undergone MRI of the cervical spine as a result of radiating pain	MRI	.69	.83	4.06	.37

MRI, magnetic resonance imaging.

1. Bogduk N. Neck pain. *Aust Fam Physician.* 1984;13:26-30.

2. Lord S, Barnsley L, Wallis B, Bogduk N. Chronic cervical zygapophyseal joint pain after whiplash. *Spine.* 1996;21:1737-1745.

3. Janda V. Evaluation of muscular imbalance. In: Liebenson C, editor. *Rehabilitation of the Spine: A Practitioner's Manual.* Baltimore: Williams and Wilkins; 1996:97-112.

4. Janda V. Muscles and motor control in cervicogenic disorders: assessment and management. In: Grant R, editor. *Physical Therapy of the Cervical and Thoracic Spine.* 2nd ed. New York: Churchill Livingstone; 1994:195-216.

5. Childs JD. *Physical Therapy of the Cervical Spine and Temporomandibular Joint.* Lacrosse: Orthopaedic Section, American Physical Therapy Association; 2003.

6. Wainner R, Fritz J, Irrgang J, Boninger M, Delitto A, Allison S. Reliability and diagnostic accuracy of the clinical examination and patient self-report measures for cervical radiculopathy. *Spine.* 2003;28:52-62.

7. Olson S, O'Connor D, Birmingham G, Broman P, Herrera L. Tender point sensitivity, range of motion, and perceived disability in subjects with neck pain. *J Orthop Sports Phys Ther.* 2000;30:13-20.

8. Hole DE, Cook JM, Bolton JE. Reliability and concurrent validity of two instruments for measuring cervical range of motion: effects of age and gender. *Man Ther.* 2000;1:36-42.

9. Youdas J, Carey J, Garrett T. Reliability of measurements of cervical spine range of motion. Comparison of three models. *Phys Ther.* 1991;71:98-106.

10. Smedmark V, Wallin M, Arvidsson I. Inter-examiner reliability in assessing passive intervertebral motion of the cervical spine. *Man Ther.* 2000;5:97-101.

11. Pool J, Hoving J, de Vet H, van Memeren H, Bouter L. The interexaminer reproducibility of physical examination of the cervical spine. *J Manipulative Physiol Ther.* 2003;27:84-90.

12. van Suijlekom H, deVet H, van den Berg S, Weber W. Interobserver reliability in physical examination of the cervical spine in patients with headache. *Headache.* 2000;40:581-586.

13. Viikari-Juntura E. Interexaminer reliability of observations in physical examinations of the neck. *Phys Ther.* 1987;67:1526-1532.

14. Bertilson B, Grunnesjo M, Strender L. Reliability of clinical tests in the assessment of patients with neck/shoulder problems. Impact of history. *Spine.* 2003;28:2222-2231.

15. Sandmark H, Nisell R. Validity of five common manual neck pain producing tests. *Scand J Rehabil Med.* 1995;27:131-136.

16. Dwyer A. Cervical zygapophyseal joint pain patterns. I: A study in normal volunteers. *Spine.* 1990;15:453-457.

17. Fukui S, Ohseto K, Shiotani M, et al. Referred pain distribution of the cervical zygapophyseal joints and cervical dorsal rami. *Pain.* 1996;68:79-83.

18. Jull G, Bogduk N, Marsland A. The accuracy of manual diagnosis for cervical zygapophyseal joint pain syndromes. *Med J Aust.* 1988;148:233-236.

19. Lauder TD, Dillingham TR, Andary M, et al. Predicting electrodiagnostic outcome in patients with upper limb symptoms: are the history and physical examination helpful? *Arch Phys Med Rehabil.* 2000;81:436-441.

20. Tong H, Haig A, Yamakawa K. The Spurling test and cervical radiculopathy. *Spine.* 2002;27:156-159.

REFERENCES

REFERENCES

21. Viikari-Juntura E, Porras M, Laasonen E. Validity of clinical tests in the diagnosis of root compression in cervical disc disease. *Spine.* 1989;14:253-257.

22. Viikari-Juntura E, Takala E, Riihimaki H, Martikainen R, Jappinen P. Predictive validity of symptoms and signs in the neck and shoulders. *J Clin Epidemiol.* 2000;53:800-808.

23. Uitvlugt G, Indenbaum S. Clinical assessment of atlantoaxial instability using the Sharp-Purser test. *Arthritis Rheum.* 1988;31:918-922.

24. Uchihara T, Furukawa T, Tsukagoshi H. Compression of brachial plexus as a diagnostic test of cervical cord lesion. *Spine.* 1994;19:2170-2173.

Thoracolumbar Spine

Chapter 5

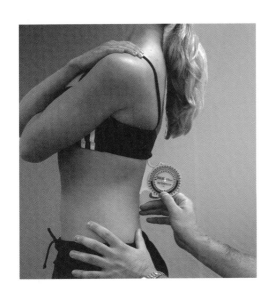

OSTEOLOGY Thoracic Vertebrae

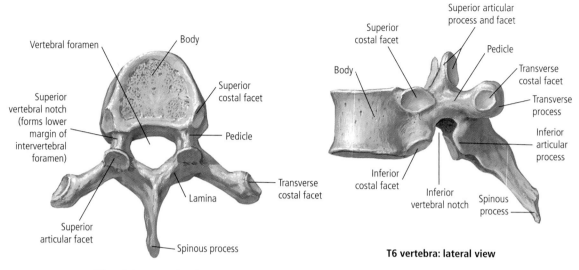

T6 vertebra: superior view

T6 vertebra: lateral view

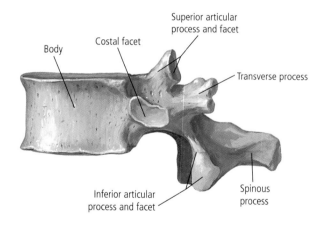

T12 vertebra: lateral view

Figure 5-1

Lumbar Vertebrae

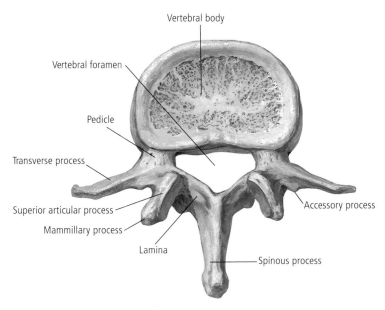

Vertebral body

Vertebral foramen

Pedicle

Transverse process

Superior articular process

Mammillary process

Lamina

Accessory process

Spinous process

L2 vertebra: superior view

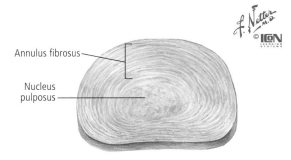

Annulus fibrosus

Nucleus pulposus

Intervertebral disc

Figure 5-2

ARTHROLOGY   Joints of the Thoracic Spine

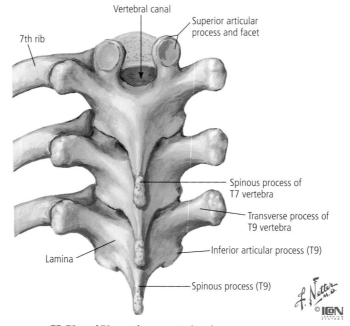

T7, T8, and T9 vertebrae: posterior view

Figure 5-3A

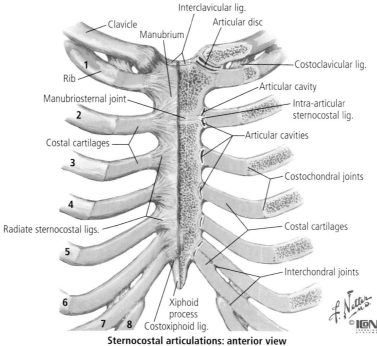

Sternocostal articulations: anterior view

Figure 5-3B

Joints of the Thoracic Spine (cont.)   **ARTHROLOGY**

Costovertebral Joints

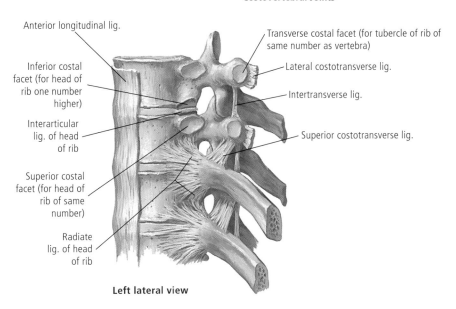

Anterior longitudinal lig.

Inferior costal facet (for head of rib one number higher)

Interarticular lig. of head of rib

Superior costal facet (for head of rib of same number)

Radiate lig. of head of rib

Transverse costal facet (for tubercle of rib of same number as vertebra)

Lateral costotransverse lig.

Intertransverse lig.

Superior costotransverse lig.

Left lateral view

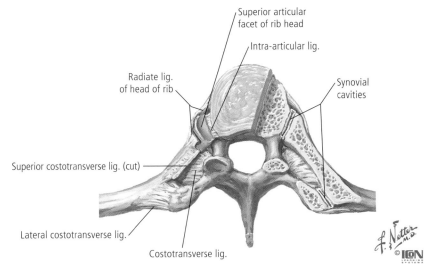

Superior articular facet of rib head

Intra-articular lig.

Radiate lig. of head of rib

Synovial cavities

Superior costotransverse lig. (cut)

Lateral costotransverse lig.

Costotransverse lig.

Transverse section: superior view

Figure 5-3C

ARTHROLOGY   Joints of the Lumbar Spine

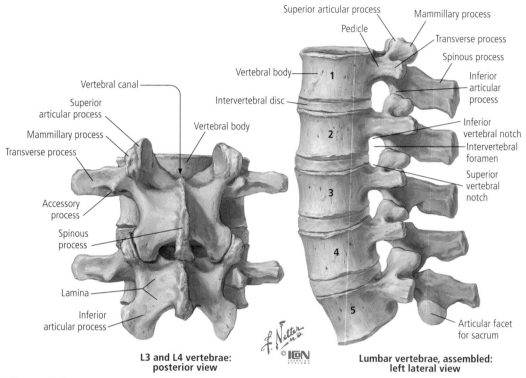

**L3 and L4 vertebrae:
posterior view**

**Lumbar vertebrae, assembled:
left lateral view**

Figure 5-4

Thoracolumbar Joints	Type and Classification	Closed Packed Position	Capsular Pattern
Zygapophyseal joints	Synovial: plane	Extension	Lumbar: significant limitation of side bending bilaterally and limitations of flexion and extension
			Thoracic: limitation of extension, side bending, and rotation; less limitation of flexion
Intervertebral joints	Amphiarthrodial	NA	NA

Spine		Type and Classification	Closed Packed Position	Capsular Pattern
Costotransverse		Synovial	NR	NR
Costovertebral		Synovial	NR	NR
Costochondral		Synchondroses	NR	NR
Interchondral		Synovial	NR	NR
Sternocostal	1st joint	Amphiarthrodial	NA	NA
	2nd–7th joint	Synovial	NR	NR

NA, not applicable; NR, not reported.

Costovertebral Ligaments

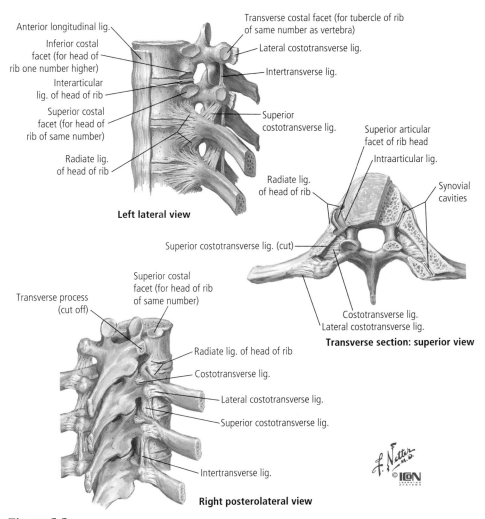

Anterior longitudinal lig.

Inferior costal facet (for head of rib one number higher)

Interarticular lig. of head of rib

Superior costal facet (for head of rib of same number)

Radiate lig. of head of rib

Transverse costal facet (for tubercle of rib of same number as vertebra)

Lateral costotransverse lig.

Intertransverse lig.

Superior costotransverse lig.

Left lateral view

Superior articular facet of rib head

Intraarticular lig.

Synovial cavities

Radiate lig. of head of rib

Superior costotransverse lig. (cut)

Costotransverse lig.
Lateral costotransverse lig.

Transverse section: superior view

Transverse process (cut off)

Superior costal facet (for head of rib of same number)

Radiate lig. of head of rib

Costotransverse lig.

Lateral costotransverse lig.

Superior costotransverse lig.

Intertransverse lig.

Right posterolateral view

Figure 5-5

Ligaments	Attachments	Function
Radiate sternocostal	Costal cartilage to the anterior and posterior surface of the sternum	Reinforces joint capsule
Interchondral ligaments	Connect adjacent borders of articulations between 6th and 7th, 7th and 8th, 8th and 9th costal cartilages	Reinforces joint capsule
Radiate head of rib	Lateral vertebral body to head of rib	Prevents separation of rib head from vertebra
Costotransverse	Posterior aspect of rib to anterior aspect of transverse process of vertebra	Prevents separation of rib from transverse process
Intra-articular	Crest of rib head to intervertebral disk	Divides joint into two cavities

LIGAMENTS   Thoracolumbar Ligaments

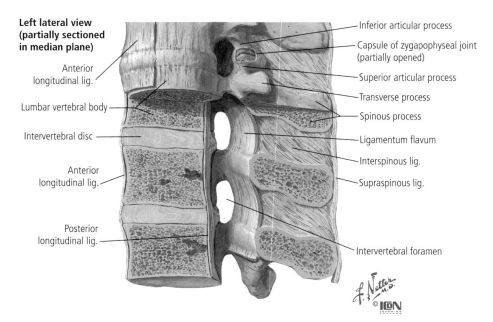

Left lateral view (partially sectioned in median plane)

- Anterior longitudinal lig.
- Lumbar vertebral body
- Intervertebral disc
- Anterior longitudinal lig.
- Posterior longitudinal lig.

- Inferior articular process
- Capsule of zygapophyseal joint (partially opened)
- Superior articular process
- Transverse process
- Spinous process
- Ligamentum flavum
- Interspinous lig.
- Supraspinous lig.
- Intervertebral foramen

Figure 5-6

Ligaments	Attachments	Function
Anterior longitudinal	Extends from anterior sacrum to anterior tubercle of C1. Connects anterolateral vertebral bodies and disks	Maintains stability and prevents excessive extension of spinal column
Posterior longitudinal	Extends from the sacrum to C2. Runs within the vertebral canal attaching the posterior vertebral bodies	Prevents excessive flexion of spinal column and posterior disc protrusion
Ligamenta flava	Binds the lamina above each vertebra to the lamina below	Prevents separation of the vertebral laminae
Supraspinous	Connects spinous processes C7-S1	Limits separation of spinous processes
Interspinous	Connects spinous processes C1-S1	Limits separation of spinous processes
Intertransverse	Connects adjacent transverse processes of vertebrae	Limits separation of transverse processes
Iliolumbar	Binds transverse processes of L5 to posterior aspect of iliac crest	Stabilizes L5 and prevents anterior shear

Thoracolumbar Ligaments (cont.)   **LIGAMENTS**

**Anterior vertebral segments:
posterior view
(pedicles sectioned)**

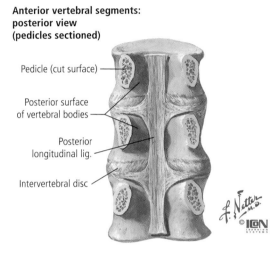

Pedicle (cut surface)

Posterior surface
of vertebral bodies

Posterior
longitudinal lig.

Intervertebral disc

**Posterior vertebral segments:
anterior view**

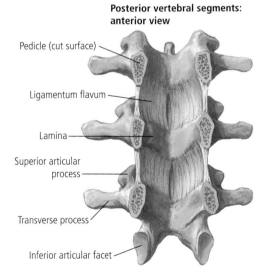

Pedicle (cut surface)

Ligamentum flavum

Lamina

Superior articular
process

Transverse process

Inferior articular facet

Figure 5-6 (cont.)

Thoracolumbar Muscles: Superficial Layers

Muscles		Proximal Attachment	Distal Attachment	Nerve and Segmental Level	Action
Latissimus dorsi		Spinous processes T6-T12, thoracolumbar fascia, iliac crest, inferior four ribs	Intertubercular groove of humerus	Thoracodorsal nerve (C6, C7, C8)	Extension, adduction, and internal rotation of humerus
Trapezius	Middle	Superior nuchal line, occipital protuberance, nuchal ligament, spinous processes T1-T12	Lateral clavicle, acromion, and spine of scapula	Accessory nerve (CN XI)	Retracts scapula
	Lower				Depresses scapula
Rhomboids	Major	Spinous processes T2-T5	Inferior medial border of scapula	Dorsal scapular nerve (C4, C5)	Retracts scapula, inferiorly rotates glenoid fossa, stabilizes scapula to thoracic wall
	Minor	Spinous processes C7-T1 and nuchal ligament	Superior medial border of scapula		
Serratus posterior superior		Spinous processes C7-T3, ligamentum nuchae	Superior surface of ribs 2–4	Intercostal nerves 2–5	Elevates ribs
Serratus posterior inferior		Spinous processes T11-L2	Inferior surface of ribs 8–12	Ventral rami of thoracic spinal nerves 9–12	Depresses ribs

CN, cranial nerve.

Thoracolumbar Muscles: Superficial Layers (cont.)

MUSCLES

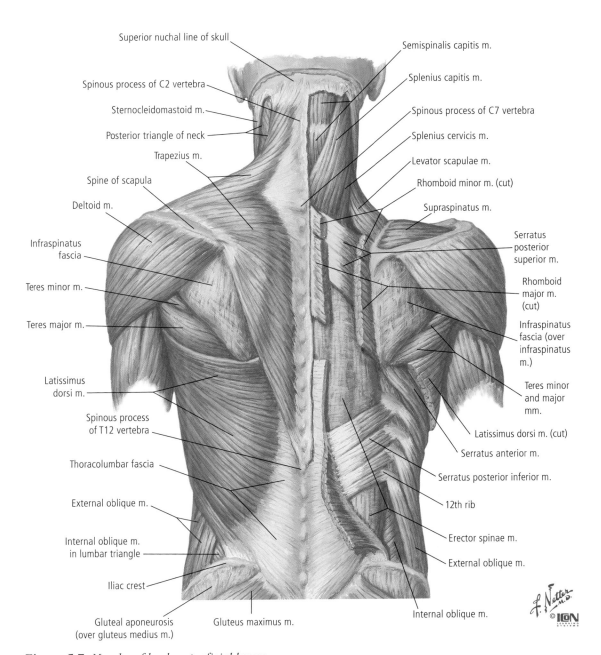

Superior nuchal line of skull

Spinous process of C2 vertebra

Sternocleidomastoid m.

Posterior triangle of neck

Trapezius m.

Spine of scapula

Deltoid m.

Infraspinatus fascia

Teres minor m.

Teres major m.

Latissimus dorsi m.

Spinous process of T12 vertebra

Thoracolumbar fascia

External oblique m.

Internal oblique m. in lumbar triangle

Iliac crest

Gluteal aponeurosis (over gluteus medius m.)

Gluteus maximus m.

Semispinalis capitis m.

Splenius capitis m.

Spinous process of C7 vertebra

Splenius cervicis m.

Levator scapulae m.

Rhomboid minor m. (cut)

Supraspinatus m.

Serratus posterior superior m.

Rhomboid major m. (cut)

Infraspinatus fascia (over infraspinatus m.)

Teres minor and major mm.

Latissimus dorsi m. (cut)

Serratus anterior m.

Serratus posterior inferior m.

12th rib

Erector spinae m.

External oblique m.

Internal oblique m.

Figure 5-7: *Muscles of back: superficial layers*

MUSCLES   **Thoracolumbar Muscles: Intermediate Layer**

Muscles	Proximal Attachment	Distal Attachment	Nerve and Segmental Level	Action
Iliocostalis thoracis	Iliac crest, posterior sacrum, spinous processes of sacrum and inferior lumbar vertebrae, supraspinous ligament	Cervical transverse processes and superior angles of lower ribs	Dorsal rami of spinal nerves	Bilaterally: extend spinal column Unilaterally: side-bend spinal column
Iliocostalis lumborum		Inferior surfaces of ribs 4–12	Dorsal rami of spinal nerves	
Longissimus thoracis		Thoracic transverse processes and superior surfaces of ribs	Dorsal rami of spinal nerves	
Longissimus lumborum		Transverse processes of lumbar vertebrae	Dorsal rami of spinal nerves	
Spinalis thoracis		Upper thoracic spinous processes	Dorsal rami of spinal nerves	

Thoracolumbar Muscles: Intermediate Layer (cont.)

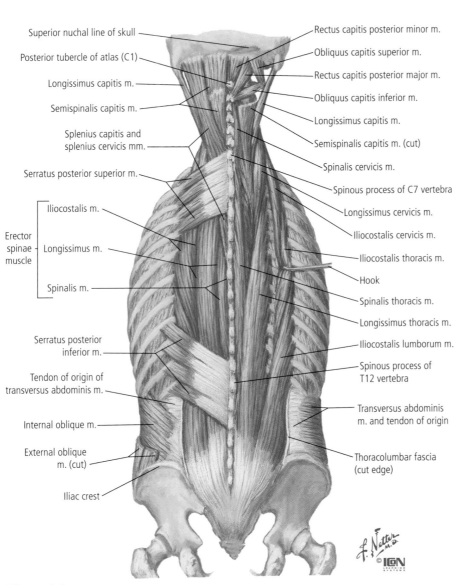

Superior nuchal line of skull

Posterior tubercle of atlas (C1)

Longissimus capitis m.

Semispinalis capitis m.

Splenius capitis and splenius cervicis mm.

Serratus posterior superior m.

Iliocostalis m.

Erector spinae muscle

Longissimus m.

Spinalis m.

Serratus posterior inferior m.

Tendon of origin of transversus abdominis m.

Internal oblique m.

External oblique m. (cut)

Iliac crest

Rectus capitis posterior minor m.

Obliquus capitis superior m.

Rectus capitis posterior major m.

Obliquus capitis inferior m.

Longissimus capitis m.

Semispinalis capitis m. (cut)

Spinalis cervicis m.

Spinous process of C7 vertebra

Longissimus cervicis m.

Iliocostalis cervicis m.

Iliocostalis thoracis m.

Hook

Spinalis thoracis m.

Longissimus thoracis m.

Iliocostalis lumborum m.

Spinous process of T12 vertebra

Transversus abdominis m. and tendon of origin

Thoracolumbar fascia (cut edge)

Figure 5-8

MUSCLES   Thoracolumbar Muscles: Deep Layer

Muscles	Proximal Attachment	Distal Attachment	Nerve and Segmental Level	Action
Rotatores	Transverse processes of vertebrae	Spinous processes of vertebrae 1 and 2, segments above origin	Dorsal rami of spinal nerves	Provides vertebral stabilization, assists with rotation and extension
Interspinalis	Superior aspect of cervical and lumbar spinous processes	Inferior aspect of spinous process superior to vertebrae of origin	Dorsal rami of spinal nerves	Causes extension and rotation of vertebral column
Intertransversarius	Cervical and lumbar transverse processes	Transverse process of adjacent vertebrae	Dorsal and ventral rami of spinal nerves	Bilaterally: stabilizes vertebral column Ipsilaterally: side-bends vertebral column
Multifidi	Sacrum, ilium, transverse processes T1-T3, articular processes C4-C7	Spinous process of vertebrae 2–4, segments above origin	Dorsal rami of spinal nerves	Stabilizes vertebrae

Thoracolumbar Muscles: Deep Layer (cont.)

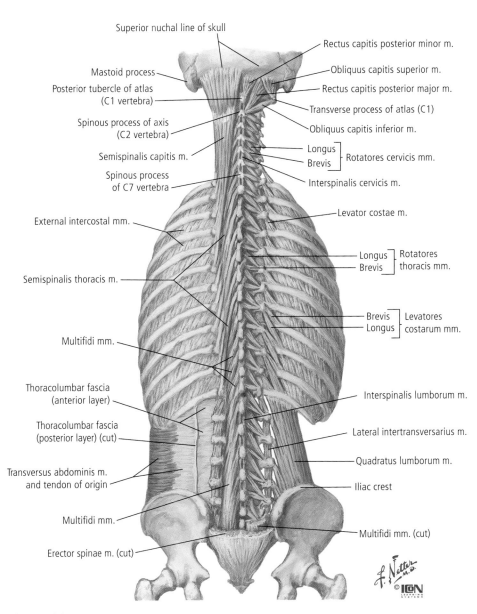

Superior nuchal line of skull

Rectus capitis posterior minor m.

Mastoid process

Obliquus capitis superior m.

Posterior tubercle of atlas (C1 vertebra)

Rectus capitis posterior major m.

Transverse process of atlas (C1)

Spinous process of axis (C2 vertebra)

Obliquus capitis inferior m.

Semispinalis capitis m.

Longus
Brevis — Rotatores cervicis mm.

Spinous process of C7 vertebra

Interspinalis cervicis m.

External intercostal mm.

Levator costae m.

Longus
Brevis — Rotatores thoracis mm.

Semispinalis thoracis m.

Brevis
Longus — Levatores costarum mm.

Multifidi mm.

Thoracolumbar fascia (anterior layer)

Interspinalis lumborum m.

Thoracolumbar fascia (posterior layer) (cut)

Lateral intertransversarius m.

Transversus abdominis m. and tendon of origin

Quadratus lumborum m.

Iliac crest

Multifidi mm.

Multifidi mm. (cut)

Erector spinae m. (cut)

Figure 5-9

MUSCLES   Muscles of Anterior Abdominal Wall

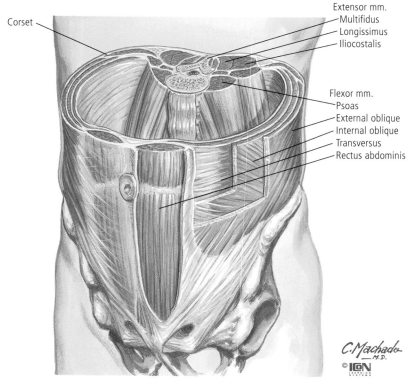

Corset

Extensor mm.
Multifidus
Longissimus
Iliocostalis

Flexor mm.
Psoas
External oblique
Internal oblique
Transversus
Rectus abdominis

C. Machado
M.D.
© ICN

Figure 5-10: *Dynamic "corset" concept of lumbar stability*

Muscles	Proximal Attachment	Distal Attachment	Nerve and Segmental Level	Action
Rectus abdominis	Pubic symphysis and pubic crest	Costal cartilage 5–7 and xiphoid process	Ventral rami T6-T12	Flexes trunk
Internal oblique	Thoracolumbar fascia, iliac crest, and lateral inguinal ligament	Inferior border of ribs 10–12, linea alba, and pubis	Ventral rami T6-L1	Flexes and rotates trunk
External oblique	External aspect of ribs 5–12	Anterior iliac crest, linea alba, and pubic tubercle	Ventral rami T6-T12 and subcostal nerve	Flexes and rotates trunk
Transversus abdominis	Internal aspect of costal cartilage 7–12, thoracolumbar fascia, iliac crest, and lateral inguinal ligament	Linea alba, pubis, and pubic crest	Ventral rami T6-L1	Supports abdominal viscera and increases intra-abdominal pressure

Thoracolumbar Fascia

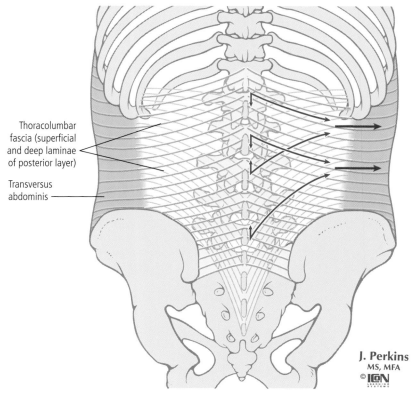

Thoracolumbar
fascia (superficial
and deep laminae
of posterior layer)

Transversus
abdominis

J. Perkins
MS, MFA
© ICN

Figure 5-11: *The transverse abdominis exerts a force through the thoracolumbar fascia, creating a stabilizing force through the lumbar spine.*[1]

The thoracolumbar fascia is a dense layer of connective tissue that runs from the thoracic region to the sacrum.[2] It comprises three separate layers—anterior, middle, and posterior. The middle and posterior layers blend together to form a dense fascia referred to as the lateral raphe.[3] The posterior layer consists of two laminae. The superficial lamina fibers are angled downward, and the deep lamina fibers are angled upward. Bergmark[4] has reported that the thoracolumbar fascia serves three purposes: to transfer forces from the muscles to the spine; to transfer forces between spinal segments; and to transfer forces from the thoracolumbar spine to the retinaculum of the erector spinae. The transverse abdominis attaches to the middle layer of the thoracolumbar fascia and exerts a force through the lateral raphe, resulting in a cephalad tension through the deep layer and a caudal tension through the superficial layer of the posterior lamina.[1-3] The result is a stabilizing force exerted through the lumbar spine, which has been reported to provide stability and assist with control of intersegmental motion of the lumbar spine.[5-7]

NERVES   Nerves of the Thoracic Spine

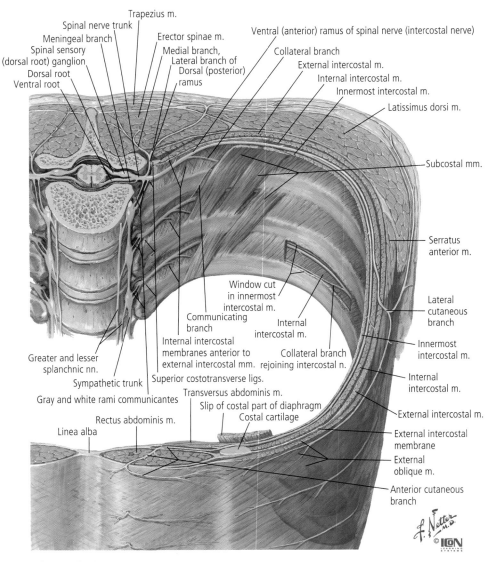

Figure 5-12

Nerve		Segmental Level	Sensory	Motor
Ventral rami	Intercostals	T1-T11	Anterior and lateral aspects of the thorax and abdomen	Intercostals, serratus posterior, levatores costarum, transversus thoracis
	Subcostals	T12		Part of external oblique
Dorsal rami		T1-T12	Posterior thorax and back	Splenius, iliocostalis, longissimus, spinalis, interspinales, intertransversarii, multifidi, semispinalis, rotatores

Nerves of the Lumbar Spine   NERVES

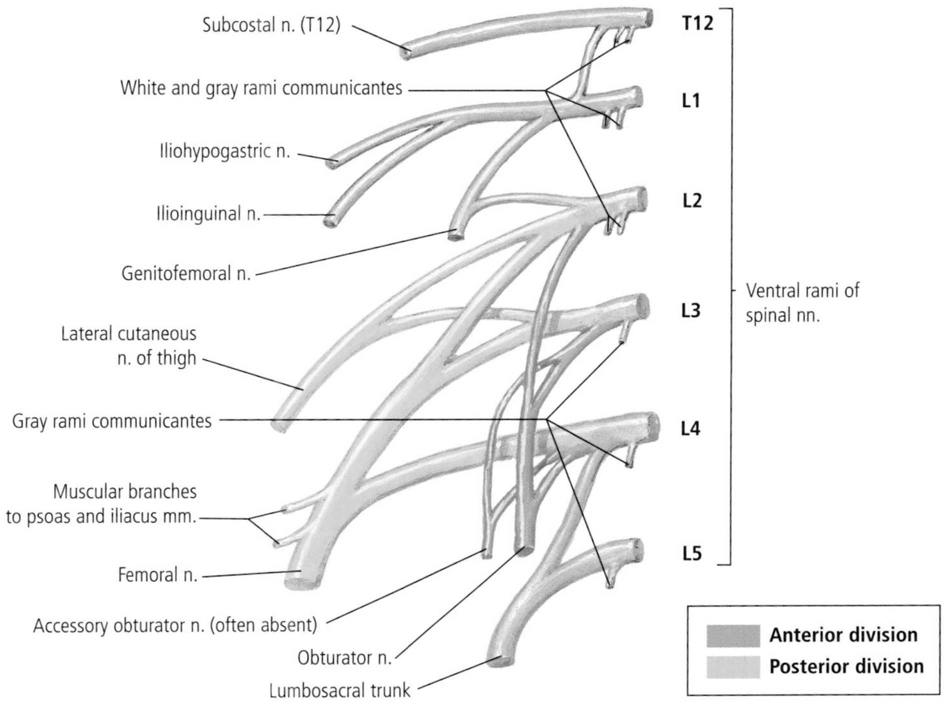

Subcostal n. (T12)

White and gray rami communicantes

Iliohypogastric n.

Ilioinguinal n.

Genitofemoral n.

Lateral cutaneous
n. of thigh

Gray rami communicantes

Muscular branches
to psoas and iliacus mm.

Femoral n.

Accessory obturator n. (often absent)

Obturator n.

Lumbosacral trunk

T12

L1

L2

L3

L4

L5

Ventral rami of
spinal nn.

Anterior division
Posterior division

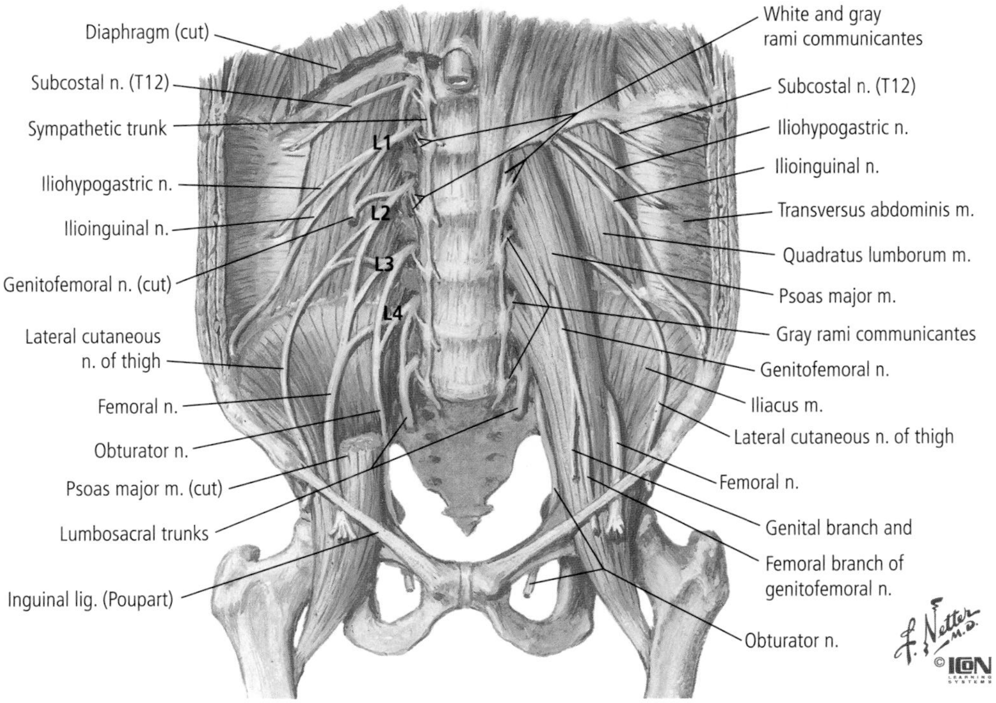

Diaphragm (cut)

Subcostal n. (T12)

Sympathetic trunk

Iliohypogastric n.

Ilioinguinal n.

Genitofemoral n. (cut)

Lateral cutaneous
n. of thigh

Femoral n.

Obturator n.

Psoas major m. (cut)

Lumbosacral trunks

Inguinal lig. (Poupart)

White and gray
rami communicantes

Subcostal n. (T12)

Iliohypogastric n.

Ilioinguinal n.

Transversus abdominis m.

Quadratus lumborum m.

Psoas major m.

Gray rami communicantes

Genitofemoral n.

Iliacus m.

Lateral cutaneous n. of thigh

Femoral n.

Genital branch and

Femoral branch of
genitofemoral n.

Obturator n.

Figure 5-13

NERVES

Nerves of the Lumbar Spine (cont.)

Nerve	Segmental Level	Sensory	Motor
Subcostal nerve	T12	Lateral hip	External oblique
Iliohypogastric nerve	T12, L1	Posterolateral gluteal region	Internal oblique, transverse abdominis
Ilioinguinal	L1	Superior medial thigh	Internal oblique, transverse abdominis
Genitofemoral	L1, L2	Superior anterior thigh	No motor
Lateral cutaneous	L2, L3	Lateral thigh	No motor
Branch to iliacus		No sensory	Iliacus
Femoral nerve	L2, L3, L4	Thigh via cutaneous nerves	Iliacus, sartorius, quadriceps femoris, articularis genu, pectineus
Obturator nerve	L2, L3, L4	Medial thigh	Adductor longus, adductor brevis, adductor magnus (adductor part), gracilis, obturator externus
Sciatic	L4, L5, S1, S2, S3	Hip joint	Knee flexors and all muscles of the lower leg and foot

Nerves of the Lumbar Spine (cont.)   NERVES

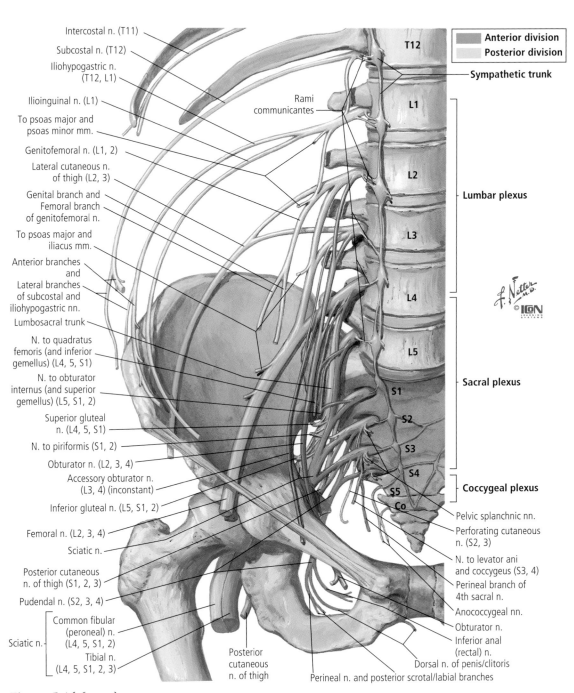

Figure 5-14 (cont.)

EXAMINATION:
HISTORY

Initial Hypotheses Based on Historical Findings

History	Initial Hypothesis
Reports of restricted motion of the lumbar spine associated with low back or buttock pain exacerbated by a pattern of movement that indicates possible opening or closing joint restriction (ie, decreased extension, side bending right, and rotation right)	Zygapophyseal joint pain syndromes[8, 9]
Reports of centralization or peripheralization of symptoms during repetitive movements, or prolonged periods in certain positions	Discogenic pain[10]
Reports of lower extremity pain/paresthesias that are greater than the low back pain. Patient may report episodes of lower extremity	Sciatica or lumbar radiculopathy[11]
Pain in the lower extremities that is exacerbated by an extension posture and relieved by flexion posture of the spine	Spinal stenosis[12]
Patient reports recurrent locking, catching, or giving way of the low back during active motion	Lumbar instability[13,14]
Reports of low back pain that is exacerbated by stretch of either ligament or muscles. Also, possibility of pain with contraction of muscular tissues	Muscle/ligamentous sprain/strain

Thoracic Zygapophyseal Joint Pain Referral Patterns

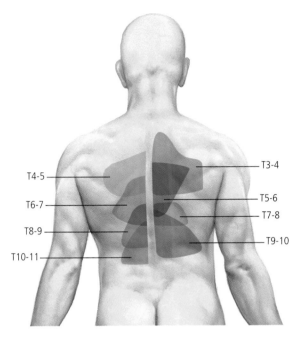

Figure 5-15A:
Zygapophyseal pain patterns of the thoracic spine, as described by Dreyfuss et al.[15]

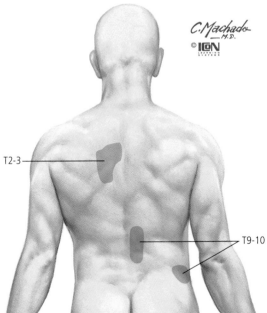

Figure 5-15B:
Zygapophyseal pain patterns of the thoracic spine, as described by Fukui et al.[16]

Lumbar Zygapophyseal Joint Pain Referral Patterns (cont.)

Prevalence of Pain Referral Patterns in Patients With Zygapophyseal Joint Pain Syndromes as Confirmed by Diagnostic Blocks[18]

Area of Pain Referral	Percentage of Patients Presenting With Pain (n=176 patients with low back pain)
Left groin	15%
Right groin	3%
Left buttock	42%
Right buttock	15%
Left thigh	38%
Right thigh	38%
Left calf	27%
Right calf	15%
Left foot	31%
Right foot	8%
In a subsequent study,[19] it was determined that in a cohort of 63 patients with chronic low back pain, the prevalence of zygapophyseal joint pain was 40%.	

Lumbar Zygapophyseal Joint Pain Referral Patterns (cont.)

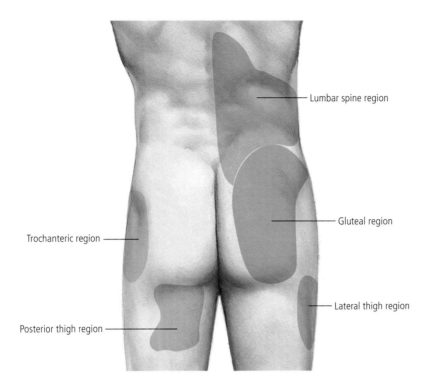

Lumbar spine region

Gluteal region

Trochanteric region

Lateral thigh region

Posterior thigh region

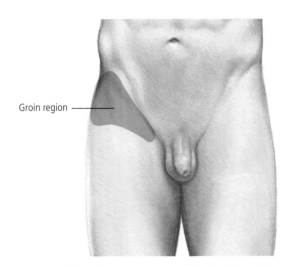

Groin region

Figure 5-16: *Zygapophyseal pain patterns of the lumbar spine, as described by Fukui et al.[17] Lumbar zygapophyseal joints L1-L2, L2-L3, and L4-L5 always refered pain to the lumbar spine region. Primary referral to the gluteal region was from L5-Sacrum (68% of the time). Levels L2-L3, L3-L4, L4-L5, and L5-S1 occasionally referred pain to the trochanteric region (10-16% of the time). Primary referral to regions lateral thigh, posterior thigh, and groin regions were most often from L3-L4, L4-L5, and L5-S1 (5-30% of the time).*

EXAMINATION: HISTORY

Reliability of the Historical Examination

Historical Question		Population	Kappa Value or % Agreement
Patient report of: *McCombe et al.[20]*	Foot pain	Group 1: 50 patients with low back pain	Inter-examiner reliability $\kappa = .12, .73$
	Leg pain	Group 2: 33 patients with low back pain	$\kappa = .53, .96$
	Thigh pain		$\kappa = .39, .78$
	Buttock pain		$\kappa = .33, .44$
	Back pain		$\kappa = -.19, .16$
Pain ever below the knee		475 patients with back pain	Test-retest among patient questionnaire Agreement 100%
Pain ever into the foot			Agreement 92%
Numbness below knee *Waddell et al.[21]*			Agreement 95%
Increased pain with: *Roach et al.[22]*	Sitting	53 subjects with a primary complaint of low back pain	Test-retest among patient questionnaire $\kappa = .46$
	Standing		$\kappa = .70$
	Walking		$\kappa = .67$
Increased pain with: *Vroomen et al.[23]*	Sitting	A random selection of 91 patients with low back pain	Inter-examiner reliability $\kappa = .49$
	Standing		$\kappa = 1.0$
	Walking		$\kappa = .56$
	Lying down		$\kappa = .41$
Pain with sitting *Van Dillen et al.[24]*		95 patients with low back pain	Inter-examiner reliability $\kappa = .99, 1.0$
Pain with bending *Van Dillen et al.[24]*			Inter-examiner reliability $\kappa = .98, .99$
Pain with bending *Roach et al.[22]*		53 subjects with a primary complaint of low back pain	Test-retest among patient questionnaire $\kappa = .65$
Pain with bending *McCombe et al.[20]*		Group 1: 50 patients with low back pain Group 2: 33 patients with low back pain	Inter-examiner reliability $\kappa = .51, .56$
Increased pain with coughing/sneezing *Vroomen et al.[23]*		A random selection of 91 patients with low back pain	Inter-examiner reliability, $\kappa = .64$

Reliability of the Historical Examination (cont.)

Historical Question	Population	Kappa Value or % Agreement
Increased pain with coughing *Roach et al.*[22]	53 subjects with a parimary complaint of low back pain	Test-retest among patient questionnaire $\kappa = .75$
Pain with pushing/lifting/carrying *Roach et al.*[22]		Test-retest among patient questionnaire $\kappa = .77, .89$
Sudden or gradual onset of pain *Waddell et al.*[21]	475 patients with back pain	Test-retest among patient questionnaire Agreement = 79%

Range of Motion

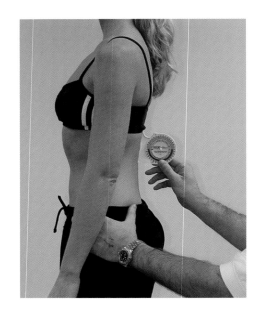

Figure 5-17A: *Inclinometer placement at the spinous process of the 12th thoracic vertebra*

Measurement	Instrumentation	Population	Pearson Correlation Coefficient (r) or ICC (95% CI)	
			Intra-examiner	Inter-examiner
Lumbar flexion Lumbar extension Side bending right Side bending left *Hunt et al.[25]*	Electronic inclinometer	45 asymptomatic individuals	r = .48 r = .53 r = .79 r = .81	r = .56 r = .37 r < .60 r < .60
Flexion Extension Left rotation Right rotation Left side bending Right side bending *Breum et al.[26]*	Back range-of-motion (BROM) instrument	47 asymptomatic students	ICC = .91 .63 .56 .57 .92 .89	ICC = .77 .35 .37 .35 .81 .89
Flexion Extension *Saur et al.[27]*	Inclinometer	54 patients with chronic low back pain (LBP)	Inter-examiner reliability, r = .88 for flexion, and .42 for extension	
Lumbar flexion *Fritz et al.[28]*	Single inclinometer	49 patients with LBP referred for flexion-extension radiographs	.60 (.33, .79)	
Lumbar extension *Fritz et al.[28]*	Single inclinometer		.61 (.37, .78)	

CI, confidence interval.

Range of Motion (cont.)

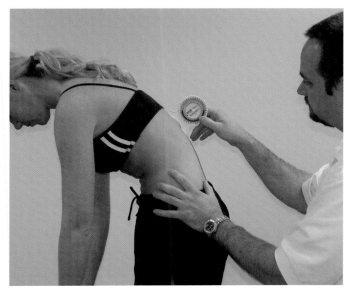

Figure 5-17B: *Measurement of thoracolumbar flexion*

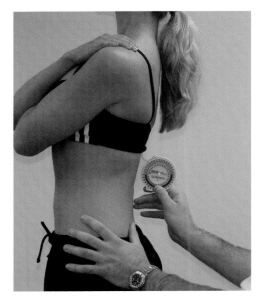

Figure 5-17C: *Measurement of thoracolumbar extension*

Identifying Segmental Levels

Procedure	Description	Population	Inter-examiner Reliability Kappa and ICC Values (95% CI)
Detection of segmental levels in the lumbar spine *Downey et al.*[29]	Patient prone. Examiner identified nominated levels of the lumbar spine and marked the specific level with a pen containing ink that could be seen only under ultraviolet light	20 patients with low back pain	κ = .69
Examiner judgment of marked segmental level *Binkley et al.*[30]	Patient prone. One spinous process was arbitrarily marked on each patient. Examiner identified the level of the marked segment	18 patients with low back pain	ICC = .69 (.53, .82)

Determination of Posteroanterior Mobility and Segmental Dysfunction

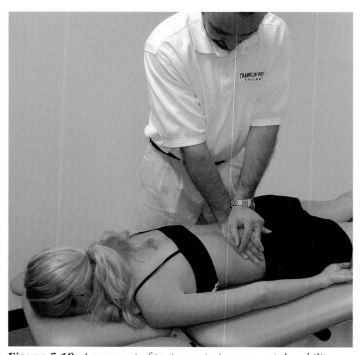

Figure 5-18: Assessment of posteroanterior segmental mobility

Determination of Posteroanterior Mobility and Segmental Dysfunction (cont.)

Procedure	Description and Positive Findings	Population	Inter-examiner Reliability Kappa Value and ICC Values (95% CI)
Determination of posteroanterior spinal stiffness Maher et al.[31]	5 raters tested lumbar spinal levels for posteroanterior mobility and graded each on an 11-point scale ranging from "markedly reduced stiffness" to "markedly increased stiffness"	40 asymptomatic patients	First study ICC = .55 (.32, .79) Second study ICC = .77 (.57, .89)
Posteroanterior mobility testing Binkley et al.[30]	Patient in prone position. Examiner evaluates posteroanterior motion mobility. Mobility is scored on a 9-point scale, ranging from "severe excess motion" to "no motion," and the presence of pain is recorded	18 patients with low back pain	ICC = .25 (.00, .39)
Segmental mobility testing Hicks et al.[32]	Patient in prone position. Examiner applies an anteriorly directed force over the spinous process of the segment to be tested. Examiner grades mobility as hypermobile, normal, or hypomobile	63 patients with current low back pain	κ = −.2 to .26, depending on level tested
Identification of a mis-aligned vertebra Keating et al.[33]	Static palpation is used to determine the relationship of one vertebra to the vertebra below	21 symptomatic and 25 asymptomatic patients	κ = −.04 to .03 with a mean of .00
Detection of a segmental lesion T11-L5/S1 French et al.[34]	2 chiropractors used visual postural analysis, pain descriptions, leg-length discrepancy, neurologic examination, motion palpation, static palpation, and any special orthopaedic tests to determine the level of segmental lesion	19 patients with chronic mechanical low back pain	κ = −.16 to .57

Pain Provocation

Procedure	Description and Positive Findings	Population	Intra-examiner Reliability	Inter-examiner Reliability
			Kappa Value (95% CI)	
Spring test T10-T7	Patient prone. Examiner applies a posteroanterior force to the spinous process of T7-L5. The pressure of each force is held for 20 seconds. Considered positive if the force produces pain	84 subjects, of whom 53% reported low back symptoms within the previous 12 months	.73 (.39, 1.0)	.12 (−.18, .41)
Spring test L2-T11			.78 (.49, 1.0)	.36 (.07, .66)
Spring test L5-L3 Hornelj et al.[35]			.56 (.18, .94)	.41 (.12, .70)
Osseous pain of each joint T11/L1–L5/S1 Keating et al.[33]	Patient prone. Examiner applies pressure over the bony structures of each joint	21 symptomatic and 25 asymptomatic patients		.34 to .65 with a mean of .48 for all levels
Intersegmental tenderness Strender et al.[36]	Patient prone. Examiner palpates the area between the spinous processes. Increased tenderness is considered positive	71 patients with low back pain		.55
Pain provocation Hicks et al.[32]	Patient prone. Examiner applies an anteriorly directed force over the spinous process of the segment to be tested. Considered positive if pain is reproduced	63 patients with current low back pain		.25 to .55 depending on the segmental level tested
Pain during mobility testing Fritz et al.[28]		49 patients with LBP referred for flexion-extension radiographs		.57 (.43, .71)

Pain Provocation During Active Movements

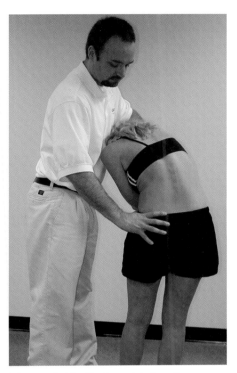

Figure 5-19: *Flexion–side bending–rotation*

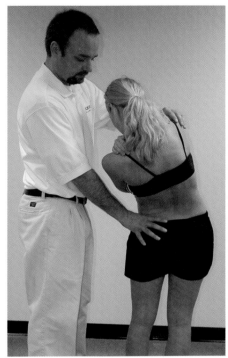

Figure 5-20: *Extension–side bending–rotation*

Movement	Procedure	Population	Kappa Value (95% CI)
Side bending	Patient standing with arms at sides. Patient is instructed to slide hand down the outside of the thigh		.60 (.40, .79)
Rotation	Patient standing with arms at sides. Patient is instructed to rotate the trunk		.17 (−.08, .42)
Side bending–rotation	Patient standing with arms at sides. Patient is instructed to move the pelvis to one side, creating a side-bend rotation to the opposite side	35 patients with low back pain	.29 (.06, .51)
Flexion–side bending–rotation	Patient standing. Examiner guides patient into lumbar flexion, then side bending, then rotation		.39 (.18, .61)
Extension–side bending–rotation *Entire table: Haswell et al.[37]*	Patient standing. Examiner guides patient into lumbar extension, then side bending, then rotation		.29 (.06, .52)

Segmental Mobility Examination

Procedure	Description and Positive Findings	Population	Intra-examiner reliability	Inter-examiner reliability
			Kappa Value and Pearson Correlational Coefficient (r) (95% CI)	
Motion palpation *Love and Brodeur*[38]	Examiner sits behind subject. The examining hand is placed horizontally on the back so that the spinous process bisects the proximal phalanges. The dorsal aspect of the palpating hand is used to determine the amount of motion at each respective segment. Examiners record the most hypomobile segment	32 asymptomatic volunteers	Ranged from −.007 to .65 (r)	Ranged from r = .021 in the first trial to r = .85 in the second trial. Association not large enough to be considered different by chance
Determination of segmental fixations *Mootz et al.*[39]	As above. However, each segment determined to exhibit a hard end-feel on examination of passive joint motion is classified as fixated	60 asymptomatic volunteers	Kappa values ranged from −.09 to .39	Kappa values ranged from −.06 to .17
Passive motion palpation *Keating et al.*[33]	Passive motion palpation is performed, and the segment is considered fixated if a hard end-feel is noted during the assessment	21 symptomatic and 25 asymptomatic subjects		Kappa values ranged from −.03 to .23, with a mean of .07
Segmental mobility testing *Strender et al.*[36]	Patient lies on one side with hips and knees flexed. Examiner assesses mobility while passively moving the patient. Examiner determines whether the mobility of the segment is decreased, normal, or increased	71 patients with low back pain		κ = .54
Hypermobility at any level *Fritz et al.*[28]	Patient is prone. Examiner applies a posteroanterior force to the spinous process of each lumbar vertebra. Mobility of each segment is judged as normal, hypermobile, or hypomobile	49 patients with LBP referred for flexion-extension radiographs	.48 (.35, .61)	
Hypomobility at any level *Fritz et al.*[28]			38 (.22, .54)	

Segmental Mobility Examination (cont.)

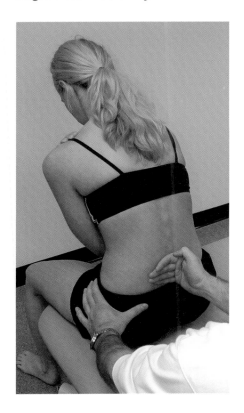

Figure 5-21: Motion palpation seated

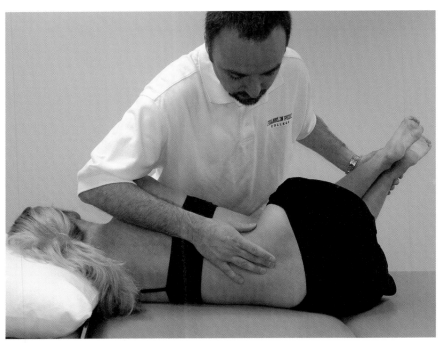

Figure 5-22: Motion palpation of side bending right

Reliability of the McKenzie Method

Procedure	Description and Positive Findings	Population	Reliability Kappa Value
Reliability of the McKenzie classification for low back pain *Riddle and Rothstein*[40]	Therapists (of whom only 32% had ever taken any form of McKenzie training) completed a McKenzie evaluation form and classified the patient as exhibiting a postural, dysfunctional, or derangement syndrome. Therapists also determined whether the patient presented with a lateral shift	363 patients referred to physical therapists for treatment of low back pain	Inter-rater reliability for classification, .26 Inter-rater reliability for lateral shift, .26
Reliability of the McKenzie classification for low back pain *Kilpkoski et al.*[41]	Two examiners with >5 years of training in the McKenzie method evaluated all patients. Therapists completed a McKenzie evaluation form and classified the patient as exhibiting a postural, dysfunctional, or derangement syndrome. Therapists also determined whether the patient presented with a lateral shift	39 patients with low back pain	Inter-examiner reliability for classification, .70 Inter-rater reliability for the presence of a lateral shift, .20
Reliability of the McKenzie evaluation *Razmjou et al.*[42]	Examination consisted of history taking, evaluation of spinal range of motion, and specified test movements	46 consecutive patients presenting with low back pain	Classification of syndrome = .70 Derangement subsyndrome = .96 Presence of lateral shift = .52 Deformity of sagittal plane = 1.0

Centralization Phenomena

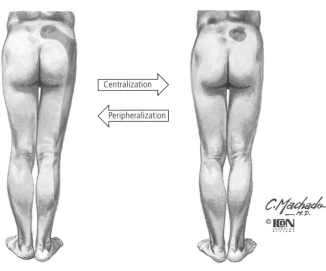

During specific movements, range of motion and movement
of pain noted. Movement of pain from peripheral to central
location (centralization) predicts outcome and appropriateness
of therapy

Figure 5-23: *Centralization of pain*

Procedure	Description and Positive Findings	Population	Reliability Kappa Value (95% CI)
Centralization and directional preference Kilpkoski et al.[41]	Two examiners with >5 years of training in the McKenzie method evaluated all patients and determined whether centralization occurred during repeated movements and, if so, the directional preference that resulted in the centralization	39 patients with low back pain	Inter-examiner reliability as to whether centralization occurred, .70 Inter-examiner reliability with regard to centralization and directional preference, .90
Judgments of centralization Fritz et al.[43]	Therapists (without formal training in McKenzie methods) and students viewed videotapes of patients being taken through an examination by one examiner. All therapists and students watching the videos were asked to make an assessment regarding change in symptoms based on movement status	12 patients receiving physical therapy for low back pain	Inter-rater reliability for physical therapists, .82 (.81, .84) Inter-rater reliability for physical therapy students, .76 (.76, .77)

RELIABILITY OF THE CLINICAL EXAMINATION

Measures of Lumbar Segmental Instability

Procedure	Description and Positive Findings	Population	Reliability Kappa Value and ICC
Painful arc in flexion	Positive if patient reports symptoms at a particular point in the movement but the symptoms are not present before or after the movement		.69 (.54, .84)
Painful arc on return from flexion	Positive if patient experiences symptoms when returning from flexed position		.61 (.44, .78)
Instability catch	Positive if patient experiences sudden acceleration or deceleration of trunk movement outside the primary plane of movement		.25 (−.10, .60)
Gower sign	Positive if patient pushes up from thighs with the hands when returning to upright from a flexed position		.00 (−1.09, 1.09)
Reversal of lumbopelvic rhythm	Positive if, on attempting to return from the flexed position, patient bends the knees and shifts the pelvis anteriorly	63 patients with current low back pain	.16 (−.15, .46)
Aberrant movement pattern	Patients who demonstrate any of the above 5 movement patterns are considered positive for an aberrant movement pattern		.60 (.47, .73)
Posterior shear test	Patient stands with arms crossed over abdomen. Examiner places one hand over patient's crossed arms, and with the other, stabilizes the pelvis. The index finger is used to palpate the L5–S1 interspace. Examiner then applies a posterior force through the patient's crossed arms. This procedure is performed at each level. A positive test is indicated by provocation of symptoms		.35 (.20, .51)
Prone instability test	Patient prone with the edge of the torso on plinth, legs over edge, and feet resting on table. Examiner performs a posteroanterior pressure and notes provocation of any symptoms. Patient then lifts the legs off the floor, posteroanterior pressure is again performed, and provocation of symptoms is reported. Positive if patient experiences symptoms with feet on floor, that disappear when feet are lifted off floor		.87 (.80, .94)

Entire table: Hicks et al.[32]

Measures of Lumbar Segmental Instability

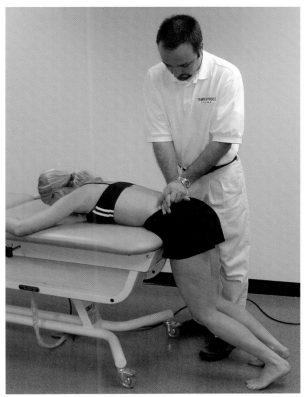

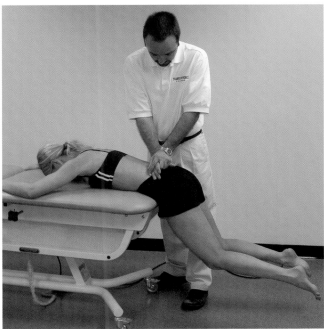

Figure 5-24A and 24B: *Prone instability test*

Straight-Leg Raise (SLR)

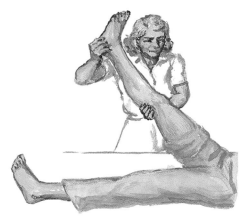

Figure 5-25

Procedure	Description and Positive Findings	Population	Reliability Kappa Value and ICC
Passive SLR *Vroomen et al.*[23]	Patient supine. Examiner passively flexes hip with knee extended. Examiner measures angle of SLR and determines whether symptoms occurred in a dermatomal fashion	91 patients with low back pain randomly selected	Inter-examiner reliability for typical dermatomal pain, $\kappa = .68$ Inter-examiner reliability for any pain in the leg, $\kappa = .36$ Inter-examiner reliability for SLR lower than 45 degrees, $\kappa = .43$
Passive SLR *Rose*[44]	Patient supine. Examiner maintains knee in extension while passively flexing hip. Hip is flexed until examiner feels resistance. Range of motion measurement is recorded	18 physiotherapy students	Inter-examiner reliability SLR right, r = .86 SLR left, r = .83
Active SLR *Mens et al.*[45]	Patient supine with legs straight and feet 20 cm apart. Patient is instructed to "try to raise your legs, one after the other, above the couch without bending the knee." The patient is asked to score the maneuver on a 6-point scale, ranging from "not difficult at all" to "unable to do."	50 females with lumbopelvic pain	Test-retest reliability, ICC = .83
Straight-leg raise *Viikari-Juntura et al.*[46]	Passive elevation of the leg with knee extended. Considered positive if pain in the low back or buttock is experienced	27 patients with low back pain	$\kappa = .32$

Lumbar Zygapophyseal Pain Syndromes

Revel and colleagues[47] have identified seven predictor variables that are capable of identifying 92% of patients presenting with zygapophyseal joint pain as confirmed by diagnostic blocks.

At least five of the following seven variables must be present to suggest the presence of a zygapophyseal pain syndrome:
1. Age >65
2. Pain not exacerbated by coughing
3. Pain not worsened on hyperextension
4. Pain not worsened by forward flexion
5. Pain not worsened by extension-rotation
6. Pain not worsened when rising from a chair
7. Pain relieved by recumbency*

*The final predictor variable must always be present to be indicative of pain arising from a zygapophyseal joint.

Lumbar Spinal Stenosis: History

Historical Question	Sensitivity	Specificity	+Likelihood Ratio (LR)	– LR
Do you get pain in your legs with walking that is relieved by sitting?	.80	.16	.95	1.27
Are you able to walk better when holding onto a shopping cart? *Fritz et al.[12]*	.63	.67	1.9	.55
Age >65	.77	.69	2.5	.33
Pain below knees?	.56	.63	1.5	.70
Pain below buttocks?	.88	.34	1.3	.35
No pain when seated	.46	.93	6.6	.58
Severe lower extremity pain?	.65	.67	2.0	.52
Symptoms improved while seated? *Katz et al.[48]*	.52	.83	3.1	.58

Lumbar Spinal Stenosis: Physical Examination

Test	Test Procedure	Determination of Findings	Population	Reference Standard	Sens (95% CI)	Spec (95% CI)	+LR (95% CI)	–LR (95% CI)
Two-stage treadmill test	Subjects ambulated on a level and inclined (15°) treadmill for 10 minutes. A 10-minute rest period sitting upright in a chair followed each treadmill test	A number of variables were recorded at baseline, including:	45 subjects with low back and lower extremity pain (26 stenotic, 19 non-stenotic)	Magnetic resonance imaging (MRI) or computed tomography (CT) scanning				
		Time to onset of symptoms			.68 (.49, .86)	.83 (.66, 1.0)	4.07 (1.40, 11.8)	.39
		Longer total walking time during the inclined test			.5 (.37, .62)	.923 (.778, 1.0)	6.46 (3.1, 13.5)	.54
Fritz et al.[12]		Prolonged recovery after level walking			.82 (.66, .98)	.68 (.48, .90)	2.59 (1.3, 5.2)	.26
Abnormal Rhomberg test	Patient stands with feet together and eyes closed for 10 seconds	Considered abnormal if compensatory movements were required to keep feet planted			.39 (.24, .54)	.91 (.81, 1.0)	4.3	.67
Katz et al.[48]								
Vibration deficit	Assessed at the first metatarsal head with a 128-Hz tuning fork	Considered abnormal if patient did not perceive any vibration	93 patients with back pain with or without radiation to the lower extremities	Retrospective chart review. Diagnoses confirmed by MRI or CT	.53 (.38, .68)	.81 (.67, .95)	2.8	.58
Pin-prick deficit	Sensation tested at the dorsomedial foot, dorsolateral foot, and medial and lateral calf	Graded as decreased or normal			.47 (.32, .62)	.81 (.67, .95)	2.5	.65
Weakness	Strength of knee flexors, extensors, and hallucis longus was tested	Graded from 0 (no movement) to 5 (normal)			.47 (.32, .62)	.78 (.64, .92)	2.1	.68
Thigh pain with 30 seconds of extension	Patient performs hip extension for 30 seconds	Positive if pain occurs in thigh after or during extension			.51 (.36, .66)	.69 (.53, .85)	1.6	.71
Absent Achilles reflex *Katz et al.*[48]	Reflex testing of the Achilles tendon	Graded from 0 (no response) to 4 (clonus)			.46 (.31, .61)	.78 (.64, .92)	2.1	.69

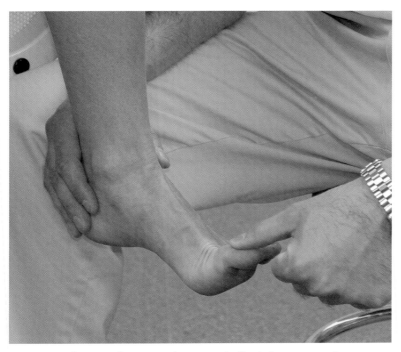

Figure 5-26: Strength testing of extensor hallucis longus muscle

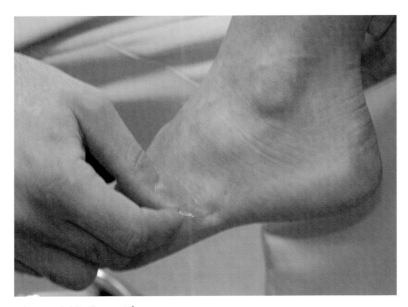

Figure 5-27: Pin-prick test

Identification of Segmental Dysfunction

Test	Test Procedure	Determination of Findings	Population	Reference Standard	Sens (95% CI)	Spec (95% CI)	+LR (95% CI)	−LR (95% CI)
Manual motion testing *Phillips and Twomey*[49]	Examiners performed passive physiologic and passive intervertebral mobility testing	Segments were graded as hypermobile, normal, or hypomobile. Pain responses were not collected	72 subjects with lumbar pain with or without referral into the lower extremities	Lumbar spinal block. Some were performed retrospectively, and some were performed prospectively	Prospective = .52 Retrospective = .48	Prospective = .8 Retrospective = .75	Prospective = 2.6 Retrospective = 1.92	Prospective = .6 Retrospective = .69
Manual motion testing *Phillips and Twomey*[49]		Segments were graded as hypermobile, normal, or hypomobile. Pain responses were collected and were used to determine the presence of a segmental dysfunction			Prospective = .95 Retrospective = .61	Prospective = 1.0 Retrospective = 1.0	Prospective = NA Retrospective = NA	Prospective = .05 Retrospective = .39
Motion palpation *Leboeuf-Yde et al.*[5]	Palpation of a motion segment during either passive or active motion	Examiners evaluated motion relative to the presence of a fixation. Patient's pain reaction was noted after motion palpation of each segment	188 individuals	Self-reported low back pain	T12-L1 = .15 L1-L2 = .35 L2-L3 and L3-L4 = .23 L4-L5 and L5-S1 = .54	T12-L1 = .89 L1-L2 = .95 L2-L3 and L3-L4 = .84 L4-L5 and L5-S1 = .77	T12-L1 = 1.36 L1-L2 = 7.0 L2-L3 = 1.44 L4-L5 and L5-S1 = 2.35	T12-L1 = .96 L1-L2 = .68 L2-L3 = .92 L4-L5 and L5-S1 = .60
Segmental hypomobility testing *Abbot and Mercer*[51]	Examiners assessed active range of motion (AROM), abnormality of segmental motion (AbnROM), passive accessory intervertebral motion (PAIVM), and passive physiologic intervertebral motion (PPIVM)	AROM, AbnROM, and PAIVM were rated as hypomobile, normal, or hypermobile. PPIVM was rated on a 5-point scale, with 0 and 1 indicating hypomobility, while 3 and 4 indicated hypermobility	9 patients with low back pain	Flexion and extension lateral radiographs. Segments were considered hypomobile if motion was more than 2 standard deviations from the mean of a normal population	AROM .75 (.36, .94) AbnROM .43 (.19, .71) PAIVM .75 (.36, .94) PPIVM .42 (.19, .71)	AROM .60 (.27, .86) AbnROM .88 (.70, .96) PAIVM .35 (.20, .55) PPIVM .89 (.71, .96)	AROM 1.88 (.57, 6.8) AbnROM 3.60 (.84, 15.38) PAIVM 1.16 (.44, 3.03) PPIVM 3.86 (.89, 16.31)	AROM .42 (.07, 1.90) AbnROM .65 (.28, 1.06) PAIVM .71 (.12, 2.75) PPIVM .64 (.28, 1.04)

Identification of Segmental Dysfunction (cont.)

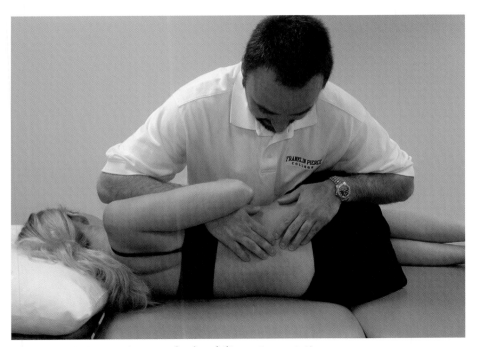

Figure 5-28: *Passive intervertebral mobility testing: rotation*

Lumbar Instability

Variables	Test Procedure	Determination of Findings	Population	Reference Standard	Sens (95% CI)	Spec (95% CI)	+LR (95% CI)	–LR (95% CI)
Age <37 years	History collected before physical examination	NA			.57 (.39, .74)	.81 (.60, .92)	3.0 (1.2, 7.7)	.53 (.33, .85)
Lumbar flexion >53°	Range of motion taken with single inclinometer	NA	49 patients with LBP referred for flexion-extension radiographs	Radiologic findings revealed either two segments with rotational/translational instability, or one segment with both rotational and translational instability	.68 (.49, .82)	.86 (.65, .94)	4.8 (1.6, 14.0)	.38 (.21, .66)
Total extension >26°	Range of motion taken with single inclinometer	NA			.50 (.33, .67)	.76 (.55, .89)	2.1 (.90, 4.9)	.66 (.42, 1.0)
Lack of hypomobility during intervertebral testing	Patient in prone, and examiner applies a posteroanterior force to the spinous process of each lumbar vertebra	Mobility of each segment was judged as normal, hypermobile, or hypomobile			.43 (.27, .61)	.95 (.77, .99)	8.6 (1.3, 63.9)	.60 (.43, .84)
Any hypermobility during intervertebral motion testing					.46 (.30, .64)	.81 (.60, .92)	2.4 (.93, 6.4)	.66 (.44, .99)

Fritz et al.[28]

Lumbar Instability (cont.)

Fritz et al.[28] investigated the accuracy of the clinical examination in 49 patients with radiographically determined lumbar instability. Results revealed that two predictor variables, including lack of hypomobility of the lumbar spine and lumbar flexion >53 degrees, demonstrated a sensitivity of .29 (.13, .46), a specificity of .98 (.91, 1.0), a +LR of 12.8 (.79, 211.6), and a –LR of .72 (.55, .94). The nomogram below represents the change from pretest probability (57% in this study) to a posttest probability of 94.3%.

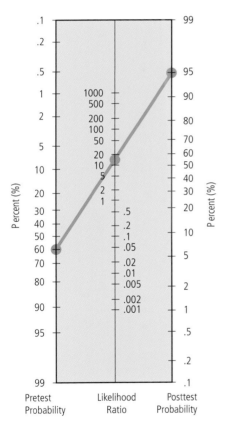

Figure 5-29: *Nomogram representing the posttest probability of lumbar instability, given the presence of hypomobility in the lumbar spine and lumbar flexion >53°.*
(Reprinted with permission from Fagan TJ. Nomogram for Baye's theorem. *N Engl J Med.* 1975;293:257. Copyright © 2005 Massachusetts Medical Society. All rights reserved.)

Lumbar Radiculopathy: History

Patient Reports of	Sensitivity	Specificity	+ LR	– LR
Weakness	.70	.41	1.19	.73
Numbness	.68	.34	1.03	.94
Tingling	.67	.31	.97	1.06
Burning *Lauder et al.*[53]	.40	.60	1.0	1.0
Paresthesias *Kerr et al.*[52]	.30	.58	.71	1.21

Lumbosacral Radiculopathy: Physical Examination

Radicular pain due to nerve root compression

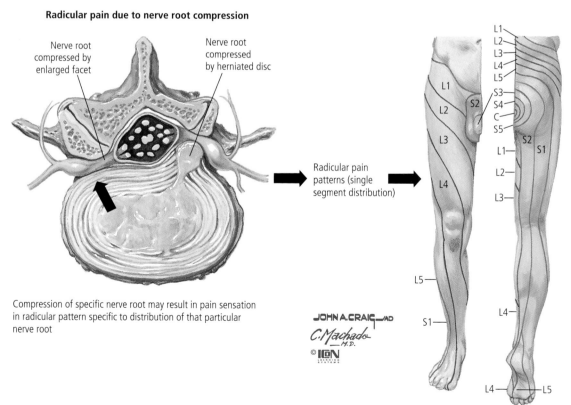

Nerve root compressed by enlarged facet

Nerve root compressed by herniated disc

Radicular pain patterns (single segment distribution)

Compression of specific nerve root may result in pain sensation in radicular pattern specific to distribution of that particular nerve root

JOHN A. CRAIG—MD
C.Machado—M.D.
©IAN

Figure 5-30: Pain patterns in lumbar disease

Lumbosacral Radiculopathy: Physical Examination (cont.)

Test		Test Procedure	Determination of Findings	Population	Reference Standard	Sens (95% CI)	Spec (95% CI)	+LR (95% CI)	LR −(95% CI)
Sensation *Lauder et al.*[53]	Vibration	NR	Considered abnormal when either vibration or pin prick was reduced on the side of the lesion	170 patients with low back and lower extremity symptoms	Electrodiagnostic testing	.50	.62	1.32	.81
	Pin prick								
Weakness	Gastrocnemius-soleus	NR	Weakness was defined as any grade less than 5/5			S1 = .47	S1 = .76	1.96	.70
	Extensor hallucis longus					L5 = .61	L5 = .55	1.36	.71
	Hip flexors					L3-L4 = .7	L3-L4 = .84	4.38	.36
	Quadricpes					L3-L4 = .40	L3-L4 = .89	3.64	.67
Reflexes	Achilles	NR	Considered abnormal when the reflex on the side of the lesion was reduced compared with the opposite side			S1 = .47	S1 = .9	4.7	.59
	Patellar					L3-L4 = .50	L3-L4 = .93	7.14	.54
If reflexes, weakness, and sensory were all found to be abnormal *Lauder et al.*[53]						.12	.97	4.0	.90
Straight-leg raise *Morris*[11]		NR	NR	25 patients with bony nerve entrapment	Surgical confirmation	.16*	NR	Unable to calculate	Unable to calculate
Straight-leg raise *Kerr et al.*[52]		Retrospective study	Retrospective chart review was performed to determine the presence of positive findings	100 patients with radiculopathy	Surgical confirmation	.98	.44	1.75	.05
Contralateral straight-leg raise						.43	.94	7.2	.61
Achilles reflex						.48	.89	4.4	.58
Extensor hallucis longus weakness						.54	.89	4.9	.52
Calf wasting						.29	.94	4.8	.76
Diminished sensation *Kerr et al.*[52]						.16	.80	.80	1.05

* Calculated by van de Hoogen et al.[54]

Detecting Disk Herniation: Straight-Leg Raise

Deville et al.[55] compiled the results of 15 studies that investigated the accuracy of the straight-leg raise (SLR) for detecting disk herniation. The SLR is performed with the patient supine, the knee fully extended, and the ankle in neutral dorsiflexion. The examiner then passively flexes the hip while maintaining the knee in extension. Once pain or paresthesia is experienced in the back or lower limb, the examiner maintains the current level of hip flexion. Sensitizing maneuvers are then added, including dorsiflexion of the ankle and flexion of the cervical spine. If these sensitizing maneuvers exacerbate the symptoms, the test is considered positive.[56] However, numerous variations of the SLR maneuver have been reported, and no consistency was noted among the studies selected for the Deville et al.[55] review. The results of each study, as well as the pooled estimates by Deville et al.,[55] are given below.

Test	Sens (95% CI)	Spec (95% CI)	+LR	−LR
Albeck[57]	.82	.21	1.0	.86
Aronson et al.[58]	.40	NR	Unable to calculate	Unable to calculate
Charnley[59]	.85	.57	1.98	.26
Edgar et al.[60]	.80	NR	Unable to calculate	Unable to calculate
Gurdjian et al.[61]	.81	.52	1.69	.37
Hakelius et al.[62]	.96	.14	1.12	.29
Hirsch et al.[63]	.91	.32	1.34	2.8
Jonsson et al.[64]	.87	.22	1.12	.59
Kerr et al.[52]	.98	.44	1.75	.05
Kortelainen et al.[65]	.94	NR	Unable to calculate	Unable to calculate
Kosteljanetz et al.[66]	.89	.14	1.03	.79
Kosteljanetz et al.[67]	.78	.48	1.5	.49
Knuttson[68]	.95	.10	1.05	.50
Shiqing et al.[56]	.94	NR	Unable to calculate	Unable to calculate
Spangfort[69]	.97	.11	1.09	.27
Pooled estimate of the above listed 15 studies as calculated by Deville et al.[55]	0.91 (.82, .94)	.26 (.16, .38)	1.2	3.5

Detecting Disk Herniation: Straight-Leg Raise (cont.)

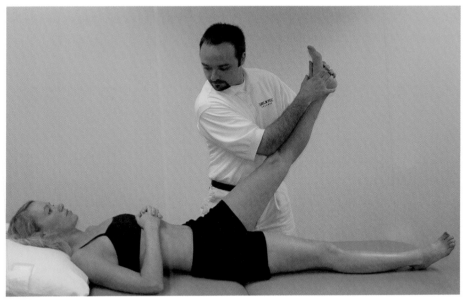

Figure 5-31A: Straight-leg raise

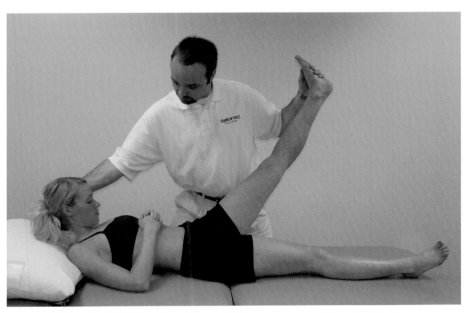

Figure 5-31B: Straight-leg raise with sensitizing maneuver of cervical flexion

Detecting Disk Herniation: Crossed Straight-Leg Raise

This test entails performing the straight-leg raise on the uninvolved lower extremity. It is considered positive if it reproduces the patient's symptoms in the involved extremity. The diagnostic accuracy as determined in 8 studies and the pooled estimates as calculated by Deville et al.[55] are shown below.

Test	Sens (95% CI)	Spec (95% CI)	+LR (95% CI)	−LR (95% CI)
Edgar et al.[60]	.44	NR	Unable to calculate	Unable to calculate
Hakelius et al.[62]	.28	.88	2.33	.82
Jonsson et al.[64]	.22	.93	3.14	.84
Kerr et al.[52]	.43	.93	6.14	.61
Kosteljanetz et al.[66]	.57	1.0	NA	.43
Knuttson[68]	.25	.93	3.57	.81
Shiqing et al.[56]	.15	NR	Unable to calculate	Unable to calculate
Spangfort[69]	.23	.88	1.92	.88
Pooled estimate for the 8 studies listed above as calculated by Deville et al.[55]	.29 (.24, .34)	.88 (.86, .90)	2.4	.80

Ankylosing Spondylitis: History

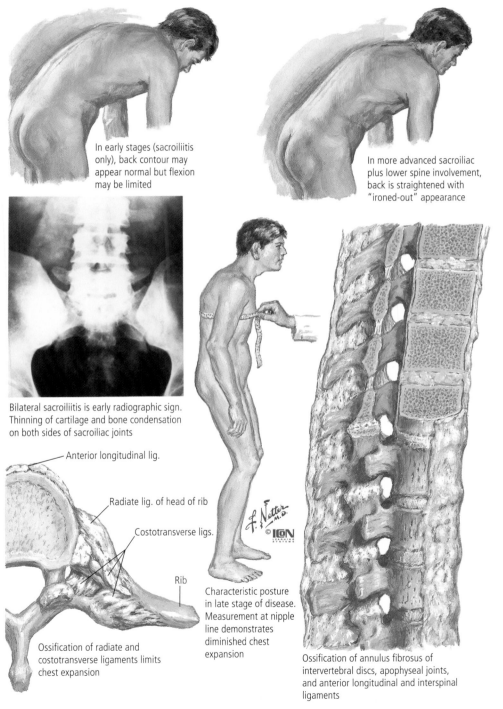

In early stages (sacroiliitis only), back contour may appear normal but flexion may be limited

In more advanced sacroiliac plus lower spine involvement, back is straightened with "ironed-out" appearance

Bilateral sacroiliitis is early radiographic sign. Thinning of cartilage and bone condensation on both sides of sacroiliac joints

Anterior longitudinal lig.

Radiate lig. of head of rib

Costotransverse ligs.

Rib

Ossification of radiate and costotransverse ligaments limits chest expansion

Characteristic posture in late stage of disease. Measurement at nipple line demonstrates diminished chest expansion

Ossification of annulus fibrosus of intervertebral discs, apophyseal joints, and anterior longitudinal and interspinal ligaments

Figure 5-32: *Ankylosing spondylitis*

Ankylosing Spondylitis: History (cont.)

Clinical Symptom	Population	Reference Standard	Sens	Spec	+LR	−LR
Pain not relieved by lying down	Randomly selected group of patients with low back pain (n=449)	New York criteria and radiographic confirmation of ankylosing spondylitis .27 patients were found to be positive	.80	.49	1.57	.41
Back pain at night			.71	.53	1.51	.55
Morning stiffness >.5 hour			.64	.59	1.56	.68
Pain or stiffness relieved by exercise			.74	.43	1.30	.60
Age of onset ≤40 years *Gran[70]*			1.0	.07	1.07	0

Ankylosing Spondylitis: Physical Examination

Test		Test Procedure	Determination of Findings	Population	Reference Standard	Sens	Spec	+LR	–LR
Measurements of chest expansion *Gran*[70]	<7 cm	NR	Measured to the closest centimeter			.63	.53	1.34	.70
	<2.5 cm					.91	.99	.91	.09
Schober test <4 cm *Gran*[70]		Patient is standing. The examiner marks a point 5 cm below and 10 cm above S2. This distance is then measured in the upright position, then in full flexion	The difference between the two measurements is calculated and recorded to the closest centimeter	Randomly selected group of patients with low back pain (n=449)	New York criteria and radiographic confirmation of ankylosing spondylitis. 27 patients were found to be positive	.30	.86	2.14	.81
Decreased lumbar lordosis *Gran*[70]		Visual observation	Individually judged by each examiner			.36	.80	1.8	.80
Direct tenderness over sacroiliac joint *Gran*[70]		Direct pressure over the joint with the patient in an upright position	Positive if patient reported pain			.27	.68	.84	1.07
L3-S1 Midline pressure *Russell et al.*[71]		Pressure is applied to the midline points between spinal segments	Provocation of pain considered a positive response	113 patients with low back pain (41 with ankylosing spondylitis)	Radiographically confirmed ankylosing spondylitis	.15*	.60*	.38	1.42
Lumbar spine pressure *Blower and Griffin*[72]		Pressure applied over the lumbar spine		66 patients with low back pain (33 with ankylosing spondylitis)	Radiographs and HLA B27 antigen testing	.33	.30	.47	2.23

* Calculated by van de Hoogen et al.[54]

REFERENCES

1. Bogduk N. *Clinical Anatomy of the Lumbar Spine and Sacrum*. 3rd ed. London: Churchill Livingstone; 1997.

2. Vleeming A, Pool-Goudzwaard A, Stoeckart R, van Winderden J, Snijders C. The posterior layer of the thoracolumbar fascia. Its function in load and transfer from spine to legs. *Spine*. 1995;20:753-758.

3. Bogduk N. The applied anatomy of the lumbar fascia. *Spine*. 1984;9:164-170.

4. Bergmark A. Stability of the lumbar spine. A study in mechanical engineering. *Acta Orthop Scand*. 1989;60:5-24.

5. Evans C, Oldreive W. A study to investigate whether golfers with a history of low back pain show a reduced endurance of transversus abdominis. *J Man Manipulative Ther*. 2000;8:162-174.

6. Kay A. An extensive literature review of the lumbar multifidus: biomechanics. *J Man Manipulative Ther*. 2001;9:17-39.

7. Norris C. Spinal stabilisation. 1. Active lumbar stabilisation—concepts. *Physiotherapy*. 1995;81:61-78.

8. Bogduk N. Neck pain. *Aust Fam Physician*. 1984;13:26-30.

9. Schwartzer A, Aprill C, Derby R, Fortin J, Kine G, Bogduk N. The relative contributions of the disc and zygopophyseal joint in chronic low back pain. *Spine*. 1994;19:801-806.

10. McKenzie R. Mechanical diagnosis and therapy for disorders of the low back. In: Twomey L, Taylor J, editors. *Physical Therapy of the Low Back*. 3rd ed. Philadelphia: Churchill Livingstone; 2000:141-165.

11. Morris EW. Diagnosis and decision making in lumbar disc prolapse and nerve entrapment. *Spine*. 1986;11:436-439.

12. Fritz J, Erhard R, Delitto A, Welch W, Nowakowski P. Preliminary results of the use of a two-stage treadmill test as a clinical diagnostic tool in the differential diagnosis of lumbar spinal stenosis. *J Spinal Disord*. 1997;10:410-416.

13. Fritz J, Erhard R, Hagen B. Segmental instability of the lumbar spine. *Phys Ther*. 1998;78:889-896.

14. O'Sullivan P. Lumbar segmental "instability": clinical presentation and specific stabilizing exercise management. *Man Ther*. 2000;5:2-12.

15. Dreyfuss P, Tibiletti C, Dreyer S. Thoracic zygopophyseal joint pain patterns. *Spine*. 1994;19:807-811.

16. Fukui S, Ohseto K, Shiotani M. Patterns of pain induced by distending the thoracic zygopophyseal joints. *Reg Anesth*. 1997;22:332-336.

17. Fukui S. Distribution of referred pain from the lumbar zygapophyseal joints and dorsal rami. *Clin J Pain*. 1997;13:303-307.

18. Schwartzer A, Aprill C, Derby R, et al. Clinical features of patients with pain stemming from the lumbar zygopophyseal joints. *Spine*. 1994;19:1132-1137.

19. Schwartzer A, Wang S, Bogduk N, McNaught P, Laurent R. Prevalence and clinical features of lumbar zygopophyseal joint pain: a study in an Australian population with chronic low back pain. *Ann Rheum Dis*. 1995;54:100-106.

20. McCombe F, Fairbank J, Cockersole B, Pynsent P. Reproducibility of physical signs in low back pain. *Spine*. 1989;14:908-918.

21. Waddell G, Main C, Morris E, et al. Normality and reliability in the clinical assessment of backache. *BMJ*. 1982;284:1519-1523.

22. Roach K, Brown M, Dunigan K, Kusek C, Walas M. Test-retest reliability of patient reports of low back pain. *J Orthop Sports Phys Ther*. 1997;26:253-259.

23. Vroomen P, de Krom M, Knottnerus J. Consistency of history taking and physical examination in patients with suspected lumbar nerve root involvement. *Spine.* 2000;25:91-97.

24. Van Dillen L, Sahrmann S, Norton B, et al. Reliability of physical examination items used for classification of patients with low back pain. *Phys Ther.* 1998;78:979-988.

25. Hunt D, Zuberbier O, Kozlowski A, et al. Reliability of the lumbar flexion, lumbar extension, and passive straight leg raise test in normal populations embedded within a complete physical examination. *Spine.* 2001;26:2714-2718.

26. Breum J, Wiberg J, Bolton J. Reliability and concurrent validity of the BROM II for measuring lumbar mobility. *J Manipulative Physiol Ther.* 1995;18:497-502.

27. Saur P, Ensink F, Frese K, Seegar D, Hildebrandt J. Lumbar range of motion: reliability and validity of the inclinometer technique in the clinical measurement of trunk flexibility. *Spine.* 1996;21:1332-1338.

28. Fritz JM, Piva S, Childs JD. Accuracy of the clinical examination to predict radiographic instability of the lumbar spine. *Euro Spine J.* In press.

29. Downey B, Taylor N, Niere K. Manipulative physiotherapists can reliably palpate nominated lumbar spinal levels. *Man Ther.* 1999;4:151-156.

30. Binkley J, Stratford P, Gill C. Interrater reliability of lumbar accessory motion mobility testing. *Phys Ther.* 1995;75:786-795.

31. Maher C, Latimer J, Adams R. An investigation of the reliability and validity of posteroanterior spinal stiffness judgments made using a reference-based protocol. *Phys Ther.* 1998;78:829-837.

32. Hicks G, Fritz J, Delitto A, Mishock J. Interrater reliability of clinical examination measures for identification of lumbar segmental instability. *Arch Phys Med Rehabil.* 2003;84:1858-1864.

33. Keating J, Bergmann T, Jacobs G, Finer B, Larson K. Interexaminer reliability of eight evaluative dimensions of lumbar segmental abnormality. *J Manipulative Physiol Ther.* 1990;13:463-470.

34. French S, Green S, Forbes A. Reliability of chiropractic methods commonly used to detect manipulable lesions in patients with chronic low back pain. *J Manipulative Physiol Ther.* 2000;23:231-238.

35. Horneij E, Hemborg B, Johnsson B, Ekdahl C. Clinical tests on impairment level related to low back pain: a study of test reliability. *J Rehabil Med.* 2002;34:176-182.

36. Strender L, Sjoblom A, Ludwig R, Taube A, Sundell K. Interexaminer reliability in physical examination of patients with low back pain. *Spine.* 1997;22:814-820.

37. Haswell K. Interexaminer reliability of symptom-provoking active sidebend, rotation and combined movement assessments of patients with low back pain. *J Man Manipulative Ther.* 2004;12:11-20.

38. Love R, Brodeur R. Inter- and intra-examiner reliability of motion palpation for the thoracolumbar spine. *J Manipulative Physiol Ther.* 1987;10:261-266.

39. Mootz R, Keating J, Kontz H, Milus T, Jacobs G. Intra- and interobserver reliability of passive motion palpation of the lumbar spine. *J Manipulative Physiol Ther.* 1989;12:440-445.

40. Riddle D, Rothstein J. Intertester reliability of McKenzie's classification of the syndrome types present in patients with low back pain. *Spine.* 1993;18:1333-1344.

41. Kilpkoski S, Airaksinen O, Kankaanpaa M, et al. Interexaminer reliability of low back pain assessment using the McKenzie method. *Spine.* 2002;27:E207-E214.

42. Razmjou H, Kramer J, Yamada R. Intertester reliability of the McKenzie evaluation in

REFERENCES

assessing patients with mechanical low-back pain. *J Orthop Sports Phys Ther*. 2000; 30:368-389.

43. Fritz J, Delitto A, Vignovic M, Busse R. Interrater reliability of judgments of the centralization phenomenon and status change during movement testing in patients with low back pain. *Arch Phys Med Rehabil*. 2000;81:57-61.

44. Rose M. The statistical analysis of the intra-observer repeatability of four clinical measurement techniques. *Physiotherapy*. 1991;77:89-91.

45. Mens J, Vleeming A, Snijders C, Koes B, Stam H. Reliability and validity of the active straight leg raise test in posterior pelvic pain since pregnancy. *Spine*. 2003;26:1167-1171.

46. Viikari-Juntra E, Takala E, Riihimaki H, Malmivaara A, Martikaimen R, Jappinen P. Standardized physical examination protocol for low back disorders: feasibility of use and validity of symptoms and signs. *J Clin Epidemiol*. 1998;51:245-255.

47. Revel M, Poiraudeau S, Auleley G, et al. Capacity of the clinical picture to characterize low back pain relieved by facet joint anesthesia: proposed criteria to identify patients with painful facet joints. *Spine*. 1998;23:1972-1976.

48. Katz J, Dalgas M, Stucki G, et al. Degenerative lumbar spinal stenosis: diagnostic value of the history and physical examination. *Arthritis Rheum*. 1995;38:1236-1241.

49. Phillips J, Twomey L. A comparison of manual diagnosis with a diagnosis established by a uni-level lumbar spinal block procedure. *Man Ther*. 1996;2:82-87.

50. Leboeuf-Yde C, van Dijk J, Franz C, et al. Motion palpation findings and self-reported low back pain in a population-based study sample. *J Manipulative Physiol Ther*. 2002;25:80-87.

51. Abbot J, Mercer S. Lumbar segmental hypomobility: criterion-related validity of clinical examination items (a pilot study). *N Z J Physiother*. 2003;31:3-9.

52. Kerr R, Cadoux-Hudson T, Adams C. The value of accurate clinical assessment in the surgical management of lumbar disc protrusion. *Neurol Neurosurg Psychiatry*. 1988;51:169-173.

53. Lauder TD, Dillingham TR, Andary M, et al. Effect of history and exam in predicting electrodiagnostic outcome among patients with suspected lumbosacral radiculopathy. *Am J Phys Med Rehabil*. 2000;79:60-68.

54. van de Hoogen HMM. On the accuracy and history, physical examination, and erythrocyte sedimentation in diagnosing low back pain in general practice. *Spine*. 1995;20:318-327.

55. Deville W, van der Windt D, Dzaferagic A, Bezemer P, Bouter L. The test of Lasègue. Systematic review of the accuracy in diagnosing herniated discs. *Spine*. 2000;25:1140-1147.

56. Shiqing X, Quanzhi Z, Dehao F. Significance of the straight leg raising test in the diagnosis and clinical evaluation of lower lumbar vertebral-disc protrusion. *J Bone Joint Surg*. 1987;69-A:517-522.

57. Albeck M. A critical assessment of clinical diagnosis of disc herniation in patients with monoradicular sciatica. *Acta Neurochir*. 1996;138:40-44.

58. Aronson H, Dunsmore R. Herniated upper lumbar discs. *J Bone Joint Surg*. 1963;45-A:311-317.

59. Charnley J. Orthopaedic signs in the diagnosis of disc protrusion. *Lancet*. 1951;260:186-192.

60. Edgar M, Park W. Induced pain patterns on passive straight-leg raising in lower lumbar disc protrusion. *J Bone Joint Surg*. 1974;56-B:658-667.

61. Gurdjian E, Webster J, Ostrowski A, Hardy W, Lindner D, Thomas L. Herniated lumbar intervertebral discs: an analysis of 1176 operated cases. *J Trauma*. 1961;1:158-176.

62. Hakelius A, Hindmarsh J. The significance of neurological signs and myelographic findings in the diagnosis of lumbar root compression. *Acta Orthop Scand*. 1972;43:239-246.

63. Hirsch C, Nachemson A. The reliability of lumbar disc surgery. *Clin Orthop*. 1963;29:189-195.

64. Jonsson B, Stromqvist B. The straight leg raising test and the severity of symptoms in lumbar disc herniation. *Spine*. 1995;20:27-30.

65. Kortelainen P, Puranen J, Koivisto E, Lahde S. Symptoms and signs of sciatica and their relation to the location of the lumbar disc herniation. *Spine*. 1985;10:88-92.

66. Kosteljanetz M, Bang F, Schmidt-Olsen S. The clinical significance of straight-leg raising (Lasegue's sign) in the diagnosis of prolapsed lumbar disc: interobserver variation and correlation with surgical finding. *Spine*. 1988;13:393-395.

67. Kosteljanetz M, Espersen J, Halaburt H, Miletec T. Predictive value of clinical and surgical findings in patients with lumbago-sciatica. *Acta Neurochir*. 1984;73:67-76.

68. Knuttson B. Comparative value of electromyographic, myelographic and clinical-neurological examinations in diagnosis of lumbar root compression syndrome. *Acta Orthop Scand*. 1961;49:107-135.

69. Spangfort E. The lumbar disc herniation: a computer aided analysis of 2504 operations. *Acta Orthop Scand*. 1972;142(suppl):5-79.

70. Gran JT. An epidemiological survey of the signs and symptoms of ankylosing spondylitis. *Clin Rheumatol*. 1985;4:161-169.

71. Russell A, Maksymowych W, LeClercq S. Clinical examination of the sacroiliac joints: a prospective study. *Arthritis Rheum*. 1981;24:1575-1577.

72. Blower P, Griffin A. Clinical sacroiliac tests in ankylosing spondylitis and other causes of low back pain—2 studies. *Ann Rheum Dis*. 1984;43:192-195.

Sacroiliac Region

Chapter 6

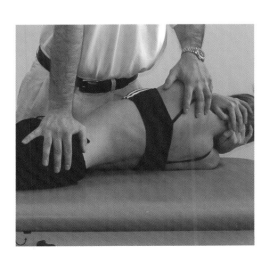

OSTEOLOGY   Sacroiliac Region

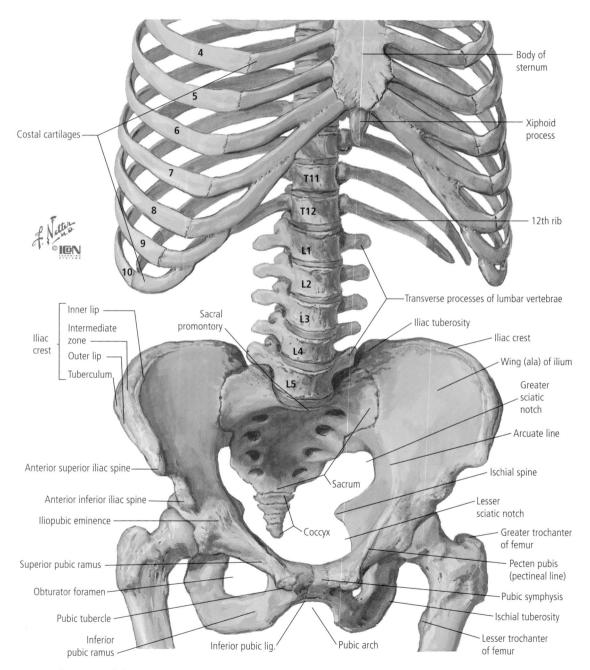

Figure 6-1: Bony framework of abdomen

Sacrum and Coccyx

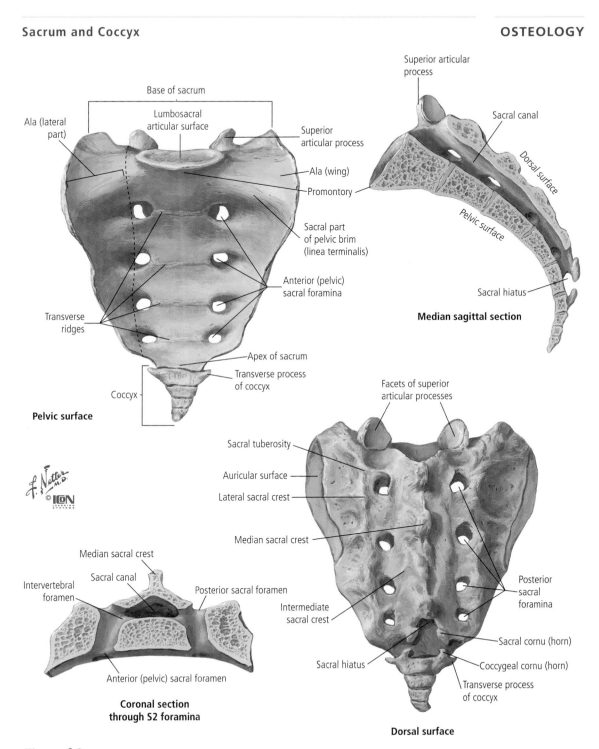

Base of sacrum

Ala (lateral part)

Lumbosacral articular surface

Superior articular process

Ala (wing)

Promontory

Sacral part of pelvic brim (linea terminalis)

Anterior (pelvic) sacral foramina

Transverse ridges

Apex of sacrum

Transverse process of coccyx

Coccyx

Pelvic surface

Superior articular process

Sacral canal

Dorsal surface

Pelvic surface

Sacral hiatus

Median sagittal section

Facets of superior articular processes

Sacral tuberosity

Auricular surface

Lateral sacral crest

Median sacral crest

Posterior sacral foramina

Intermediate sacral crest

Sacral cornu (horn)

Coccygeal cornu (horn)

Transverse process of coccyx

Sacral hiatus

Dorsal surface

Median sacral crest

Sacral canal

Intervertebral foramen

Posterior sacral foramen

Anterior (pelvic) sacral foramen

Coronal section through S2 foramina

Figure 6-2

OSTEOLOGY   Hip (Coxal) Bone

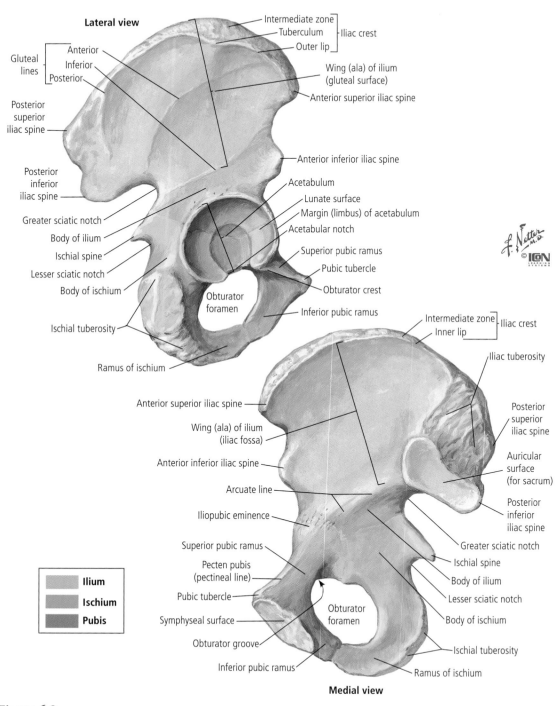

Lateral view

Intermediate zone
Tuberculum — Iliac crest
Outer lip

Gluteal lines
Anterior
Inferior
Posterior

Wing (ala) of ilium
(gluteal surface)

Anterior superior iliac spine

Posterior superior iliac spine

Anterior inferior iliac spine

Posterior inferior iliac spine

Acetabulum
Lunate surface
Margin (limbus) of acetabulum
Acetabular notch

Greater sciatic notch
Body of ilium
Ischial spine
Lesser sciatic notch
Body of ischium

Superior pubic ramus
Pubic tubercle
Obturator crest

Ischial tuberosity
Obturator foramen
Inferior pubic ramus

Ramus of ischium

Anterior superior iliac spine

Wing (ala) of ilium
(iliac fossa)

Anterior inferior iliac spine

Arcuate line

Iliopubic eminence

Superior pubic ramus

Pecten pubis
(pectineal line)

Pubic tubercle

Symphyseal surface

Obturator groove

Inferior pubic ramus

Intermediate zone
Inner lip — Iliac crest

Iliac tuberosity

Posterior superior iliac spine

Auricular surface
(for sacrum)

Posterior inferior iliac spine

Greater sciatic notch
Ischial spine
Body of ilium
Lesser sciatic notch
Body of ischium

Obturator foramen

Ischial tuberosity

Ramus of ischium

Ilium
Ischium
Pubis

Medial view

Figure 6-3

Sex Differences of Pelvis   OSTEOLOGY

**Female pelvis/female pelvic
inlet: anterior view**

Sacroiliac joint
Sacral promontory
Conjugate (~11 cm)
Transverse (~13 cm)] Diameters of
Oblique (~12.5 cm)] pelvic inlet
Ischial spine
Iliopubic eminence
Pubic symphysis
Ischial tuberosity

Pubic arch

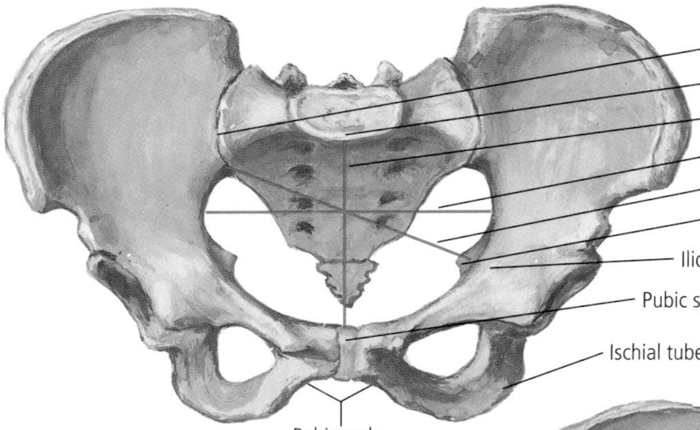

**Male pelvis/male pelvic
inlet: anterior view**

All measurements slightly shorter in
  relation to body size than in female
Pelvic inlet oriented more antero-
  posteriorly than in female, where
  it tends to be transversely oval
Pubic symphysis deeper (taller)
Pubic arch (subpubic angle) narrower
Ischial tuberosities less far apart
Iliac wings less flared

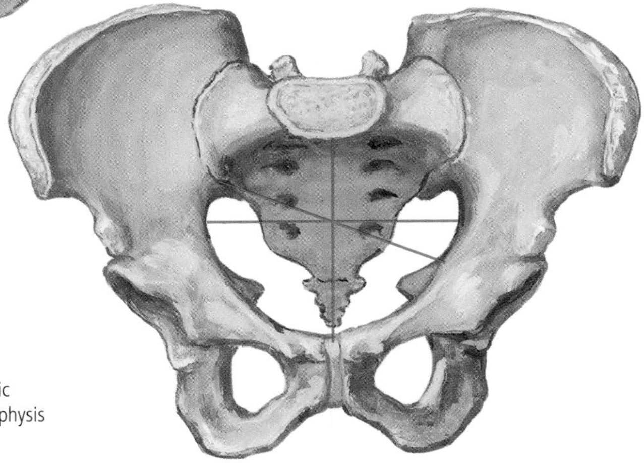

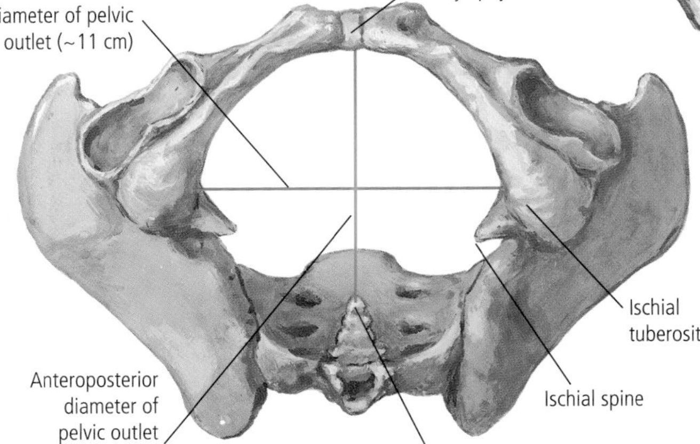

Pubic
symphysis

Transverse
diameter of pelvic
outlet (~11 cm)

Sacral
promontory

Conjugate
diameter
of pelvic inlet
(~11 cm)

Plane of pelvic inlet

Plane of pelvic outlet

Ischial
tuberosity

Ischial spine

Anteroposterior
diameter of
pelvic outlet
(varies 9.5–11.5 cm
because of mobility
of coccyx)

Tip of coccyx

Pubic
symphysis

Anteroposterior
diameter of
pelvic outlet
(9.5–11.5 cm)

**Female pelvis/female pelvic outlet:
inferior view**

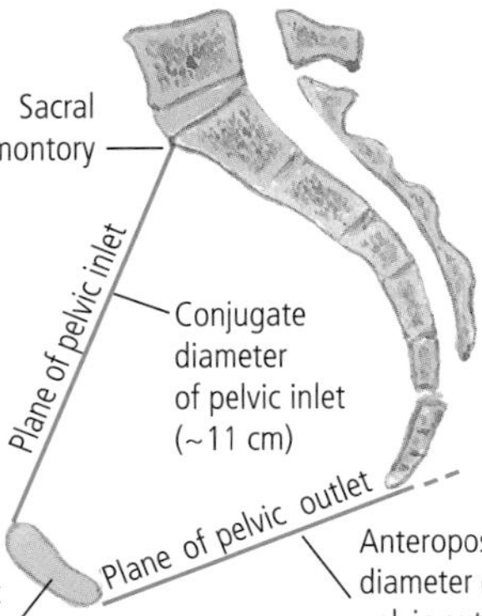

Female: sagittal section

Figure 6-4

ARTHROLOGY Sacroiliac Joint

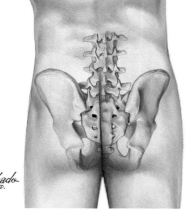

Sacroiliac Region		Type and Classification	Closed Packed Position	Capsular Pattern
Sacroiliac joint		Plane synovial	Has not been described	Considered a capsular pattern if pain is provoked when joints are stressed
Lumbosacral	Apophyseal joints	Plane synovial	Extension	Equal limitations of side bending, flexion, and extension
	Intervertebral joint	Amphiarthrodial	NA	NA

NA, not applicable.

Figure 6-5: *Sacroiliac joint*
Just the sacrum and innominate as a
functional unit

Sacroiliac Region Ligaments

Sacroiliac Region Ligaments	Attachments	Function
Posterior sacroiliac	Iliac crest to tubercles of S1-S4	Limits movement of sacrum on iliac bones
Anterior sacroiliac	Anterosuperior aspect of sacrum to anterior ala of ilium	Limits movement of sacrum on iliac bones
Sacrospinous	Inferior lateral border of sacrum to ischial spine	Limits gliding and rotary movement of sacrum on iliac bones
Sacrotuberous	Middle lateral border of sacrum to ischial tuberosity	Limits gliding and rotary movement of sacrum on iliac bones
Posterior sacrococcygeal	Posterior aspect of inferior sacrum to posterior aspect of coccyx	Reinforces sacrococcygeal joint
Anterior sacrococcygeal	Anterior aspect of inferior sacrum to anterior aspect of coccyx	Reinforces sacrococcygeal joint
Lateral sacrococcygeal	Lateral aspect of inferior sacrum to lateral aspect of coccyx	Reinforces sacrococcygeal joint
Anterior longitudinal	From anterior sacrum to anterior tubercle of C1. Connects anterolateral vertebral bodies and disks	Maintains stability of vertebral body joints and prevents hyperextension of vertebral column

Sacroiliac Region Ligaments (cont.)

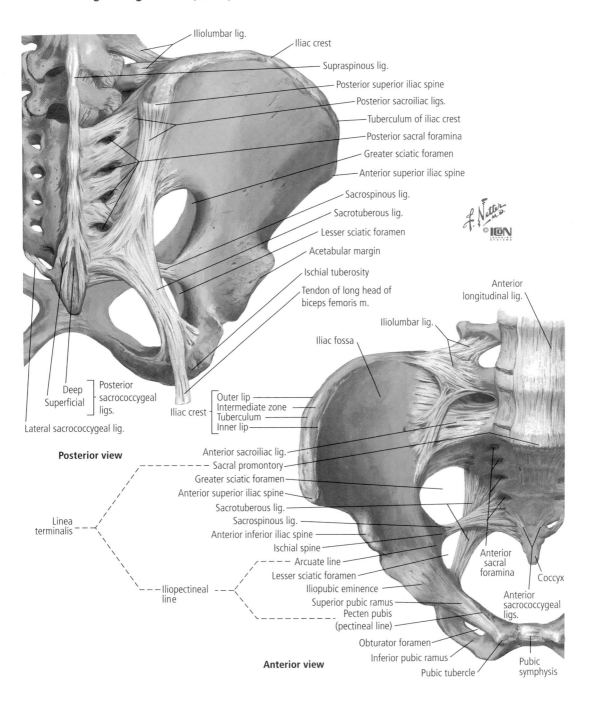

Iliolumbar lig.

Iliac crest

Supraspinous lig.

Posterior superior iliac spine

Posterior sacroiliac ligs.

Tuberculum of iliac crest

Posterior sacral foramina

Greater sciatic foramen

Anterior superior iliac spine

Sacrospinous lig.

Sacrotuberous lig.

Lesser sciatic foramen

Acetabular margin

Ischial tuberosity

Tendon of long head of biceps femoris m.

Anterior longitudinal lig.

Iliolumbar lig.

Iliac fossa

Deep
Superficial

Posterior sacrococcygeal ligs.

Iliac crest

Outer lip
Intermediate zone
Tuberculum
Inner lip

Lateral sacrococcygeal lig.

Posterior view

Linea terminalis

Iliopectineal line

Anterior sacroiliac lig.

Sacral promontory

Greater sciatic foramen

Anterior superior iliac spine

Sacrotuberous lig.

Sacrospinous lig.

Anterior inferior iliac spine

Ischial spine

Arcuate line

Lesser sciatic foramen

Iliopubic eminence

Superior pubic ramus

Pecten pubis (pectineal line)

Obturator foramen

Inferior pubic ramus

Pubic tubercle

Anterior sacral foramina

Coccyx

Anterior sacrococcygeal ligs.

Pubic symphysis

Anterior view

Figure 6-6

MUSCLES   Sacroiliac Region Muscles

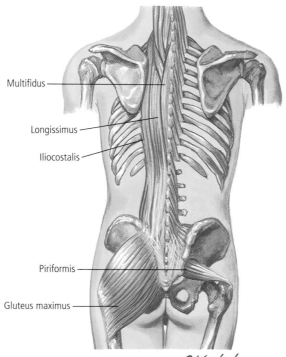

Multifidus

Longissimus

Iliocostalis

Piriformis

Gluteus maximus

C. Machado
M.D.
©ICON

Figure 6-7: *Posterior view of spine and associated musculature*

Sacroiliac Region Muscles	Proximal Attachment	Distal Attachment	Nerve and Segmental Level	Action
Gluteus maximus	Posterior border of ilium, posterior aspect of sacrum and coccyx, and sacrotuberous ligament	Iliotibial tract of fascia lata and gluteal tuberosity of femur	Inferior gluteal nerve (L5, S1, S1)	Extension, external rotation, and some abduction of the hip joint
Piriformis	Anterior aspect of sacrum and sacrotuberous ligament	Greater trochanter of femur	Ventral rami S1, S2	External rotation of extended hip
Multifidi	Sacrum, ilium, transverse processes T1-T3, articular processes C4-C7	Spinous processes of vertebrae 2–4 segments above origin	Dorsal rami of spinal nerves	Stabilizes vertebrae
Longissimus	Iliac crest, posterior sacrum, spinous processes of sacrum and inferior lumbar vertebrae, supraspinous ligament	Transverse processes of lumbar vertebrae	Dorsal rami of spinal nerves	Bilaterally: extends vertebral column Unilaterally: side-bends spinal column
Iliocostalis		Ribs 4–12		

Sacroiliac Dysfunction

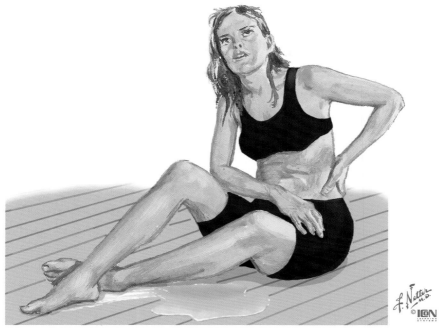

Figure 6-8: *Fall on buttock: common cause of sacroiliac injury*

Considerable controversy has surrounded the contribution of the sacroiliac joint in low back pain syndromes. Recent research suggests that the sacroiliac joint can be a contributor to low back pain and disability.[1-3] Only one study[1] to date has investigated the diagnostic utility of components of the historical examination in comparison with a reference standard of diagnostic sacroiliac blocks.

Question	Positive if	Sens	Spec	+LR	−LR
Pain with standing?	Pain is relieved with standing	.07	.98	3.5	.95
Pain with walking?	Pain is relieved with walking	.13	.77	.57	1.13
Pain with sitting?	Pain is relieved with sitting	.07	.8	.35	1.16
Pain with lying down?	Pain is relieved with lying down	.53	.49	1.04	.96
Coughing/sneezing aggravates symptoms?	Pain is aggravated with coughing/sneezing	.45	.47	.85	1.17
Bowel movements aggravate symptoms?	Pain is aggravated with bowel movements	.38	.63	1.03	.98
Wearing of heels/ boots aggravates symptoms?	Pain is aggravated with wearing of heels/boots	.26	.56	.59	1.32
Job activities aggravate symptoms? *Dreyfuss et al.[1]*	Pain is aggravated by job activities	.2	.74	.77	1.08

LR. likelihood ratio.

NERVES   Sacroiliac Region Nerves

Nerve	Segmental Level	Sensory	Motor
Superior gluteal	L4, L5, S1	No sensory	Tensor fascia lata, gluteus medius, gluteus minimus
Inferior gluteal	L5, S1, S2	No sensory	Gluteus maximus
Nerve to piriformis	S1, S2	No sensory	Piriformis
Sciatic	L4, L5, S1, S2, S3	Hip joint	Knee flexors and all muscles of leg and foot
Nerve to quadratus femoris	L5, S1, S2	No sensory	Quadratus femoris, inferior gemellus
Nerve to obturator internus	L5, S1, S2	No sensory	Obturator internus, superior gemellus
Posterior cutaneous	S2, S3	Posterior thigh	No motor
Perforating cutaneous	S2, S3	Inferior gluteal region	No motor
Pudendal	S2, S3, S4	Genitals	Perineal muscles, external urethral sphincter, external anal sphincter
Nerve to levator ani	S3, S4	No sensory	Levator ani
Perineal branch	S1, S2, S3	Genitals	No motor
Anococcygeal	S4, S5, C0	Skin in the coccygeal region	No motor
Coccygeal	S3, S4	No sensory	Coccygeus
Pelvic splanchnic	S2, S3, S4	No sensory	Pelvic viscera

Sacroiliac Region Nerves (cont.)   **NERVES**

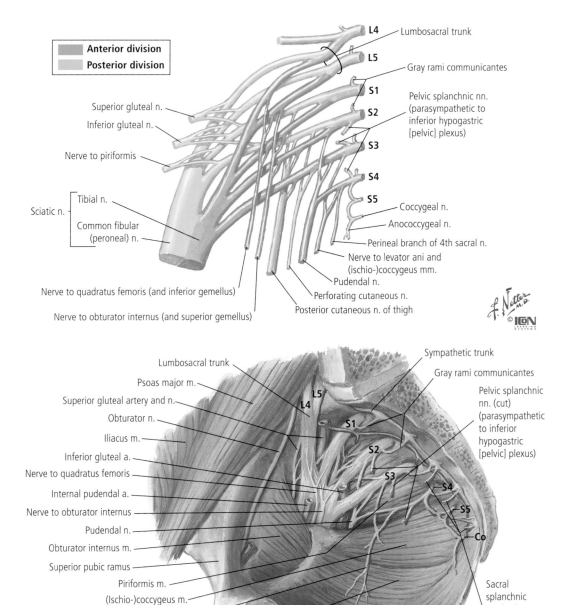

Anterior division
Posterior division

L4 — Lumbosacral trunk
L5
S1 — Gray rami communicantes
S2 — Pelvic splanchnic nn.
(parasympathetic to
inferior hypogastric
[pelvic] plexus)
S3
S4
S5 — Coccygeal n.
— Anococcygeal n.
— Perineal branch of 4th sacral n.
Nerve to levator ani and
(ischio-)coccygeus mm.
Pudendal n.
Perforating cutaneous n.
Posterior cutaneous n. of thigh

Superior gluteal n.
Inferior gluteal n.
Nerve to piriformis
Sciatic n. — Tibial n.
Common fibular
(peroneal) n.
Nerve to quadratus femoris (and inferior gemellus)
Nerve to obturator internus (and superior gemellus)

Lumbosacral trunk
Psoas major m.
Superior gluteal artery and n.
Obturator n.
Iliacus m.
Inferior gluteal a.
Nerve to quadratus femoris
Internal pudendal a.
Nerve to obturator internus
Pudendal n.
Obturator internus m.
Superior pubic ramus
Piriformis m.
(Ischio-)coccygeus m.
Nerve to levator ani m.
Levator ani m.

Sympathetic trunk
Gray rami communicantes
Pelvic splanchnic
nn. (cut)
(parasympathetic
to inferior
hypogastric
[pelvic] plexus)

Sacral
splanchnic
nn. (cut)
(sympathetic
to inferior
hypogastric
[pelvic] plexus)

L4 L5 S1 S2 S3 S4 S5 Co

Figure 6-9: Schema (top) and medial and slightly anterior view of hemisected pelvis (bottom)

**PAIN
REFERRAL
PATTERNS**

Sacroiliac Joint Pain Referral Patterns

Slipman and colleagues[5] investigated pain referral patterns in 50 patients with sacroiliac pain verified by diagnostic injection. Results demonstrated referral patterns in the following anatomic regions.

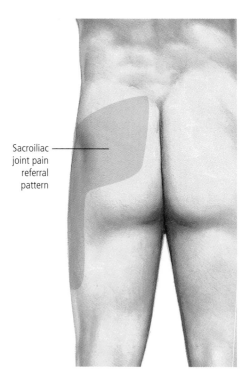

Sacroiliac joint pain referral pattern

Anatomic Region	Percentage of Patients With Pain
Upper back	6
Low back	72
Buttock	94
Groin	14
Abdomen	2
Thigh	48
Lower leg	28
Ankle	14
Foot	12

Figure 6-10: *Composite referral map illustrating area of referral after fluoroscopically guided injections of a contrast material followed by Xylocaine in 10 asymptomatic individuals.[4]*

Dreyfuss and colleagues[1] performed a prospective study to determine the diagnostic utility of both the history and the physical examination in determining pain of sacroiliac origin. The diagnostic properties for the patient-reported location of pain are provided below.

Patient Report of Pain Location	Sens	Spec	+LR	−LR
Groin pain	.19	.63	.51	1.29
Buttock pain	.80	.14	.9	1.42
Patient points to PSIS as main area of pain	.76	.47	1.4	.51
Pain with sitting *Dreyfuss* et al.[1]	.03	.90	.3	1.07

PSIS, posterior superior iliac spine.

Prone Knee Bend Test

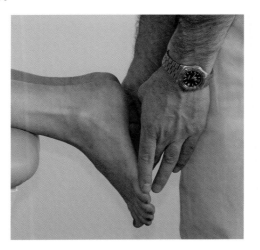

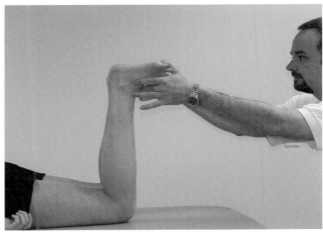

Figure 6-12: *Prone knee bend test*

Motion Palpation	Description and Positive Findings	Population	Inter-examiner Reliability Kappa Values
Prone knee bend test *Flynn et al.*[9]	Patient in prone. Examiner, looking at heels, assesses leg lengths. Knees are passively flexed to 90 degrees, and leg lengths again assessed. Considered positive if a change in leg lengths occurs between positions	71 patients referred to physical therapy with a diagnosis related to the lumbosacral spine and a chief complaint of pain or numbness in the lumbar spine, buttock, or lower extremity	.21
Prone knee bend test *Potter and Rothstein*[7]		17 patients with back pain referred to a physical therapy outpatient clinic	Agreement 23.53% Kappa values not reported
Prone knee bend test *Riddle et al.*[6]		65 patients currently receiving treatment for low back pain	.26

RELIABILITY OF THE CLINICAL EXAMINATION

Static Palpation

Motion Palpation		Description and Positive Findings	Population	Reliability Kappa Values
Sitting PSIS test Riddle et al.[6]		Patient seated. Examiner palpates inferior aspect of each PSIS. Positive for sacroiliac (SI) joint dysfunction if inequality of PSIS is found	65 patients currently receiving treatment for low back pain	Inter-examiner reliability = .37
Palpation of PSIS levels in sitting Potter and Rothstein[7]			17 patients with back pain referred to a physical therapy outpatient clinic	Agreement 35% Kappa values not reported
Palpation of PSIS levels Flynn et al.[8]	Sitting	Examiner palpates right and left PSIS. Positive if one PSIS is higher than the other	71 patients referred to physical therapy with a diagnosis related to the lumbosacral spine and a chief complaint of pain or numbness in the lumbar spine, buttock, or lower extremity	Sitting = .23 Standing = .13
	Standing			
Palpation of iliac crest levels Potter and Rothstein[7]	Sitting	Examiner places radial border of the hand on top of iliac crests. Positive if one hand is higher than the other	17 patients with back pain referred to a physical therapy outpatient clinic	Sitting agreement 41% Standing agreement 35% Kappa values not reported
	Standing			
Iliac crest symmetry in standing Flynn et al.[8]		Examiner palpates right and left iliac crest. Positive if one crest is higher than the other	71 patients referred to physical therapy with a diagnosis related to the lumbosacral spine and a chief complaint of pain or numbness in the lumbar spine, buttock, or lower extremity	Inter-examiner reliability = .23
Palpation of: O'Haire and Gibbons[9]	PSIS	Examiner determines whether the landmarks are: 1. Right higher than left 2. Left higher than right 3. Right equal to left	10 asymptomatic female volunteers	Inter-examiner reliability PSIS = .33 SS = .24 SILA = .69 Inter-examiner reliability PSIS = .04 SS = .07 SILA = .08
	Sacral sulcus (SS)			
	Sacral inferior lateral angle (SILA)			

Static Palpation (cont.)

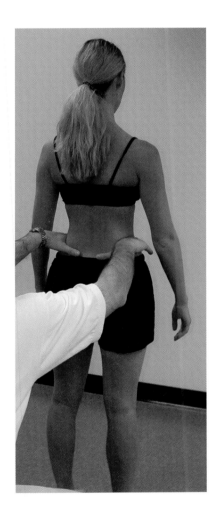

Figure 6-11: Assessment of iliac crest symmetry in standing

Motion Palpation: Standing Flexion Test

Motion Palpation	Description and Positive Findings	Population	Inter-examiner Reliability Kappa Values
Standing flexion test *Riddle et al.*[6]		65 patients currently receiving treatment for low back pain	.32
Standing flexion test *Potter and Rothstein*[7]	Patient standing. Examiner palpates inferior slope of PSIS. Patient is asked to forward bend completely. Positive for SI hypomobility if one PSIS moves more cranially than the contralateral side	17 patients with back pain referred to a physical therapy outpatient clinic	Agreement 43.75% (Kappa values not reported)
Standing flexion test *Vincent-Smith and Gibbons*[10]		14 asymptomatic graduate students	.52
Standing flexion test *Toussaint et al.*[11] *and Toussaint et al.*[12]		480 male construction workers. 50 had low back pain the day of the examination; 236 reported experiencing low back pain within the previous 12 months	Kappa values ranged from .31 to .68
Standing flexion test *Flynn et al.*[8]		71 patients referred to physical therapy with a diagnosis related to the lumbosacral spine and a chief complaint of pain or numbness in the lumbar spine, buttock, or lower extremity	.08

Motion Palpation: Standing Flexion Test (cont.)

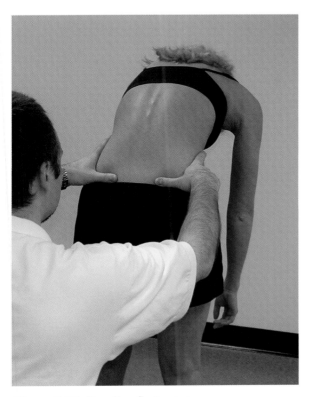

Figure 6-13: *Standing flexion test*

Motion Palpation: Gillet Test

Motion Palpation	Description and Positive Findings	Population	Reliability Kappa Values (95% CI)
Gillet test Carmichael[13]	1. L5 spinous process and PSIS 2. S1 tubercle and PSIS 3. S3 tubercle and PSIS 4. Sacral apex and posteromedial margin of the ischium	Patient standing. Examiner palpates landmarks, then asks patient to raise the ipsilateral leg. Mobility is graded as normal or fixated	54 asymptomatic college students	Intra-examiner mean value for all tests: .31 Inter-examiner mean value for all tests: .02
Gillet test Meijne et al.[14]		Patient standing. Examiner palpates the following landmarks: 1. L5 spinous process and PSIS 2. S1 spinous process and PSIS 3. S3 spinous process and PSIS 4. Sacral hiatus and caudolateral just below the ischial spine The patient is instructed to raise the ipsilateral leg of the side of palpation. If the lateral landmark does not move caudad or moves cephalward relative to the medial landmark, the SI joint is considered hypomobile	38 male students. Nine during the first testing procedure and 12 during the second were considered symptomatic	Intra-examiner reliability of examiner 1 = .08 (.01, .14) Intra-examiner reliability of examiner 2 = .03 (−.11, .04) Inter-examiner reliability = −.05 (−.06, −.12)
Gillet test Dreyfuss et al.[1]		Patient standing. Examiner palpates the S2 spinous process with one thumb and the PSIS with the other and asks the patient to flex the hip and knee on the side being tested. Positive if the PSIS fails to move posteroinferiorly with respect to S2	85 patients with sacroiliac joint block confirmation of SI pain	κ = .22
Gillet test Flynn et al.[8]		Patient standing. Examiner palpates ipsilateral PSIS and spinous process of S2. Patient is instructed to flex the knee and hip on the side being tested. Positive if the PSIS fails to move posteriorly and inferiorly relative to S2	71 patients referred to physical therapy with a diagnosis related to the lumbosacral spine and a chief complaint of pain or numbness in the lumbar spine, buttock, or lower extremity	κ = .59
Gillet test Potter and Rothstein[7]			17 patients with back pain referred to a physical therapy outpatient clinic	Agreement 47% (Kappa values not reported)
Gillet test Herzog et al.[15]		Procedure as above. Joint motion is considered normal if the sacrum moves in an anterior/inferior direction and the ilium moves in a posterior/inferior direction	11 subjects identified by a chiropractor as having sacroiliac dysfunction	Intra-examiner agreement: Positive finding 68% Negative finding 79% Correct side 72% Inter-examiner agreement: Positive finding 65% Correct side 61%

CI, confidence interval.

Pain Provocation Tests: Distraction Test

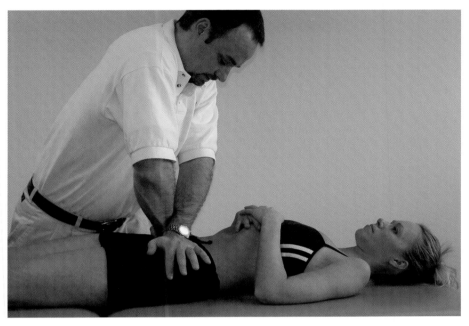

Figure 6-14: *Distraction test*

Pain Provocation	Description and Positive Findings	Population	Inter-examiner Reliability Kappa Values (95% CI)
Distraction test *Laslett and Williams[16]*	Patient supine. Examiner applies pressure to both anterior superior iliac spines in a posterolateral direction. Positive if pain is reproduced.	51 patients with low back pain with or without radiation into the lower limb	.69
Distraction test *Kokmeyer et al.[17]*		59 patients with low back pain	.45 (.10, −.78)
Distraction test *Flynn et al.[8]*		71 patients referred to physical therapy with a diagnosis related to the lumbosacral spine and a chief complaint of pain or numbness in the lumbar spine, buttock, or lower extremity	.26

Pain Provocation Tests: Compression Test

Pain Provocation	Description and Positive Findings	Population	Inter-examiner Reliability Kappa Values (95% CI)
Compression test *Laslett and Williams[16]*	Patient sidelying. Examiner compresses pelvis with pressure applied over the iliac crest and directed at the opposite iliac crest. Positive if symptoms are reproduced.	51 patients with low back pain with or without radiation into the lower limb	.73
Compression test *Kokmeyer et al.[17]*		59 patients with low back pain	.57 (.21,. 93)
Compression test *Flynn et al.[8]*		71 patients referred to physical therapy with a diagnosis related to the lumbosacral spine and a chief complaint of pain or numbness in the lumbar spine, buttock, or lower extremity	.26

Pain Provocation Tests: Gaenslen Test

Pain Provocation	Description and Positive Findings	Population	Inter-examiner Reliability Kappa Values (95% CI)
Gaenslen test *Flynn et al.[8]*	Patient supine with both legs extended. The leg being tested is passively brought into full knee flexion, while the opposite hip remains in extension. Overpressure is then applied to the flexed extremity. Positive if pain is reproduced	71 patients referred to physical therapy with a diagnosis related to the lumbosacral spine and a chief complaint of pain or numbness in the lumbar spine, buttock, or lower extremity	.54
Gaenslen test *Laslett and Williams[16]*		51 patients with low back pain with or without radiation into the lower limb	.76
Gaenslen test *Kokmeyer et al.[17]*		59 patients with low back pain	.60 (.33, −.88)

Pain Provocation Tests: Patrick Test

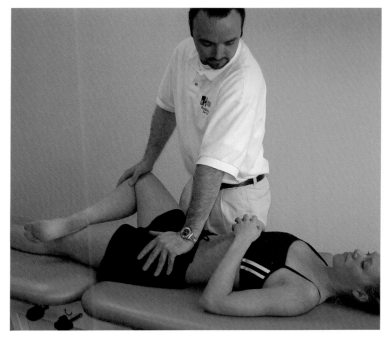

Figure 6-15: *Patrick test*

Pain Provocation	Description and Positive Findings	Population	Inter-examiner Reliability Kappa Values (95% CI)
Patrick test *Flynn et al.[8]*	The patient's hip is flexed, abducted, and externally rotated by placement of the lateral malleolus on the knee of the contralateral leg. The pelvis is stabilized, and overpressure is applied to the medial aspect of the knee. Positive if buttock or groin pain is reproduced	71 patients referred to physical therapy with a diagnosis related to the lumbosacral spine and a chief complaint of pain or numbness in the lumbar spine, buttock, or lower extremity	.60
Patrick sign *Kokmeyer et al.[17]*		59 patients with low back pain	.61 (.31, −.91)
Patrick test *Dreyfuss et al.[1]*		85 patients with sacroiliac joint block confirmation of SI pain	.62

RELIABILITY OF THE CLINICAL EXAMINATION

Pain Provocation Tests: Sacral Thrust Test

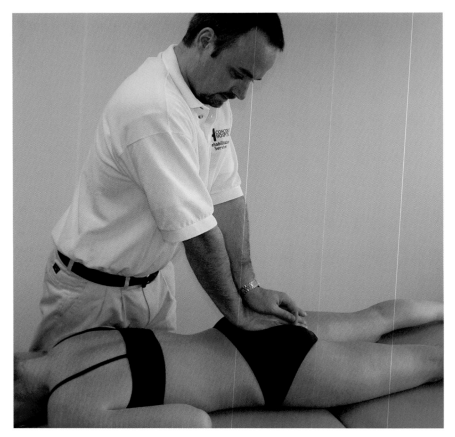

Figure 6-16: *Sacral thrust test*

Pain Provocation	Description and Positive Findings	Population	Inter-examiner Reliability Kappa Values
Sacral thrust test *Flynn et al.[8]*	Patient prone. Examiner delivers an anteriorly directed thrust over the sacrum. Positive if pain is reproduced	71 patients referred to physical therapy with a diagnosis related to the lumbosacral spine and a chief complaint of pain or numbness in the lumbar spine, buttock, or lower extremity	.41
Sacral thrust test *Laslett and Williams[16]*		51 patients with low back pain with or without radiation into the lower limb	.56
Midline sacral thrust *Dreyfuss et al.[1]*		85 patients with sacroiliac joint block confirmation of SI pain	.30

Pain Provocation Tests: Thigh Thrust

Pain Provocation	Description and Positive Findings	Population	Inter-examiner Reliability Kappa Values (95% CI)
Thigh thrust or posterior shear test Flynn et al.[8]	Patient supine. Examiner flexes (90°) and adducts the hip. Examiner then applies posteriorly directed force through the femur at varying angles of abduction/adduction. Positive if buttock pain is reproduced	71 patients referred to physical therapy with a diagnosis related to the lumbosacral spine and a chief complaint of pain or numbness in the lumbar spine, buttock, or lower extremity	.70
Thigh thrust or posterior shear test Laslett and Williams[16]		51 patients with low back pain with or without radiation into the lower limb	.88
Thigh thrust or posterior shear test Kokmeyer et al.[17]		59 patients with low back pain	.67 (.46, .88)
Thigh thrust Dreyfuss et al.[1]		85 patients with sacroiliac joint block confirmation of SI pain	.64

Palpation and Patient Identification of Location of Pain

Measurement	Population	Reference Standard	Sens	Spec	+LR	−LR
Sacral sulcus tenderness, and the patient points to the PSIS as the main site of pain *Dreyfuss et al.[1]*			.49	.60	1.2	.85
Sacral sulcus tenderness plus groin pain *Dreyfuss et al.[1]*	85 consecutive patients with low back pain referred for sacroiliac joint blocks. 40 patients responded to the anesthetic block	Intra-articular injection of local anesthetics into sacroiliac joint	.11	.73	.4	1.22
Patient points to PSIS as main site of pain but also complains of groin pain *Dreyfuss et al.[1]*			.16	.85	1.1	.99
Sacral sulcus tenderness plus patient identifies PSIS as main site of pain plus groin pain *Dreyfuss et al.[1]*			.13	.86	.9	1.01

Pain Provocation Test: Patrick Test

Test	Description and Positive Findings	Population	Reference Standard	Sens	Spec	+LR	−LR
Patrick test *Broadhurst and Bond[18]*	The patient's hip is flexed, abducted, and externally rotated by placement of the lateral malleolus on the knee of the contralateral leg. The pelvis is stabilized, and overpressure is applied to the medial aspect of the knee. Positive if buttock or groin pain is reproduced	40 patients who were suspected of having sacroiliac joint dysfunction based on history	Double-blind block of the sacroiliac joint	.77	1.0	NA	.23
Patrick test *Dreyfuss et al.[1]*		85 consecutive patients with low back pain referred for sacroiliac joint blocks. 40 patients responded to the anesthetic block	Intra-articular injection of local anesthetics into sacroiliac joint	.69	.16	.82	1.94

Thigh Thrust

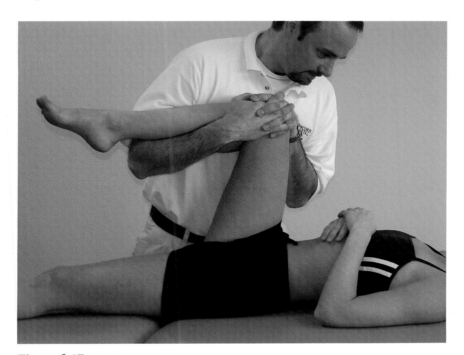

Figure 6-17

Test	Description and Positive Findings	Population	Reference Standard	Sens	Spec	+LR	−LR
Posterior shear test (thigh thrust) *Broadhurst and Bond[18]*	Patient supine. Examiner flexes (90°) and adducts the hip. The examiner then applies posteriorly directed force through the femur at varying angles of abduction/adduction. Positive if buttock pain is reproduced	40 patients who were suspected of having sacroiliac joint dysfunction based on history	Double-blind block of the sacroiliac joint	.80	1.0	NA	.2
Thigh thrust *Dreyfuss et al.[1]*		85 consecutive patients with low back pain referred for sacroiliac joint blocks. 40 patients responded to the anesthetic block	Intra-articular injection of local anesthetics into sacroiliac joint	.36	.50	.7	1.28

Compression Test

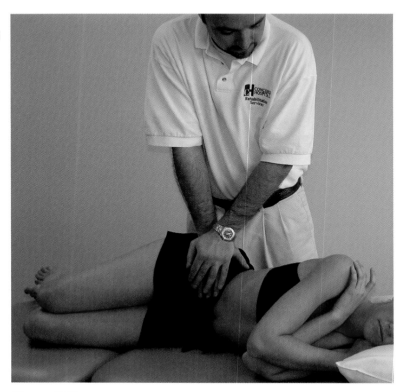

Figure 6-18

Test	Description and Positive Findings	Population	Reference Standard	Sens	Spec	+LR	−LR
Compression test to identify ankylosing spondylitis *Blower and Griffin*[19]	Patient sidelying. Firm downward pressure is applied to the contralateral ilium. Positive if patient complains of pain over sacrum or into buttocks	66 patients with low back pain (33 with ankylosing spondylitis)	Radiographs and HLA B27 antigen testing	0.0	1.0	NA	1.0
Lateral pelvic compression test to identify ankylosing spondylitis *Russell et al.*[20]	Procedure as above. Positive if pain is provoked	113 patients with low back pain (41 with ankylosing spondylitis)	Radiographically confirmed ankylosing spondylitis	.70	.90	7.0	.33

* Sensitivity and specificity data calculated by van der Wuff et al.[21] Likelihood ratios calculated by the author of this text.

Sacral Thrust Test

Test	Description and Positive Findings	Population	Reference Standard	Sens	Spec	+LR	−LR
Midsacral thrust *Dreyfuss et al.[1]*	Patient prone. Examiner delivers an anteriorly directed thrust over the sacrum. Positive if pain is reproduced	85 consecutive patients with low back pain referred for sacroiliac joint blocks. 40 patients responded to the anesthetic block	Intra-articular injection of local anesthetics into sacroiliac joint	.53	.29	.75	1.62
Sacral thrust test *Blower and Griffin[19]*		66 patients with low back pain (33 with ankylosing spondylitis)	Radiographs and HLA B27 antigen testing	.27*	1.0*	NA	.73
Compression test *Russell et al.[20]*		113 patients with low back pain (41 with ankylosing spondylitis)	Radiographically confirmed ankylosing spondylitis	.30*	.90*	3.0	.78

* Sensitivity and specificity data calculated by van der Wuff et al.[21] Likelihood ratios calculated by the author of this text.

DIAGNOSTIC UTILITY OF THE CLINICAL EXAMINATION

Gaenslen Test

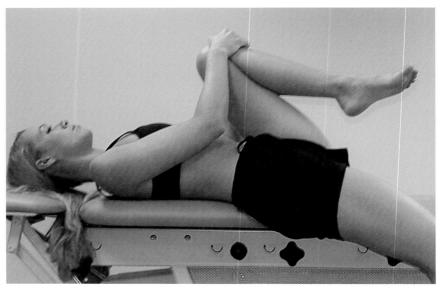

Figure 6-19

Test	Description and Positive Findings	Population	Reference Standard	Sens	Spec	+LR	−LR
Gaenslen test Dreyfuss et al.[1]	Patient supine with both legs extended. The leg being tested is passively brought into full knee flexion, while the opposite hip remains in extension. Overpressure is then applied to the flexed extremity. Positive if pain is reproduced	85 consecutive patients with low back pain referred for sacroiliac joint blocks. 40 patients responded to the anesthetic block	Intra-articular injection of local anesthetics into sacroiliac joint	.71	.26	1.0	1.12
Gaenslen test Russell et al.[20]		113 patients with low back pain (41 with ankylosing spondylitis)	Radiographically confirmed ankylosing spondylitis	.21*	.72*	.75	1.10

* Sensitivity and specificity data calculated by van der Wuff et al.[21] Likelihood ratios calculated by the author of this text.

Gillet Test

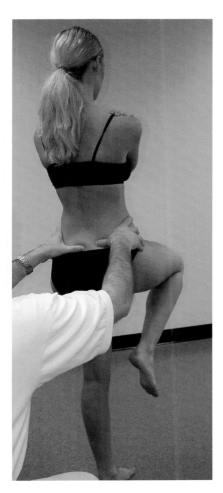

Figure 6-20

The Gillet test was described by Dreyfuss et al..[1] The patient stands with feet spread 12 inches apart while the examiner palpates the S2 spinous process with one thumb and the posterior superior iliac spine with the other. The patient is asked to flex the hip and knee on the side of palpation. The test is considered positive if the PSIS fails to move in a posteroinferior direction relative to S2. When compared with a reference standard of anesthetic sacroiliac joint blocks, in a patient population with low back pain, the Gillet test has demonstrated sensitivity of 0.43, specificity of 0.68, +LR of 1.3, and –LR of 0.84.

**DIAGNOSTIC
UTILITY OF
THE CLINICAL
EXAMINATION**

Spring Test

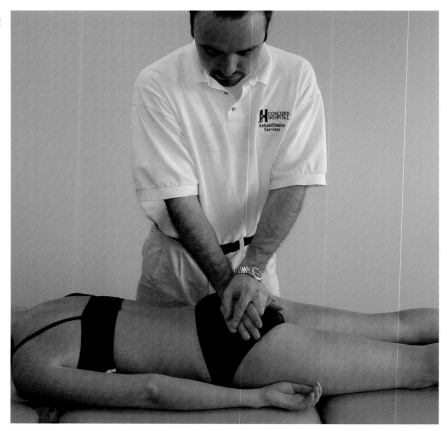

Figure 6-21

The Spring test (joint play assessment) was described by Dreyfuss et al.[1] The therapist's hands are placed over the sacrum, and a posteroanterior thrust is applied while the therapist monitors the spring at the end range of motion. The asymptomatic side is compared with the symptomatic side. This test has demonstrated sensitivity of 0.75, specificity of .35, +LR of 1.2, and –LR of 0.71.

Resisted Abduction of the Hip

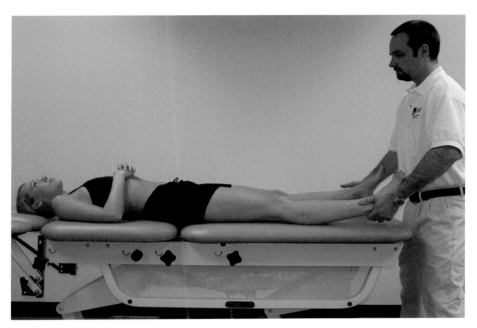

Figure 6-22: *Resisted abduction test*

Resisted abduction of the hip test is advocated by Broadhurst and Bond[18] for patients with knee or hip replacement. The patient is supine with the leg fully extended and abducted to 30°. The therapist then resists abduction. A positive test is indicated by the reproduction of pain. The diagnostic utility of this test was compared with a double-blind block of the sacroiliac joint in 40 patients with sacroiliac joint dysfunction. The test demonstrated sensitivity of 0.87, specificity of 1.0, and –LR of .13. The +LR could not be calculated as a result of the excellent specificity.

DIAGNOSTIC UTILITY OF THE CLINICAL EXAMINATION

Clusters of Tests for Identifying Sacroiliac Dysfunction: Sacroiliac Pain Provocation Tests

Test	Description and Positive Findings	Population	Reference Standard	Sens	Spec	+LR	−LR
Standing flexion test *Levangie*[22]	Patient standing. Examiner palpates inferior slope of PSIS. Patient is asked to forward-bend completely. Positive for SI hypomobility if one PSIS moves more cranially than the contralateral side	219 patients being treated for low back pain or another condition not related to the low back	Compared findings of patients who complained of low back pain with those of patients being treated for other physical impairments not related to the back	.82	.88	6.83	.20
Sitting PSIS palpation *Levangie*[22]	Patient seated. Examiner palpates inferior aspect of each PSIS. Positive for SI joint dysfunction if inequality of PSIS is found						
Supine long sitting test *Levangie*[22]	Patient supine. Lengths of medial malleoli are compared. Patient is asked to long sit, and lengths of medial malleoli are again compared. Positive if one leg appears shorter in supine, then lengthens when the patient comes into long sitting						
Prone knee flexion test *Levangie*[22]	Patient in prone. Examiner, looking at heels, assesses leg lengths. Knees are passively flexed to 90° and leg lengths are again assessed. Considered positive if a change in leg lengths occurs between positions						
Distraction *Laslett et al.*[23]	Procedures all previously described in this chapter. Positive if test procedure reproduced symptoms. Three of four tests needed to be positive to indicate sacroiliac joint dysfunction	48 patients with buttock pain with or without lower extremity symptoms	Sacroiliac joint anesthetic block	.91 (.62, −.98)	.78 (.61, .89)	4.16 (2.16, 8.39)	.12 (.02, .49)
Thigh thrust *Laslett et al.*[23]							
Gaenslen test *Laslett et al.*[23]							
Sacral thrust *Laslett et al.*[23]							
Compression *Laslett et al.*[23]							

Clusters of Tests for Identifying Sacroiliac Dysfunction: Sacroiliac Pain Provocation Tests (cont.)

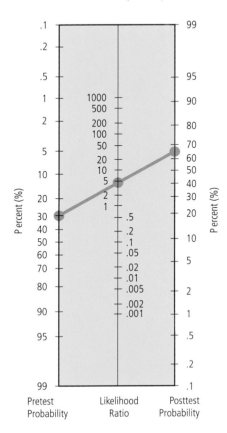

Figure 6-23: Nomogram representing the changes from pretest to posttest probability using the cluster of tests identified by Laslett et al.[23] for detecting sacroiliac dysfunction. Considering a 33% pretest probability and a +LR of 4.16, the posttest probability that the patient presents with sacroiliac dysfunction is 67%. (Adapted with permission from Fagan TJ. Nomogram for Baye's theorem. *N Engl J Med.* 1975;293:257. Copyright © 2005 Massachusetts Medical Society. All rights reserved.)

DIAGNOSTIC UTILITY OF THE CLINICAL EXAMINATION

Cluster of Tests for Sacroiliac Dysfunction After the McKenzie Evaluation to Rule Out Discogenic Pain

Laslett et al.[23] assessed the diagnostic utility of the McKenzie method of mechanical assessment combined with the following sacroiliac tests: *distraction, thigh thrust, Gaenslen, sacral thrust, and compression.* The McKenzie assessment consisted of flexion in standing, extension in standing, right and left side gliding, flexion in lying, and extension in lying. The movements were repeated in sets of 10, and centralization and peripheralization were recorded. If it was determined that repeated movements resulted in centralization, the patient was considered to present with pain of discogenic origin. After the McKenzie method was used to rule out persons who presented with discogenic pain, in terms of diagnostic utility, the cluster of these tests exhibited a sensitivity of .91 (95% CI: .62, .98), specificity of .87 (95% CI : .68, .96), +LR of 6.97 (95% CI: 2.16, 8.39), and –LR of .11 (95% CI: .02, .44).

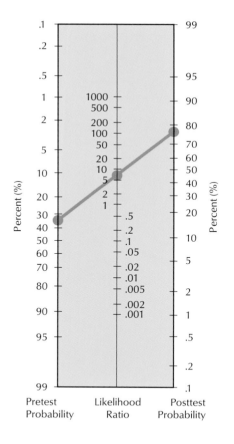

Figure 6-24: *Nomogram representing the changes from pretest to posttest probability with the use of the above cluster of tests for detecting sacroiliac dysfunction after the exclusion of patients determined to have pain of discogenic origin, as determined by the McKenzie assessment. Considering a 33% pretest probability and a +LR of 6.97, the posttest probability that the patient presents with sacroiliac dysfunction is 77%.* (Adapted with permission from Fagan TJ. Nomogram for Baye's theorem. *N Engl J Med.* 1975;293:257. Copyright © 2005 Massachusetts Medical Society. All rights reserved.)

Identifying Patients Likely to Benefit from Spinal Manipulation

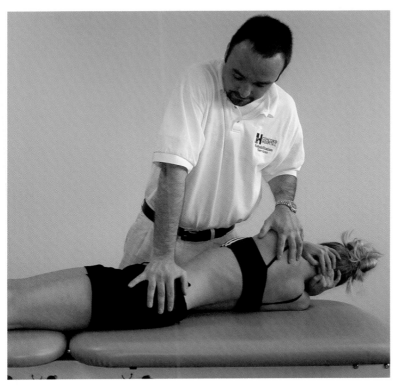

Figure 6-25: Spinal manipulation technique used by Flynn and colleagues.[8] The patient is passively side-bent toward the side to be manipulated (away from the therapist). The therapist then rotates the patient away from the side to be manipulated (toward the therapist) and delivers a quick thrust through the anterior superior iliac spine in a posteroinferior direction.

Flynn and colleagues[8] investigated the effects of a spinal manipulation technique in a heterogeneous population of patients with low back pain. They identified a number of variables that were associated with a successful outcome after manipulation. A logistic regression equation was used to identify a cluster of signs and symptoms leading to a clinical prediction rule that could significantly enhance the likelihood that patients who will achieve a successful outcome with spinal manipulation could be identified. Five variables formed the clinical prediction. These variables included *duration of symptoms less than 16 days, a Fear-Avoidance Beliefs[24] work subscale score less than 19, at least one hip with greater than 35° of internal rotation range of motion, hypomobility of at least one segment in the lumbar spine, and no symptoms distal to the knee.* The number of predictor variables present significantly alters the posttest probability that the patient will have a successful outcome with manipulation.

Identifying Patients Likely to Benefit from Spinal Manipulation (cont.)

Number of Variables Present	Sensitivity	Specificity	Positive Likelihood Ratio	Probability of Success Assuming a Pretest Probability of Success at 45%
5	0.19 (0.09–0.35)	1.0 (0.91–1.0)	Infinite (2.02–infinite)	—
4+	0.63 (0.45–0.77)	0.97 (0.87–1.0)	24.38 (4.63–139.41)	95
3+	0.94 (0.80–0.98)	0.64 (0.48–0.77)	2.61 (1.78–4.15)	68
3+	1.0 (0.89–1.0)	0.15 (0.07–0.30)	1.18 (1.09–1.42)	49
1+	1.0 (0.89–1)	0.03 (0.005–0.13)	1.03 (1.01–1.01)	48

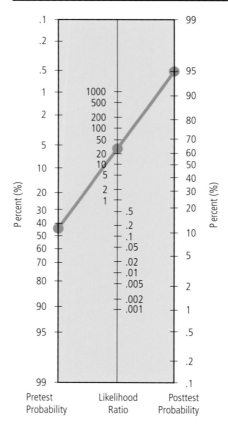

Figure 6-26: Nomogram representing the changes from pretest to posttest likelihood that a patient with low back pain who satisfies four of five criteria for the rule will have a successful outcome after spinal manipulation. The pretest likelihood that any patient with low back pain would respond favorably to sacroiliac manipulation was determined to be 45%. However, if the patient presents with four of the five predictor variables identified by Flynn et al.[8] (+LR 24), the posttest probability that the patient will respond positively to spinal manipulation increases dramatically to 95%. (Adapted with permission from Fagan TJ. Nomogram for Baye's theorem. *N Engl J Med.* 1975;293:257. Copyright © 2005 Massachusetts Medical Society. All rights reserved.)

Identifying Patients Likely to Benefit from Spinal Manipulation (cont.)

The clinical prediction rule identified by Flynn and colleagues[8] has recently been validated by Childs et al.[25] Childs and colleagues tested the validity of the clinical prediction rule when applied in a separate patient population by a variety of clinicians with varying levels of clinical experience who were practicing in different settings. Consecutive patients with low back pain were randomly assigned to receive either spinal manipulation or a lumbar stabilization program. Results of the study demonstrated that patients who satisfied the clinical prediction rule and received spinal manipulation had significantly better outcomes than did patients who did not meet the clinical prediction rule but still received spinal manipulation, or the group who met the clinical prediction rule but received lumbar stabilization exercises. The positive likelihood ratio for the clinical prediction rule was 13.2 (95% CI: 3.4, 52.1), inferring that a patient who satisfies at least four of the five criteria will have a posttest probability of success of 92% if treated with spinal manipulation. In addition, the negative likelihood ratio for patients who met fewer than three of the criteria was 0.10 (95% CI: 0.03, 0.41), inferring that patients who satisfied fewer than three criteria would have only a 7% posttest probability of success if treated with spinal manipulation. The results of Childs et al.[25] support the findings of Flynn et al.[8] and significantly increase clinician confidence in using the clinical prediction rule in decision making regarding the use of manipulation in the management of individual patients with low back pain.

REFERENCES

1. Dreyfuss P, Michaelsen M, Pauza K, McLarty J, Bogduk N. The value of medical history and physical examination in diagnosing sacroiliac joint pain. *Spine*. 1996;21:2594-2602.

2. Maigne J-Y, Aivaliklis A, Piefer F. Results of sacroiliac joint double block and value of sacroiliac pain provocation tests in 54 patients with low back pain. *Spine*. 1996;21:1889-1892.

3. Schwarzer A, Aprill C, Bogduk N. The sacroiliac joint in chronic low back pain. *Spine*. 1995;20:31-37.

4. Fortin J, Dwyer A, West S, Pier J. Sacroiliac joint: pain referral maps upon applying a new injection/arthrography technique. *Spine*. 1994;19:1475-1482.

5. Slipman C, Jackson H, Lipetz J, Chan K, Lenrow D, Vresilovic E. Sacroiliac joint pain referral zones. *Arch Phys Med Rehabil*. 2000;81:334-338.

6. Riddle D, Freburger J. Evaluation of the presence of sacroiliac joint dysfunction using a combination of tests: a multicenter intertester reliability study. *Phys Ther*. 2002;82:772-781.

7. Potter N, Rothstein J. Intertester reliability for selected clinical tests of the sacroiliac joint. *Phys Ther*. 1985;65:1671-1675.

8. Flynn T, Fritz J, Whitman J, et al. A clinical prediction rule for classifying patients with low back pain who demonstrate short-term improvement with spinal manipulation. *Spine*. 2002;27:2835-2843.

9. O'Haire C, Gibbons P. Inter-examiner and intraexaminer agreement for assessing sacroiliac anatomical landmarks using palpation and observation: pilot study. *Man Ther*. 2000;5:13-20.

10. Vincent-Smith B, Gibbons P. Inter-examiner and intra-examiner reliability of the standing flexion test. *Man Ther*. 1999;4:87-93.

11. Toussaint R, Gawlik C, Rehder U, Ruther W. Sacroiliac dysfunction in construction workers. *J Manipulative Physiol Ther*. 1999;22:134-139.

REFERENCES

12. Toussaint R, Gawlik C, Rehder U, Ruther W. Sacroiliac joint diagnosis in the Hamburg Construction Workers study. *J Manipulative Physiol Ther.* 1999;22:139-143.

13. Carmichael J. Inter- and intra-examiner reliability of palpation for sacroiliac joint dysfunction. *J Manipulative Physiol Ther.* 1987;10:164-171.

14. Meijne W, van Neerbos K, Aufdemkampe G, van der Wuff P. Intraexaminer and interexaminer reliability of the Gillet test. *J Manipulative Physiol Ther.* 1999;22:4-9.

15. Herzog W, Read L, Conway P, Shaw L, McEwen M. Reliability of motion palpation procedures to detect sacroiliac joint fixations. *J Manipulative Physiol Ther.* 1989;12:86-92.

16. Laslett M, Williams M. The reliability of selected pain provocation tests for sacroiliac joint pathology. *Spine.* 1994;19:1243-1249.

17. Kokmeyer D, van der Wuff P, Aufdemkampe G, Fickenscher T. The reliability of multitest regimens with sacroiliac pain provocation tests. *J Manipulative Physiol Ther.* 2002;25:42-48.

18. Broadhurst N, Bond M. Pain provocation tests for the assessment of sacroiliac joint dysfunction. *J Spinal Disord.* 1998;11:341-345.

19. Blower P, Griffin A. Clinical sacroiliac tests in ankylosing spondylitis and other causes of low back pain—2 studies. *Ann Rheum Dis.* 1984;43:192-195.

20. Russell A, Maksymowych W, LeClercq S. Clinical examination of the sacroiliac joints: a prospective study. *Arthritis Rheum.* 1981;24:1575-1577.

21. van der Wuff P, Hagmeijer R, Meyne W. Clinical tests of the sacroiliac joint. *Man Ther.* 2000;5:30-36.

22. Levangie P. Four clinical tests of sacroiliac joint dysfunction: the association of test results with innominate torsion among patients with and without low back pain. *Phys Ther.* 1999;79:1043-1057.

23. Laslett M, Young S, Aprill C, McDonald B. Diagnosing painful sacroiliac joints: a validity study of a McKenzie evaluation and sacroiliac provocation tests. *Aust J Physiother.* 2003;49:89-97.

24. Waddel G. Fear-Avoidance Beliefs Questionnaire (FABQ), the role of fear-avoidance beliefs in chronic low back pain and disability. *Pain.* 1993;52:157-168.

25. Childs JD, Fritz JM, Flynn TW, et al. A clinical prediction rule to identify patients likely to benefit from spinal manipulation: a validation study. *Ann Intern Med.* 2004;141:920-928.

Hip and Pelvis

Chapter 7

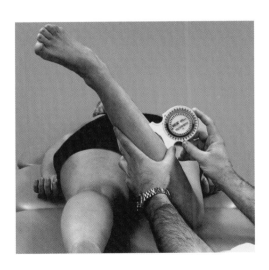

OSTEOLOGY   Hip (Coxal) Bone

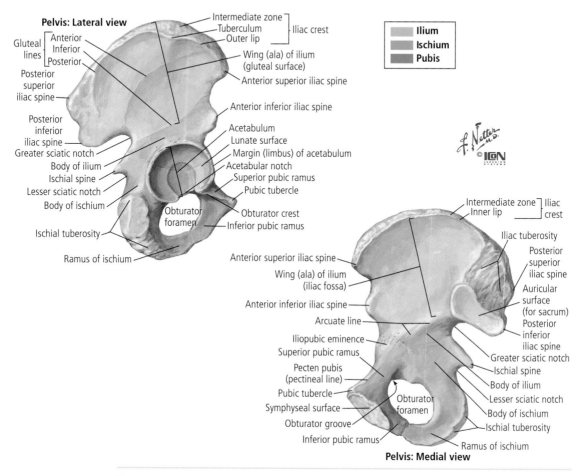

Femur

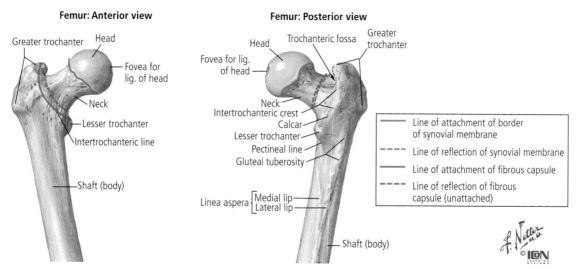

Figure 7-1: Pelvis and Femur

Hip and Pelvis Joints

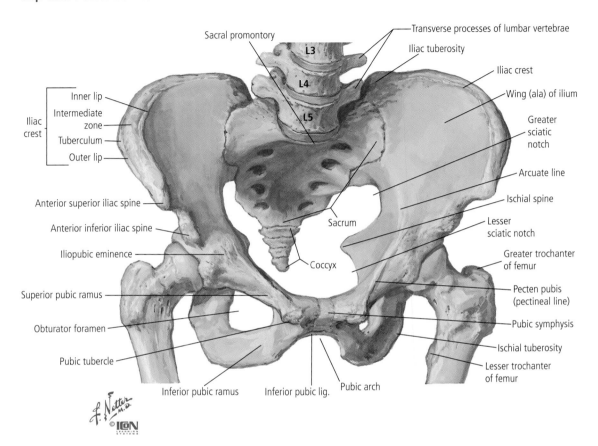

Sacral promontory

Transverse processes of lumbar vertebrae

L3

Iliac tuberosity

L4

Iliac crest

L5

Wing (ala) of ilium

Inner lip

Intermediate zone

Tuberculum

Outer lip

Iliac crest

Greater sciatic notch

Arcuate line

Anterior superior iliac spine

Ischial spine

Anterior inferior iliac spine

Sacrum

Lesser sciatic notch

Iliopubic eminence

Greater trochanter of femur

Superior pubic ramus

Coccyx

Pecten pubis (pectineal line)

Obturator foramen

Pubic symphysis

Ischial tuberosity

Pubic tubercle

Lesser trochanter of femur

Inferior pubic ramus

Inferior pubic lig.

Pubic arch

Figure 7-2

Joint	Type and Classification	Closed Packed Position	Capsular Pattern
Femoroacetabular	Synovial: spheroidal	Full extension, some internal rotation, and abduction	Internal rotation and abduction > flexion and extension
Pubic symphysis	Amphiarthrodial	NA	NA
Sacroiliac	Synovial: plane	Not documented	Considered a capsular pattern if pain is produced when joints are stressed

NA, not applicable.

LIGAMENTS

Ligaments of Hip and Pelvis

Posterior view

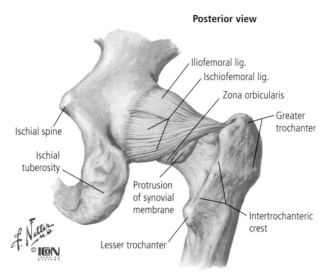

Iliofemoral lig.

Ischiofemoral lig.

Zona orbicularis

Greater trochanter

Ischial spine

Ischial tuberosity

Protrusion of synovial membrane

Intertrochanteric crest

Lesser trochanter

Figure 7-3

Hip Ligaments	Attachments	Function
Iliofemoral	Anterior inferior iliac spine to intertrochanteric line of femur	Limit hip extension
Ischiofemoral	Posterior inferior acetabulum to apex of greater tubercle	Limit internal rotation, external rotation, and extension
Pubofemoral	Obturator crest of pubic bone to blend with capsule of hip and iliofemoral ligament	Limit hip hyperabduction
Ligament of head of femur	Margin of acetabular notch and transverse acetabular ligament to head of femur	Carry blood supply to head of femur
Pubic Symphysis Ligaments	**Attachments**	**Function**
Superior pubic ligament	Connects superior aspects of pubic crests	Reinforce superior aspect of joint
Inferior pubic ligament	Connects inferior aspects of pubic crests	Reinforce inferior aspect of joint
Posterior pubic ligament	Connects posterior aspects of pubic crests	Reinforce inferior aspect of joint

Ligaments of Hip and Pelvis (cont.)

Anterior view

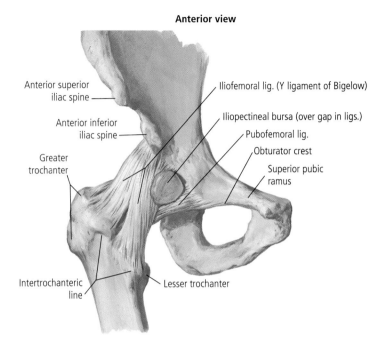

Anterior superior iliac spine

Anterior inferior iliac spine

Greater trochanter

Intertrochanteric line

Lesser trochanter

Iliofemoral lig. (Y ligament of Bigelow)

Iliopectineal bursa (over gap in ligs.)

Pubofemoral lig.

Obturator crest

Superior pubic ramus

**Joint opened:
lateral view**

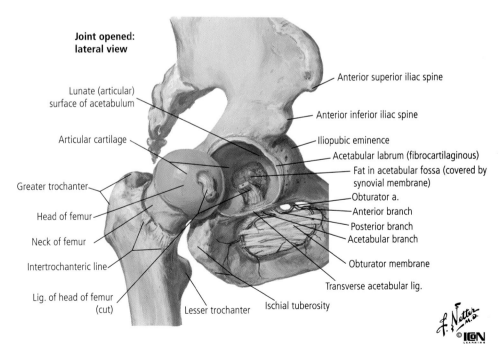

Lunate (articular) surface of acetabulum

Articular cartilage

Greater trochanter

Head of femur

Neck of femur

Intertrochanteric line

Lig. of head of femur (cut)

Lesser trochanter

Ischial tuberosity

Anterior superior iliac spine

Anterior inferior iliac spine

Iliopubic eminence

Acetabular labrum (fibrocartilaginous)

Fat in acetabular fossa (covered by synovial membrane)

Obturator a.

Anterior branch

Posterior branch

Acetabular branch

Obturator membrane

Transverse acetabular lig.

Figure 7-3 (cont.)

Posterior Muscles of Hip and Thigh

Muscle		Proximal Attachment	Distal Attachment	Nerve and Segmental Level	Action
Gluteus maximus		Posterior border of ilium, dorsal aspect of sacrum and coccyx, and sacrotuberous ligament	Iliotibial tract of fascia lata and gluteal tuberosity of femur	Inferior gluteal nerve (L5, S1, S2)	Extension, external rotation, and some abduction of the hip joint
Gluteus medius		External superior border of ilium and gluteal aponeurosis	Lateral aspect of greater trochanter of femur	Superior gluteal nerve (L5, S1)	Hip abduction and internal rotation; maintain level pelvis in single limb stance
Gluteus minimus		External surface of ilium and margin of greater sciatic notch	Anterior aspect of greater trochanter of femur		
Piriformis		Anterior aspect of sacrum and sacrotuberous ligament	Superior greater trochanter of femur	Ventral rami S1, S2	External rotation of extended hip, stabilize femoral head in acetabulum
Superior gemellus		Ischial spine	Trochanteric fossa of femur	Nerve to obturator internus (L5, S1)	
Inferior gemellus		Ischial tuberosity		Nerve to quadratus femoris (L5, S1)	
Obturator internus		Internal surface of obturator membrane, border of obturator foramen		Nerve to obturator internus (L5, S1)	
Quadratus femoris		Lateral border of ischial tuberosity	Quadrate tubercle of femur	Nerve to quadratus femoris (L5, S1)	Extend rotation of hip; steadies femoral head in acetabulum
Hamstrings	Semitendinosus	Ischial tuberosity	Superomedial aspect of tibia	Tibial division of sciatic nerve (L5, S1, S2)	Hip extension, knee flexion, medial rotation of tibia in knee flexion
	Semimembranosus		Posterior aspect of medial condyle of tibia		
	Biceps femoris	Long head: ischial tuberosity Short head: linea aspera and lateral supracondylar line of femur	Head of fibula, lateral condyle of tibia	Long head: tibial portion of sciatic nerve (L5, S1, S2) Short head: common fibular portion of sciatic nerve (L5, S1, S2)	Knee flexion, hip extension, and external rotation of tibia in knee flexion

Posterior Muscles of Hip and Thigh

MUSCLES

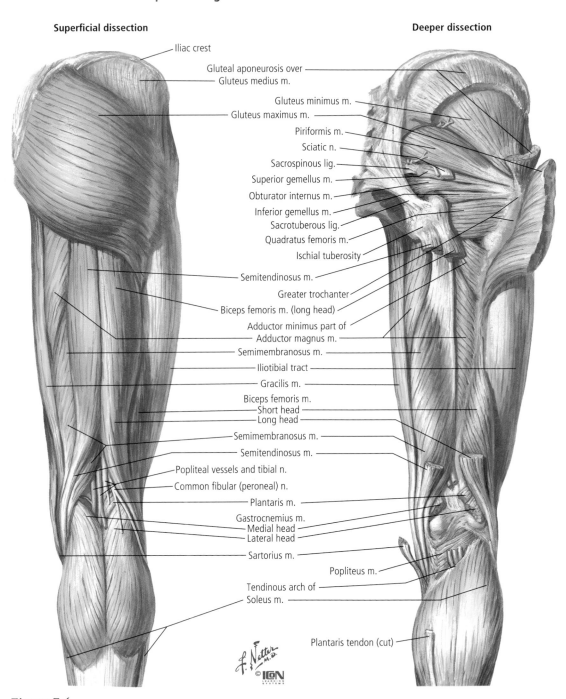

Superficial dissection

Deeper dissection

- Iliac crest
- Gluteal aponeurosis over
- Gluteus medius m.
- Gluteus minimus m.
- Gluteus maximus m.
- Piriformis m.
- Sciatic n.
- Sacrospinous lig.
- Superior gemellus m.
- Obturator internus m.
- Inferior gemellus m.
- Sacrotuberous lig.
- Quadratus femoris m.
- Ischial tuberosity
- Semitendinosus m.
- Greater trochanter
- Biceps femoris m. (long head)
- Adductor minimus part of
- Adductor magnus m.
- Semimembranosus m.
- Iliotibial tract
- Gracilis m.
- Biceps femoris m.
- Short head
- Long head
- Semimembranosus m.
- Semitendinosus m.
- Popliteal vessels and tibial n.
- Common fibular (peroneal) n.
- Plantaris m.
- Gastrocnemius m.
- Medial head
- Lateral head
- Sartorius m.
- Popliteus m.
- Tendinous arch of
- Soleus m.
- Plantaris tendon (cut)

Figure 7-4

MUSCLES Anterior Muscles of Thigh

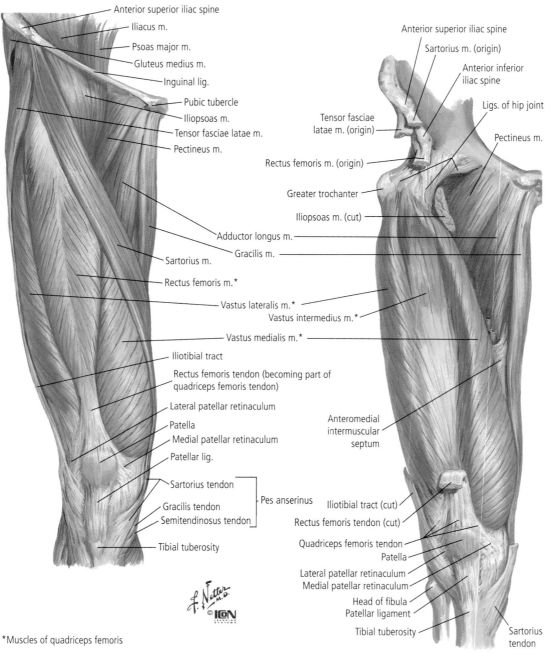

Anterior superior iliac spine
Iliacus m.
Psoas major m.
Gluteus medius m.
Inguinal lig.
Pubic tubercle
Iliopsoas m.
Tensor fasciae latae m.
Pectineus m.

Sartorius m.
Rectus femoris m.*

Vastus lateralis m.*
Vastus intermedius m.*

Vastus medialis m.*

Iliotibial tract
Rectus femoris tendon (becoming part of quadriceps femoris tendon)

Lateral patellar retinaculum
Patella
Medial patellar retinaculum
Patellar lig.

Sartorius tendon

Gracilis tendon ⎤ Pes anserinus
Semitendinosus tendon ⎦

Tibial tuberosity

Adductor longus m.
Gracilis m.

Anterior superior iliac spine
Sartorius m. (origin)
Anterior inferior iliac spine

Ligs. of hip joint

Tensor fasciae latae m. (origin)

Pectineus m.

Rectus femoris m. (origin)

Greater trochanter

Iliopsoas m. (cut)

Anteromedial intermuscular septum

Iliotibial tract (cut)
Rectus femoris tendon (cut)
Quadriceps femoris tendon
Patella
Lateral patellar retinaculum
Medial patellar retinaculum
Head of fibula
Patellar ligament
Tibial tuberosity
Sartorius tendon

*Muscles of quadriceps femoris

Figure 7-5

Muscle		Proximal Attachment	Distal Attachment	Nerve and Segmental Level	Action
Psoas	Major	Lumbar transverse processes	Lesser trochanter of femur	L1-L4	Flexes the hip, assists with external rotation and abduction
	Minor	Lateral bodies of T12-L1	Iliopectineal eminence and arcuate line of ileum	L1-L2	Flexion of pelvis on lumbar spine
Iliacus		Superior iliac fossa, iliac crest, and ala of sacrum	Lateral tendon of psoas major and lesser trochanter of femur	Femoral nerve (L1-L4)	Flexes the hip, assists with external rotation and abduction
Adductors	Longus	Inferior to pubic crest	Linea aspera of femur	Obturator nerve (L2, L3, L4)	Hip adduction
	Brevis	Inferior ramus of pubis	Pectineal line and linea aspera of femur	Obturator nerve (L2, L3, L4)	Hip adduction
	Magnus	Adductor part: inferior pubic ramus, ramus of ischium; Hamstring part: ischial tuberosity	Adductor part: gluteal tuberosity, linea aspera; Hamstring part: adductor tubercle of femur	Adductor part: obturator nerve (L2, L3, L4); Hamstring part: tibial part of sciatic nerve (L4)	Hip adduction; Adductor part: hip flexion; Hamstring part: hip extension
Gracilis		Inferior ramus of pubis	Superomedial aspect of tibia	Obturator nerve (L2, L3)	Hip adduction and flexion; assists with hip internal rotation
Pectineus		Superior ramus of pubis	Pectineal line of femur	Femoral nerve and obturator nerve (L2, L3, L4)	Hip adduction and flexion; assists with hip internal rotation
Tensor fasciae latae		Anterior superior iliac spine and anterior aspect of iliac crest	Iliotibial tract	Superior gluteal nerve (L4, L5)	Hip abduction, internal rotation and flexion; aids in maintaining knee extension
Rectus femoris		Anterior inferior iliac spine	Patellar to tibial tuberosity	Femoral nerve (L2, L3, L4)	Hip flexion and knee extension
Sartorius		Anterior superior iliac spine	Superomedial aspect of tibia	Femoral nerve (L2, L3)	Flexes, abducts, and externally rotates hip, flexes knee
Obturator externus		Margin of obturator foramen and obturator membrane	Trochanteric fossa of femur	Obturator nerve (L3, L4)	Provides hip external rotation, steadies head of femur in acetabulum

NERVES   **Nerves of Thigh**

Nerve	Segmental Level	Sensory	Motor
Obturator	L2, L3, L4	Medial thigh	Adductor longus, adductor brevis, adductor magnus (adductor part), gracilis, obturator externus
Saphenous	Femoral nerve	Medial leg and foot	No motor
Femoral	L2, L3, L4	Thigh via cutaneous nerves	Iliacus, sartorius, quadriceps femoris, articularis genu, pectineus
Lateral cutaneous of thigh	L2, L3	Lateral thigh	No motor
Posterior cutaneous of thigh	S2, S3	Posterior thigh	No motor
Inferior cluneal	Dorsal rami L1, L2, L3	Buttock region	No motor
Sciatic	L4, L5, S1, S2, S3	Hip joint	Knee flexors and all muscles of lower leg and foot
Superior gluteal	L4, L5, S1	No sensory	Tensor fasciae latae, gluteus medius, gluteus minimus
Inferior gluteal	L5, S1, S2	No sensory	Gluteus maximus
Nerve to quadratus femoris	L5, S1, S2	No sensory	Quadratus femoris, inferior gemellus
Pudendal	S2, S3, S4	Genitals	Perineal muscles, external urethral sphincter, external anal sphincter

Nerves of Thigh (cont.)

Deep dissection

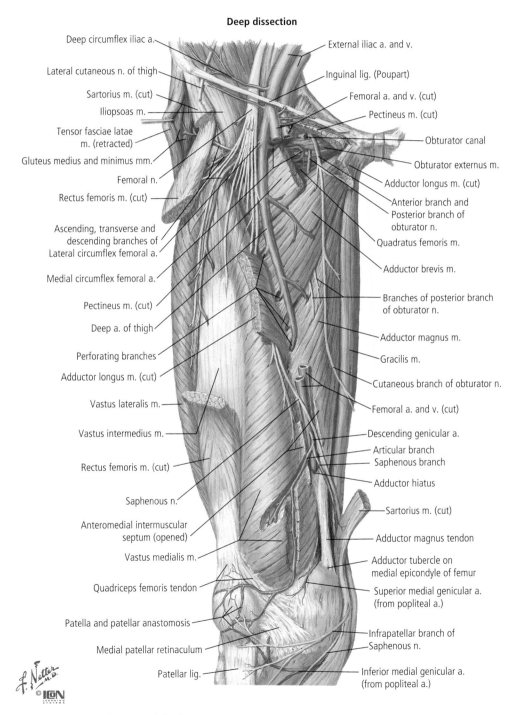

Deep circumflex iliac a.

Lateral cutaneous n. of thigh

Sartorius m. (cut)

Iliopsoas m.

Tensor fasciae latae m. (retracted)

Gluteus medius and minimus mm.

Femoral n.

Rectus femoris m. (cut)

Ascending, transverse and descending branches of Lateral circumflex femoral a.

Medial circumflex femoral a.

Pectineus m. (cut)

Deep a. of thigh

Perforating branches

Adductor longus m. (cut)

Vastus lateralis m.

Vastus intermedius m.

Rectus femoris m. (cut)

Saphenous n.

Anteromedial intermuscular septum (opened)

Vastus medialis m.

Quadriceps femoris tendon

Patella and patellar anastomosis

Medial patellar retinaculum

Patellar lig.

External iliac a. and v.

Inguinal lig. (Poupart)

Femoral a. and v. (cut)

Pectineus m. (cut)

Obturator canal

Obturator externus m.

Adductor longus m. (cut)

Anterior branch and Posterior branch of obturator n.

Quadratus femoris m.

Adductor brevis m.

Branches of posterior branch of obturator n.

Adductor magnus m.

Gracilis m.

Cutaneous branch of obturator n.

Femoral a. and v. (cut)

Descending genicular a.

Articular branch

Saphenous branch

Adductor hiatus

Sartorius m. (cut)

Adductor magnus tendon

Adductor tubercle on medial epicondyle of femur

Superior medial genicular a. (from popliteal a.)

Infrapatellar branch of Saphenous n.

Inferior medial genicular a. (from popliteal a.)

Figure 7-6 Arteries and nerve of thigh: Anterior views

NERVES   Nerves of Thigh (cont.)

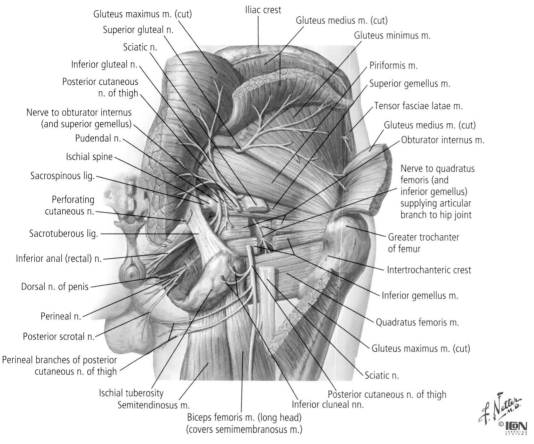

Figure 7-7: *Nerves of hips and buttocks*

EXAMINATION: HISTORY   Initial Hypotheses Based on Historical Findings

History	Initial Hypothesis
Reports of pain at the lateral thigh. Pain exacerbated when transferring from sitting to standing	Greater trochanteric bursitis[1] Muscle strain[2]
Age >60. Reports of pain and stiffness in the hip with possible radiation into the groin	Osteoarthritis[3]
Reports of clicking and/or catching in the hip joint. Pain exacerbated by full flexion or extension	Labral tear[4]
Reports of a repetitive or overuse injury	Muscle sprain/strain[2]
Deep, aching throb in the hip or groin. Possible history of prolonged steroid use	Avascular necrosis[4]
Pain in the gluteal region with occasional radiation into the posterior thigh and calf	Piriformis syndrome[5] Hamstring strain[2, 4] Ischial bursitis[2]

Passive Range-of-Motion Measurements

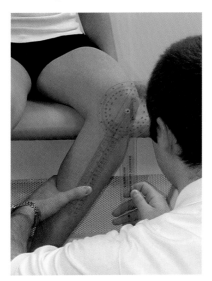

Figure 7-8A: *Measurement of passive range-of-motion external rotation*

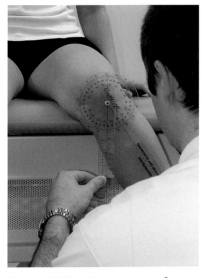

Figure 7-8B: *Measurement of passive range-of-motion internal rotation*

PROM Measurements	Instrumentation	Population	Reliability ICC (95% CI)	
Flexion Extension Abduction Adduction External rotation Internal rotation Total hip motion *Holm et al.[6]*	Goniometer	25 subjects with radiologically verified osteoarthritis of the hip	Intra-examiner reliability .82 .94 .86 .50 .90 .90 .85	
Flexion Internal rotation External rotation Abduction Extension Adduction *Klassabo et al.[7]*		168 patients, 50 with no hip osteoarthritis (OA), 77 with unilateral hip OA, and 40 with bilateral hip OA based on radiologic reports	Intra-examiner reliability .92 .90 .58 .78 .56 .62	
Hip flexion right Hip flexion left *Lin et al.[8]*		106 patients with OA of the hip or knee confirmed by a rheumatologist or orthopaedic surgeon	Intra-examiner reliability .82 (.26, .95) .83 (.33, .96)	
Flexion External rotation Internal rotation Extension *Browder et al.[9]*		17 patients with unilateral hip pain and suspected intra-articular pathology	Inter-examiner reliability	
			Involved hip .58 .58 Poor Poor	Uninvolved hip .79 .71 .68 .61

**RELIABILITY
OF THE
CLINICAL
EXAMINATION**

Range-of-Motion Measurements

ROM Measurements	Instrumentation	Population	Variability Between Measurements in Degrees or ICC
PROM Extension Flexion Internal rotation External rotation Adduction Abduction AROM Flexion Internal rotation External rotation Adduction Abduction *Bierma-Zeinstra et al.*[10]	Goniometer	9 asymptomatic persons	Variability Between Measurements in Degrees Intra-examiner 2.8 3.5 4.4 3.2 2.2 2.9 3.0 4.4 3.0 2.2 4.2
PROM Internal rotation External rotation AROM Internal rotation External rotation *Bierma-Zeinstra et al.*[10]			ICC Inter-examiner 4.9 5.2 4.8 4.1
Passive hip flexion *Cliborne et al.*[11]	Gravity inclinometer	22 patients with knee osteoarthritis and 17 asymptomatic subjects	ICC Intra-examiner .94 (95% CI: .89, .97)

AROM, active range of motion.

Range-of-Motion Measurements (cont.)

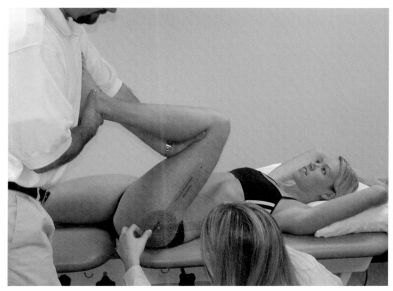

***Figure* 7-9A:** *Passive range-of-motion measurement of hip flexion*

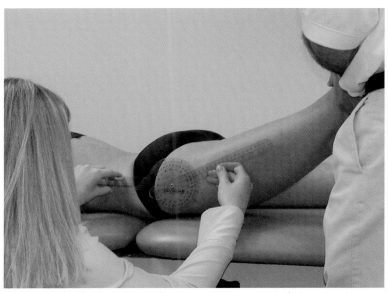

***Figure* 7-9B:** *Passive range-of-motion measurement of hip extension*

RELIABILITY OF THE CLINICAL EXAMINATION

Range-of-Motion Measurements: Iliotibial Band Length

PROM Measurements	Test Procedure	Instrumentation	Population	Reliability ICC
Ober test *Reese and Bandy[12]*	Patient sidelying. Examiner flexes knee to be examined to 90° and abducts and extends hip until hip is in line with trunk. Examiner allows gravity to adduct hip as much as possible		61 asymptomatic persons	Intra-examiner reliability .90
Modified Ober test *Melchione and Sullivan[13]*	Patient sidelying. Examiner maintains knee in extension while abducting and extending hip until hip is in line with trunk. Examiner allows gravity to adduct hip as much as possible	Inclinometer	10 patients experiencing anterior knee pain	Inter-examiner reliability .73 Intra-examiner reliability .94
Modified Ober *Reese and Bandy[12]*			61 asymptomatic persons	Intra-examiner reliability .91

Range-of-Motion Measurements: Iliotibial Band Length (cont.)

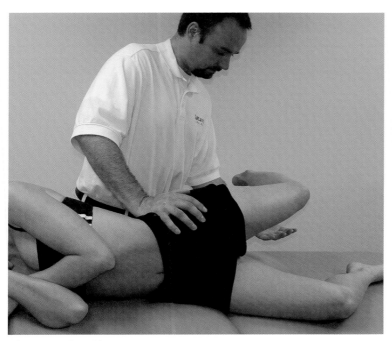

Figure 7-10A: Ober test

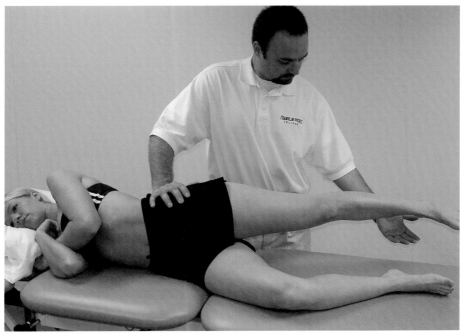

Figure 7-10B: Modified Ober test

RELIABILITY OF THE CLINICAL EXAMINATION

Miscellaneous Tests of the Hip of Patients with Suspected Intra-articular Pathology

Test		Description and Positive Results	Population	Inter-examiner Reliability Kappa Value
Hip joint mobility	Anterior	Patient prone. Examiner fully extends hip and applies anterior force over head of femur. Mobility is judged as hypermobile, normal, or hypomobile. Pain responses recorded		Anterior mobility .45 Anterior mobility with pain provocation .85
	Posterior	Patient supine. Examiner passively brings hip into 90° of flexion, internal rotation, and adduction and applies a posteriorly directed force through the femur. Mobility judged as hypermobile, normal, or hypomobile. Pain responses recorded		Posterior mobility .37 Posterior mobility with pain provocation .65
Browder et al.[9]			17 patients with unilateral hip pain and suspected intra-articular pathology	
Flexion–adduction– internal rotation test (Click test) *Browder et al.*[9]		Patient sidelying. Examiner stabilizes pelvis while passively moving the patient's hip through 50° to 100° of hip flexion and adduction while internally rotating the hip. The presence of a click or reproduction of symptoms is considered a positive test		.48
Thomas test *Browder et al.*[9]		Patient supine at end of plinth holding both knees to chest. Patient releases knee to be tested, and the leg is allowed to extend. If hip does not reach 0° of extension, it was considered to be hypomobile. Overpressure is then applied, and provocation of symptoms is recorded		With provocation .55 Determination of mobility Poor

Miscellaneous Tests of the Hip of Patients with Suspected Intra-articular Pathology (cont.)

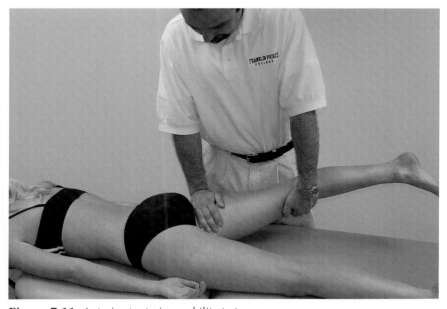

Figure 7-11: *Anterior-posterior mobility test*

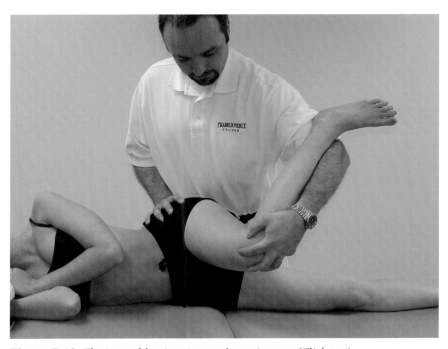

Figure 7-12: *Flexion–adduction–internal rotation test (Click test)*

RELIABILITY OF THE CLINICAL EXAMINATION

Muscle Length Measurements

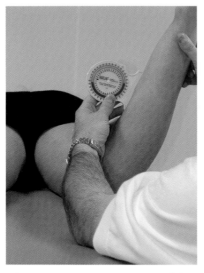

Figure 7-13A: *Measurement of the length of external rotators of the hip with a bubble inclinometer*

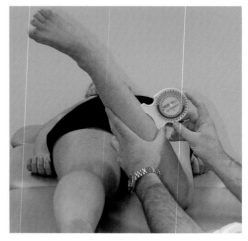

Figure 7-13B: *Measurement of the length of internal rotators of the hip with a bubble inclinometer*

Muscle Length Measurements	Description	Instrumentation	Population	Intra-examiner Reliability ICC
Short hip extensors	Patient supine. Examiner brings hip passively into flexion while the PSIS is palpated on the ipsilateral side. As soon as the posterior superior iliac spine (PSIS) moves posteriorly, the movement is ceased and the measurement recorded			.87
Short hip flexors	Patient supine with lower limbs over the plinth. Both hips are flexed; examiner slowly lowers the side being tested. When limb ceases to move, measurement is recorded	Inclinometer	11 asymptomatic individuals	.98
External rotators of the hip	Patient prone. Examiner passively flexes knee to 90°. Examiner palpates contralateral PSIS and passively internally rotates limb. When rotation of pelvis occurs, measurement is taken			.99
Internal rotators of the hip *Bullock-Saxton and Bullock[14]*	Same as above, except examiner takes hip into external rotation			.98

Detecting Osteoarthritis of the Hip: Utility of the Historical Examination

Hip Joint Involvement in Osteoarthritis

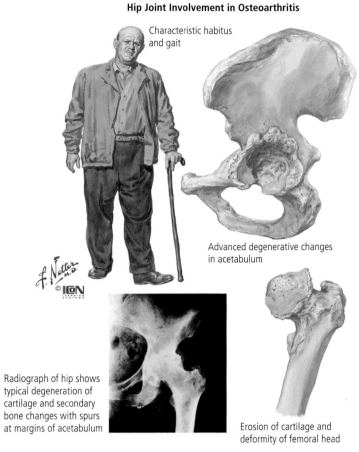

Characteristic habitus and gait

Advanced degenerative changes in acetabulum

Radiograph of hip shows typical degeneration of cartilage and secondary bone changes with spurs at margins of acetabulum

Erosion of cartilage and deformity of femoral head

Figure 7-14: *Hip joint involvement in osteoarthritis*

Historical Question		Population	Reference Standard	Sens	Spec	+LR	−LR
Pain distribution	Lateral thigh			.57	.44	1.02	.98
	Groin			.39	.46	.72	1.3
	Radiates to the knee			.64	.16	.76	2.25
Pain with prolonged ambulation?		201 patients with hip pain	Clinical diagnosis of hip OA by physician	.97	.12	1.10	.25
Reports of reduced LE function				.93	.22	1.19	.32
Morning stiffness in the hip less than or equal to 60 minutes?				.91	.41	1.54	.22
Family history of OA? Altman et al.[3]				.34	.84	2.94	.79

LE, Lower extremity

DIAGNOSTIC UTILITY OF THE CLINICAL EXAMINATION

Detecting Osteoarthritis of the Hip: Range of Motion

Motion		Population	Reference Standard	Sens	Spec	+LR	−LR
Flexion ≤115				.96	.18	1.17	.22
Internal rotation <15 *Altman et al.[3]*				.66	.72	2.35	.47
Hip pain and hip IR <15 hip flexion ≤115		201 patients with hip pain	Clinical diagosis of hip OA by physician	.86	.75	3.40	.19
Hip pain with IR >50 years of age, morning stiffness ≤60 minutes *Altman[3]*				.86	.75	3.40	.19
Number of planes with restricted movement *Birrell et al.[15]*	0	195 patients presenting with first-time episodes of hip pain	Radiographic evidence of OA Mild to moderate OA	1.0	0	1.0	NA
	1			.86	.54	1.87	.26
	2			.57	.77	2.48	.56
	3			.33	.93	4.71	.72
Number of planes with restricted movement *Birrell et al.[15]*	0	195 patients presenting with first-time episodes of hip pain	Radiographic evidence of OA Severe OA	1.0	0	1.0	NA
	1			1.0	.42	1.72	NA
	2			.81	.69	2.61	.28
	3			.54	.88	4.5	.52

Detecting Osteoarthritis of the Hip: Range of Motion

Movement	Population	Reference Standard	Sens	Spec	+LR	−LR
Flexion	201 patients with hip pain	Clinical diagnosis of hip OA by physician	.80	.40	1.33	.50
Extension			.64	.50	1.28	.72
Abduction			.76	.44	1.36	.54
Adduction			.68	.54	1.48	.59
Internal rotation			.82	.39	1.34	.46
External rotation			.79	.37	1.25	.57
Altman et al[3]						

Determining Iliosacral Dysfunction: The Long Sitting Test

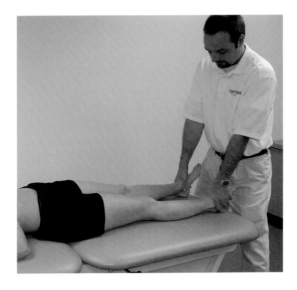

Figure 7-15A: Palpation of the inferior border of the medial malleoli in supine

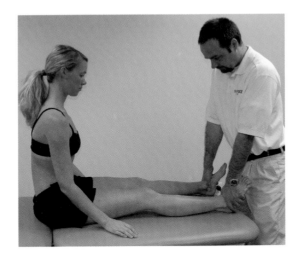

Figure 7-15B: Palpation of the inferior border of the medial malleoli in long sitting

Test	Description and Positive Findings	Population	Reference Standard	Sens	Spec	+LR	−LR
Long sitting test *Bemis and Caniel*[18]	Patient supine. Examiner palpates inferior border of medial malleoli and makes a determination of symmetry. Patient assumes the long sitting position, and examiner again records symmetry of the malleoli. Considered positive if asymmetric malleoli lengths reverse from supine to long sit	51 asymptomatic patients	Classified as having or not having iliosacral dysfunction based on the assessment of PSIS heights, the standing flexion test, and the sitting flexion test	.17	.38	.27	2.18

Detecting Osteoarthritis of the Hip: The Cyriax Capsular Pattern

A few studies[7, 16] have investigated the diagnostic utility of the Cyriax capsular pattern (greater limitation of flexion and internal rotation than of abduction, little if any limitation of adduction and external rotation) in detecting the presence of OA of the hip. Biji et al.[16] demonstrated that hip joints with OA had significantly lower range-of-motion values in all planes when compared with hip joints without OA. However, the magnitude of the range limitations did not follow the Cyriax capsular pattern. Similarly, Klassabo et al.[7] did not detect a correlation between hip OA and the Cyriax capsular pattern. In fact, they identified 138 patterns of passive range-of-motion restrictions, depending on the established norms used (the mean for symptom-free hips or Kaltenborn's published norms).

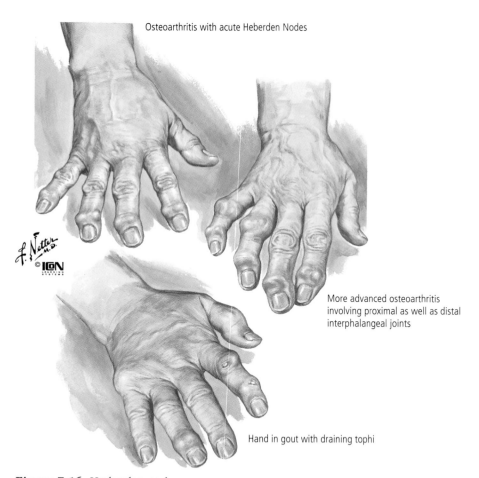

Osteoarthritis with acute Heberden Nodes

More advanced osteoarthritis involving proximal as well as distal interphalangeal joints

Hand in gout with draining tophi

Figure 7-16: Herberden nodes

Detecting Osteoarthritis of the Hip: The Cyriax Capsular Pattern (cont.)

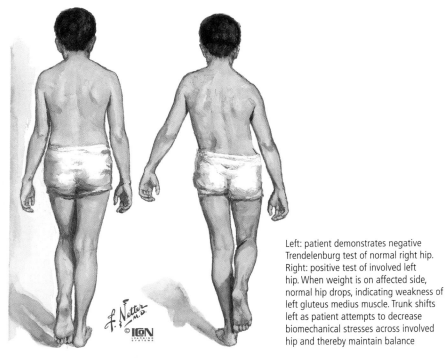

Left: patient demonstrates negative Trendelenburg test of normal right hip. Right: positive test of involved left hip. When weight is on affected side, normal hip drops, indicating weakness of left gluteus medius muscle. Trunk shifts left as patient attempts to decrease biomechanical stresses across involved hip and thereby maintain balance

Figure 7-17: Trendelenburg test

Altman and colleagues[3] have reported that the presence of both Herberden nodes and a Trendelenburg sign can be indicative of OA of the hip. They determined that the presence of Herberden nodes resulted in a sensitivity of .58, a specificity of .73, a +LR of 2.1, and a –LR of .57.

Detecting Acetabular Labral Tears

Test	Description and Positive Findings	Population	Reference Standard	Sens (95% CI)	Spec (95% CI)	+LR	–LR
Patient complaints of clicking in the hip *Narvani et al.*[17]	NA			1 (.48, 1)	.85 (.55, .98)	6.67	0
Internal rotation–flexion–axial compression maneuver *Narvani et al.*[17]	Patient supine. Examiner flexes and internally rotates the hip, then applies an axial compression force through the femur. Provocation of pain is considered positive	18 patients with hip pain	Diagnosis determined via magnetic resonance arthrography	.75 (.19, .99)	.43 (.18, .72)	1.32	.58
Thomas test *Narvani et al.*[17]	Patient supine. Examiner extends involved extremity from the flexed position. Provocation of symptoms is considered positive			.25	Not stated	NA	NA

Detecting Acetabular Labral Tears

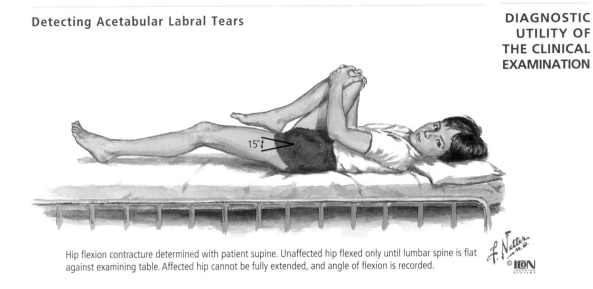

Hip flexion contracture determined with patient supine. Unaffected hip flexed only until lumbar spine is flat against examining table. Affected hip cannot be fully extended, and angle of flexion is recorded.

Figure 7-18: *Thomas test*

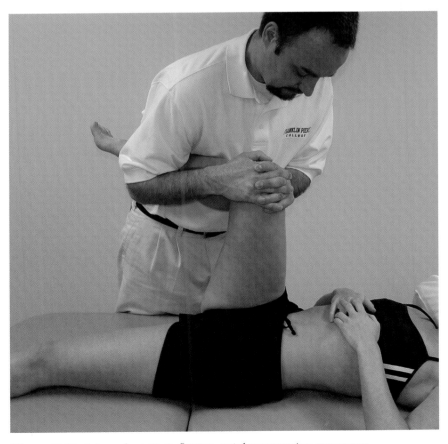

Figure 7-19: *Internal rotation–flexion–axial compression maneuver*

Detecting Hip Disease: Flexion-Adduction Test

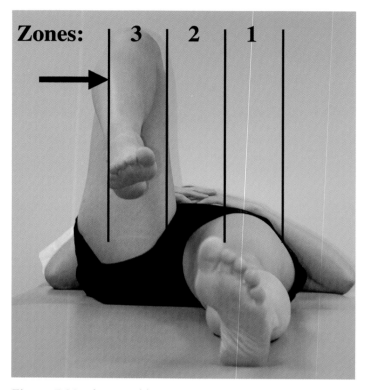

Figure 7-20: *Flexion-adduction test.*

Test	Description	Determination of Positive Finding	Population	Reference Standard	Findings
Flexion-adduction test *Woods and Macnicol[19]*	Patient supine with hip flexed to 90° and in neutral rotation. The hip is then allowed to adduct	In a normal population, the knee should adduct to zone 1. Pathologic changes allow adduction to only zone 2 or 3	87 patients attending an orthopaedic clinic with reports of hip pain	Confirmation of hip disease through examination and investigative procedures	Demonstrated that the test possessed diagnostic utility for detecting the affected extremity

Avascular Necrosis of the Hip

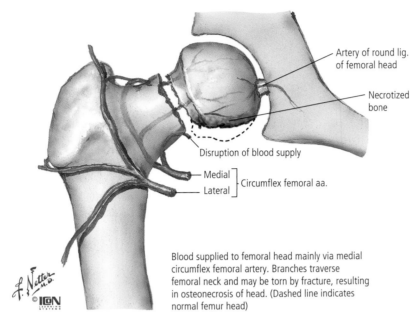

Artery of round lig.
of femoral head

Necrotized
bone

Disruption of blood supply

Medial ⎤
⎦ Circumflex femoral aa.
Lateral ⎦

Blood supplied to femoral head mainly via medial
circumflex femoral artery. Branches traverse
femoral neck and may be torn by fracture, resulting
in osteonecrosis of head. (Dashed line indicates
normal femur head)

Figure 7-21: *Osteonecrosis*

Motion and Finding	Population	Reference Standard	Sens (95% CI)	Spec (95% CI)	+LR	−LR
PROM extension <15	176 asymptomatic HIV-infected patients	MRI confirmation of avascular necrosis (AVN) of the hip. Ten were identified as having AVN	.19 (0, .38)	.92 (.89, .95)	2.38	.88
PROM abduction <45			.31 (.9, .54)	.85 (.82, .89)	2.07	.81
PROM internal rotation <15			.50 (.26, .75)	.67 (.62, .72)	1.52	.75
PROM external rotation <60			.38 (.14, .61)	.73 (.68, .77)	.48	.85
Pain with internal rotation *Joe et al.*[20]			.13 (0, .29)	.86 (.83, .89)	.93	1.01

HIV, human immunodeficiency virus; MRI, magnetic resonance imaging.

Detecting Developmental Dysplasia of the Hip in Infants: Limited Hip

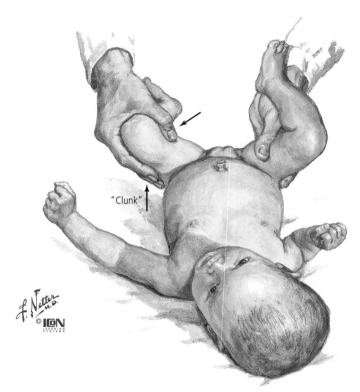

Figure 7-22: *Recognition of congenital dislocation of the hip*

Test		Description and Positive Findings	Population	Reference Standard	Sens (95% CI)	Spec (95% CI)	+LR	−LR
Limited hip abduction test *Jari et al.[21]*	Unilateral limitation	Passive abduction of the hips performed with both hips flexed to 90°	1107 infants	Ultrasound verification of clinical instability of the hip	.70 (.60, .69)	.90 (.88, .92)	7.0	.33
	Bilateral limitation	Considered positive if abduction is more than 20° greater than on the contralateral side			.43 (.50, .64)	.90 (.88, .92)	4.3	.63

Detecting Piriformis Syndrome: The FAIR Test

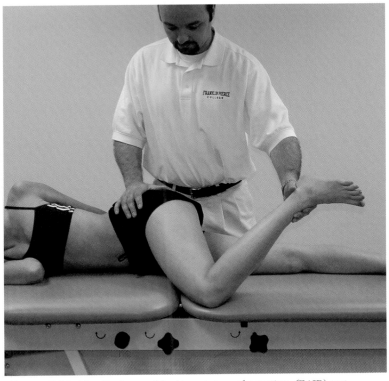

Figure 7-23: *The flexion, adduction, internal rotation (FAIR) test*

Piriformis syndrome, or compression of the sciatic nerve as it passes under the piriformis muscle, has been considered a diagnosis of exclusion.[5, 22] Recently, the FAIR (flexion, adduction, internal rotation) test has been demonstrated to detect compression of the sciatic nerve at the piriformis. The FAIR position entails placing the patient sidelying with the involved extremity up. The patient's involved extremity is then brought into a position of flexion, adduction, and internal rotation. If pain is elicited at the intersection of the sciatic nerve and the piriformis during this test, the result is considered positive. The FAIR test has been demonstrated to have a sensitivity of .88, a specificity of .83, a +LR of 5.2, and a −LR of .14.[5, 22]

1. Hertling D, Kessler RM. The hip. In: Hertling D, Kessler RM, editors. *Management of Common Musculoskeletal Disorders: Physical Therapy Principles and Methods.* 3rd ed. Philadelphia: Lippincott; 1996:285-314.

2. Pecina MM, Bojanic I. *Overuse Injuries of the Musculoskeletal System.* Boca Raton: CRC Press; 1993.

3. Altman R, Alarcon G, Appelrouth D, et al. The American College of Rheumatology criteria for the classification and reporting of osteoarthritis of the hip. *Arthritis Rheum.* 1991;34:505-514.

REFERENCES

4. Hartley A. *Practical Joint Assessment*. St. Louis: Mosby; 1995.

5. Fishman L, Dombi G, Michaelson C, et al. Piriformis syndrome: diagnosis, treatment and outcome—a 10-year study. *Arch Phys Med Rehabil*. 2002;83:295-301.

6. Holm I, Bolstad B, Lutken T, Ervik A, Rokkum M, Steen H. Reliability of goniometric measurements and visual estimates of hip ROM in patients with osteoarthritis. *Physiother Res Int*. 2000;5:241-248.

7. Klassabo M, Harms-Ringdahl K, Larsson G. Examination of passive ROM and capsular patterns in the hip. *Physiother Res Int*. 2003;8:1-12.

8. Lin Y-C, Davey R, Cochrane T. Tests for physical function of the elderly with knee and hip osteoarthritis. *Scand J Med Sci Sports*. 2001;11:280-286.

9. Browder D, Enseki K, Fritz J. Intertester reliability of hip range of motion measurements and special tests. *J Orthop Sports Phys Ther*. 2004; 34:A1.

10. Bierma-Zeinstra S, Bohnen A, Ramlal R, Ridderikhoff J. Comparison between two devices for measuring hip joint motions. *Clin Rehabil*. 1998;12:497-505.

11. Cliborne AV, Wainner RS, Rhon DI, et al. Clinical hip tests and a functional squat test in patients with knee osteoarthritis: reliability, prevalence of positive test findings, and short-term response to hip mobilization. *J Orthop Sports Phys Ther*. 2004;34:676-685.

12. Reese N, Bandy W. Use of an inclinometer to measure flexibility of the iliotibial band using the Ober test and the Modified Ober test: difference in magnitude and reliability of measurements. *J Orthop Sports Phys Ther*. 2003;33:326-330.

13. Melchione WE, Sullivan M. Reliability of measurments obtained by use of an instrument designed to indirectly measure iliotibial band length. *J Orthop Sports Phys Ther*. 1993;18:511-515.

14. Bullock-Saxton J, Bullock M. Repeatability of muscle length measures around the hip. *Physiother Can*. 1994;46:105-109.

15. Birrell F, Croft P, Cooper C, Hosie G, Macfarlane G, Silman A. Predicting radiographic hip osteoarthritis from range of movement. *Rheumatology*. 2001;40:506-512.

16. Biji D, Dekker J, van Baar M, et al. Validity of Cyriax's concept *capsular pattern* for the diagnosis of osteoarthritis of hip and/or knee. *Scand J Rheumatol*. 1998;27:347-351.

17. Narvani A, Tsirdis E, Kendall S, Chaudhuri R, Thomas P. A preliminary report on prevalence of acetabular labral tears in sports patients with groin pain. *Knee Surg Sports Traumatol Arthrosc*. 2003;11:403-408.

18. Bemis T, Caniel M. Validation of the long sitting test on subjects with iliosacral dysfunction. *J Orthop Sports Phys Ther*. 1987;8:336-345.

19. Woods D, Macnicol M. The flexion-adduction test: an early sign of hip disease. *J Pediatr Orthop*. 2001;10:180-185.

20. Joe G, Kovacs J, Miller K, et al. Diagnosis of avascular necrosis of the hip in asymptomatic HIV-infected patients: clinical correlation of physical examination with magnetic resonance imaging. *J Back Musculoskel Rehabil*. 2002;16:135-139.

21. Jari S, Paton R, Srinivasan M. Unilateral limitation of abduction of the hip: a valuable clinical sign for DDH? *J Bone Joint Surg*. 2002;84-B:104-107.

22. Fishman L, Zybert P. Electrophysiologic evidence of piriformis syndrome. *Arch Phys Med Rehabil*. 1992;73:359-364.

Knee

Chapter 8

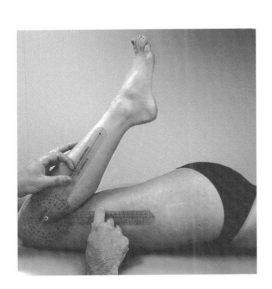

ANATOMY   **Knee**

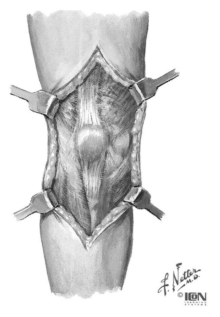

Figure 8-1

Patella

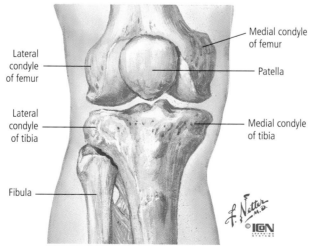

Lateral
condyle
of femur

Medial condyle
of femur

Patella

Lateral
condyle
of tibia

Medial condyle
of tibia

Fibula

Figure 8-2

Femur

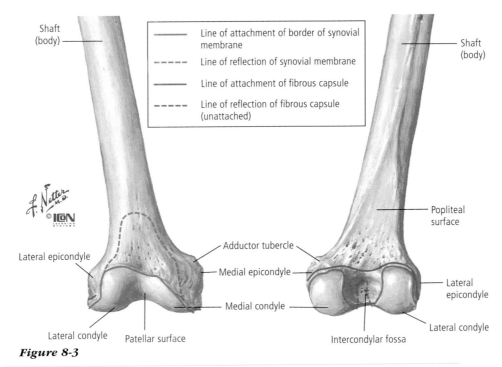

	Line of attachment of border of synovial membrane
	Line of reflection of synovial membrane
	Line of attachment of fibrous capsule
	Line of reflection of fibrous capsule (unattached)

Shaft (body)

Shaft (body)

Popliteal surface

Lateral epicondyle

Adductor tubercle

Medial epicondyle

Lateral epicondyle

Medial condyle

Lateral condyle — Patellar surface

Lateral condyle

Intercondylar fossa

Figure 8-3

Tibia and Fibula

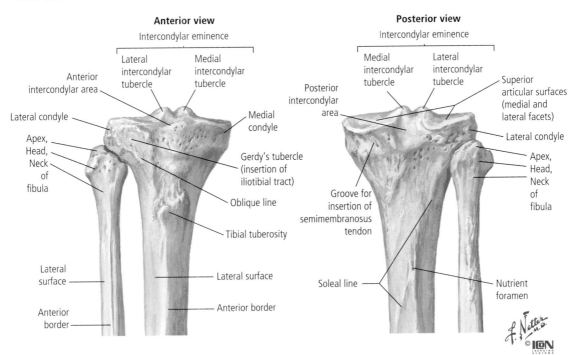

Anterior view

Intercondylar eminence

Lateral intercondylar tubercle

Medial intercondylar tubercle

Anterior intercondylar area

Lateral condyle

Apex, Head, Neck of fibula

Medial condyle

Gerdy's tubercle (insertion of iliotibial tract)

Oblique line

Tibial tuberosity

Lateral surface

Lateral surface

Anterior border

Anterior border

Posterior view

Intercondylar eminence

Medial intercondylar tubercle

Lateral intercondylar tubercle

Posterior intercondylar area

Superior articular surfaces (medial and lateral facets)

Lateral condyle

Apex, Head, Neck of fibula

Groove for insertion of semimembranosus tendon

Soleal line

Nutrient foramen

Figure 8-4

ARTHROLOGY   Sagittal Knee

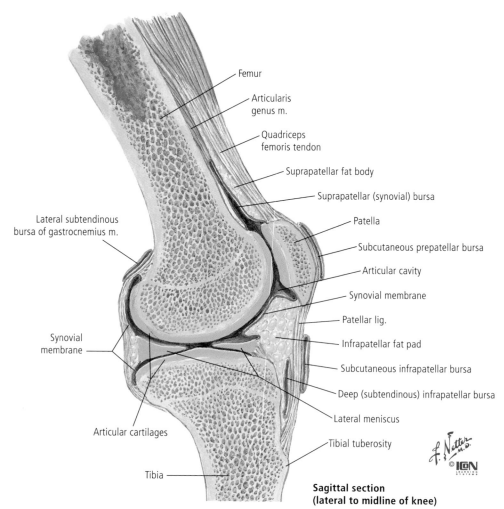

Femur

Articularis genus m.

Quadriceps femoris tendon

Suprapatellar fat body

Suprapatellar (synovial) bursa

Patella

Subcutaneous prepatellar bursa

Articular cavity

Synovial membrane

Patellar lig.

Infrapatellar fat pad

Subcutaneous infrapatellar bursa

Deep (subtendinous) infrapatellar bursa

Lateral meniscus

Tibial tuberosity

Lateral subtendinous bursa of gastrocnemius m.

Synovial membrane

Articular cartilages

Tibia

Sagittal section (lateral to midline of knee)

Figure 8-5

Joints	Type and Classification	Closed Packed Position	Capsular Pattern
Tibiofemoral	Double condyloid	Full extension	Flexion restricted more than extension
Proximal tibiofibular	Synovial: plane	NR	NR
Patellofemoral	Synovial: plane	Full flexion	NR

NR, not reported.

Posterior Ligaments of Knee

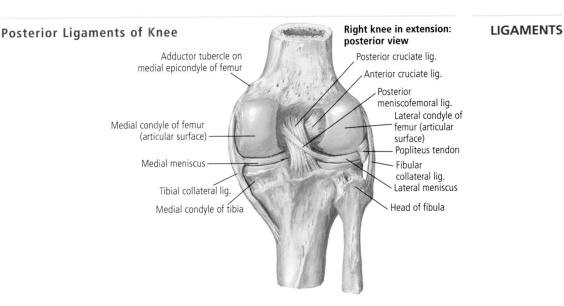

Right knee in extension: posterior view

- Adductor tubercle on medial epicondyle of femur
- Posterior cruciate lig.
- Anterior cruciate lig.
- Posterior meniscofemoral lig.
- Medial condyle of femur (articular surface)
- Lateral condyle of femur (articular surface)
- Popliteus tendon
- Medial meniscus
- Fibular collateral lig.
- Lateral meniscus
- Tibial collateral lig.
- Medial condyle of tibia
- Head of fibula

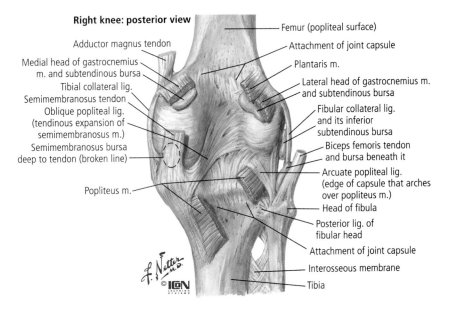

Right knee: posterior view

- Adductor magnus tendon
- Femur (popliteal surface)
- Attachment of joint capsule
- Medial head of gastrocnemius m. and subtendinous bursa
- Plantaris m.
- Tibial collateral lig.
- Lateral head of gastrocnemius m. and subtendinous bursa
- Semimembranosus tendon
- Oblique popliteal lig. (tendinous expansion of semimembranosus m.)
- Fibular collateral lig. and its inferior subtendinous bursa
- Semimembranosus bursa deep to tendon (broken line)
- Biceps femoris tendon and bursa beneath it
- Arcuate popliteal lig. (edge of capsule that arches over popliteus m.)
- Popliteus m.
- Head of fibula
- Posterior lig. of fibular head
- Attachment of joint capsule
- Interosseous membrane
- Tibia

Figure 8-6

Ligaments	Attachments	Function
Posterior meniscofemoral	Lateral meniscus to PCL and medial femoral condyle	Reinforce posterior lateral meniscal attachment
Oblique popliteal	Posterior aspect of medial tibial condyle to posterior aspect of fibrous capsule	Strengthen posterior portion of joint capsule
Arcuate popliteal	Posterior fibular head over tendon of popliteus to posterior capsule	Strengthen posterior portion of joint capsule
Posterior ligament of fibular head	Posterior fibular head to inferior lateral tibial condyle	Reinforce posterior joint capsule

PCL, posterior cruciate ligament

LIGAMENTS Interior and Anterior Ligaments of Knee

Right knee in flexion: anterior view

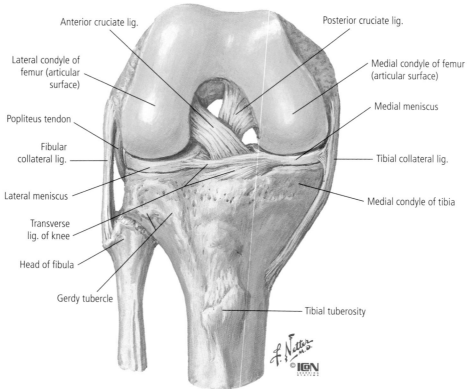

Anterior cruciate lig.

Posterior cruciate lig.

Lateral condyle of femur (articular surface)

Medial condyle of femur (articular surface)

Medial meniscus

Popliteus tendon

Fibular collateral lig.

Tibial collateral lig.

Lateral meniscus

Medial condyle of tibia

Transverse lig. of knee

Head of fibula

Gerdy tubercle

Tibial tuberosity

Figure 8-7

Ligaments	Attachments	Function
Anterior cruciate	Anterior intracondylar aspect of tibial plateau to posteromedial side of lateral femoral condyle	Prevent posterior translation of femur on tibia and anterior translation of tibia on femur
Posterior cruciate	Posterior intracondylar aspect of tibial plateau to anterolateral side of medial femoral condyle	Prevent anterior translation of femur on tibia and posterior translation of tibia on femur
Fibular collateral	Lateral epicondyle of femur to lateral aspect of fibular head	Protect joint from varus stress
Tibial collateral	Femoral medial epicondyle to medial condyle of tibia	Protect joint from valgus stress
Transverse ligament of knee	Anterior edges of menisci	Attach media and lateral menisci

Interior and Anterior Ligaments of Knee (cont.)

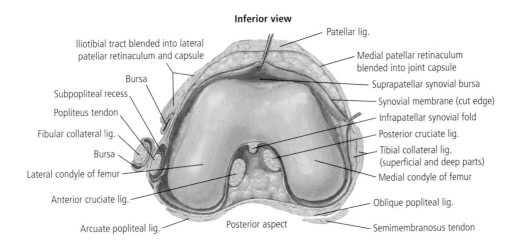

Inferior view

Iliotibial tract blended into lateral patellar retinaculum and capsule

Bursa

Subpopliteal recess

Popliteus tendon

Fibular collateral lig.

Bursa

Lateral condyle of femur

Anterior cruciate lig.

Arcuate popliteal lig.

Posterior aspect

Patellar lig.

Medial patellar retinaculum blended into joint capsule

Suprapatellar synovial bursa

Synovial membrane (cut edge)

Infrapatellar synovial fold

Posterior cruciate lig.

Tibial collateral lig. (superficial and deep parts)

Medial condyle of femur

Oblique popliteal lig.

Semimembranosus tendon

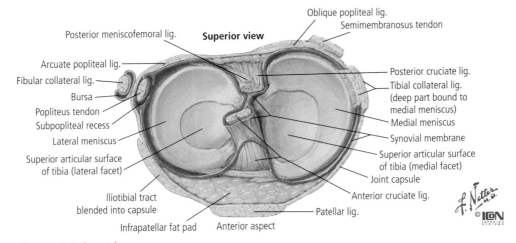

Superior view

Oblique popliteal lig.

Semimembranosus tendon

Posterior meniscofemoral lig.

Arcuate popliteal lig.

Fibular collateral lig.

Bursa

Popliteus tendon

Subpopliteal recess

Lateral meniscus

Superior articular surface of tibia (lateral facet)

Iliotibial tract blended into capsule

Infrapatellar fat pad

Anterior aspect

Posterior cruciate lig.

Tibial collateral lig. (deep part bound to medial meniscus)

Medial meniscus

Synovial membrane

Superior articular surface of tibia (medial facet)

Joint capsule

Anterior cruciate lig.

Patellar lig.

Figure 8-7 (cont.)

MUSCLES Anterior Muscles of Knee

Muscles		Proximal Attachments	Distal Attachments	Nerve and Segmental Level	Action
Quadriceps	Rectus femoris	AIIS and ileum just superior to acetabulum	Base of patella and by patellar ligament to tibial tuberosity	Femoral nerve (L2, L3, L4)	Extend knee; rectus femoris also flexes hip and stabilizes head of femur in acetabulum
	Vastus lateralis	Greater trochanter and linea aspera of femur			
	Vastus medialis	Intertrochanteric line and linea aspera			
	Vastus intermedius	Anterolateral aspect of shaft of femur			
Articularis genu		Anteroinferior aspect of femur	Synovial membrane of knee joint	Femoral nerve (L3, L4)	Pulls synovial membrane superiorly during knee extension to prevent pinching of membrane

AIIS, anterior inferior iliac spine.

Anterior Muscles of Knee (cont.)

Right knee in extension

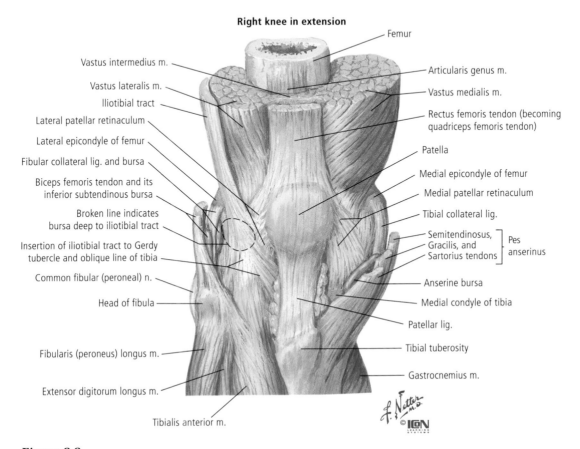

Femur

Vastus intermedius m.

Vastus lateralis m.

Iliotibial tract

Lateral patellar retinaculum

Lateral epicondyle of femur

Fibular collateral lig. and bursa

Biceps femoris tendon and its inferior subtendinous bursa

Broken line indicates bursa deep to iliotibial tract

Insertion of iliotibial tract to Gerdy tubercle and oblique line of tibia

Common fibular (peroneal) n.

Head of fibula

Fibularis (peroneus) longus m.

Extensor digitorum longus m.

Tibialis anterior m.

Articularis genus m.

Vastus medialis m.

Rectus femoris tendon (becoming quadriceps femoris tendon)

Patella

Medial epicondyle of femur

Medial patellar retinaculum

Tibial collateral lig.

Semitendinosus, Gracilis, and Sartorius tendons — Pes anserinus

Anserine bursa

Medial condyle of tibia

Patellar lig.

Tibial tuberosity

Gastrocnemius m.

Figure 8-8

MUSCLES   Lateral and Medial Muscles of Knee

Muscles			Proximal Attachments	Distal Attachments	Nerve and Segmental Level	Action
Hamstrings	Semimembranosus		Ischial tuberosity	Medial aspect of superior tibia	Tibial branch of sciatic nerve (L4, L5, S1, S2)	Flex and medially rotate knee, extend and medially rotate hip
	Semitendinosus		Ischial tuberosity	Posterior aspect of medial condyle of tibia		
	Biceps femoris	Short head	Lateral linea aspera and proximal two thirds of supracondylar line of femur	Lateral head of fibula and lateral tibial condyle	Fibular branch of sciatic nerve (L5, S1, S2)	Flex and laterally rotate knee
		Long head	Ischial tuberosity		Tibial branch of sciatic nerve (L5, S1-S3)	Flex and laterally rotate knee, extend and laterally rotate hip
Gracilis			Body and ramus of pubis	Medial aspect of superior tibia	Obturator nerve (L2, L3)	Adduct hip, flex and medially rotate knee
Sartorius			ASIS and anterior iliac crest	Superomedial aspect of tibia	Femoral nerve (L2, L3)	Flex, abduct, and externally rotate hip; flex knee
Gastrocnemius	Lateral head		Lateral femoral condyle	Posterior calcaneus	Tibial nerve (S1, S2)	Plantarflex ankle and flex knee
	Medial head		Superior aspect of medial femoral condyle			
Popliteus			Lateral femoral condyle and lateral meniscus	Superior to soleal line on posterior tibia	Tibial nerve (L4, L5, S1)	Weak knee flexion and unlocking of knee joint
Plantaris			Lateral supracondylar line of femur and oblique popliteal ligament	Posterior calcaneus	Tibial nerve (S1, S2)	Weak assist in knee flexion and ankle plantarflexion

ASIS, anterior superior iliac spine.

Lateral and Medial Muscles of Knee (cont.)   **MUSCLES**

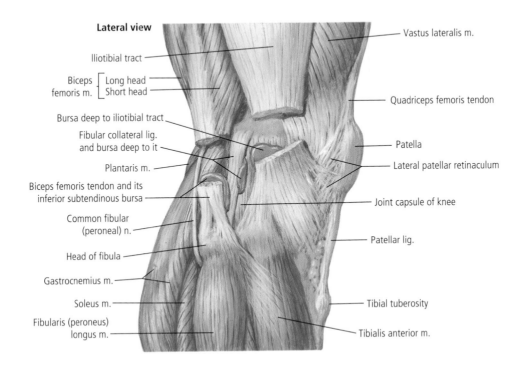

Lateral view

- Vastus lateralis m.
- Iliotibial tract
- Biceps femoris m. — Long head / Short head
- Quadriceps femoris tendon
- Bursa deep to iliotibial tract
- Fibular collateral lig. and bursa deep to it
- Patella
- Plantaris m.
- Lateral patellar retinaculum
- Biceps femoris tendon and its inferior subtendinous bursa
- Joint capsule of knee
- Common fibular (peroneal) n.
- Patellar lig.
- Head of fibula
- Gastrocnemius m.
- Soleus m.
- Tibial tuberosity
- Fibularis (peroneus) longus m.
- Tibialis anterior m.

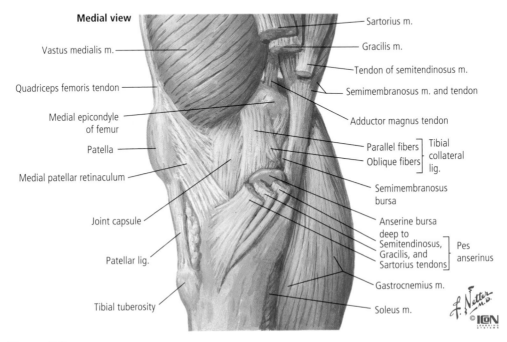

Medial view

- Sartorius m.
- Vastus medialis m.
- Gracilis m.
- Tendon of semitendinosus m.
- Quadriceps femoris tendon
- Semimembranosus m. and tendon
- Medial epicondyle of femur
- Adductor magnus tendon
- Patella
- Parallel fibers / Oblique fibers — Tibial collateral lig.
- Medial patellar retinaculum
- Semimembranosus bursa
- Joint capsule
- Anserine bursa deep to Semitendinosus, Gracilis, and Sartorius tendons — Pes anserinus
- Patellar lig.
- Gastrocnemius m.
- Tibial tuberosity
- Soleus m.

Figure 8-9

NERVES   Nerves of Thigh and Knee

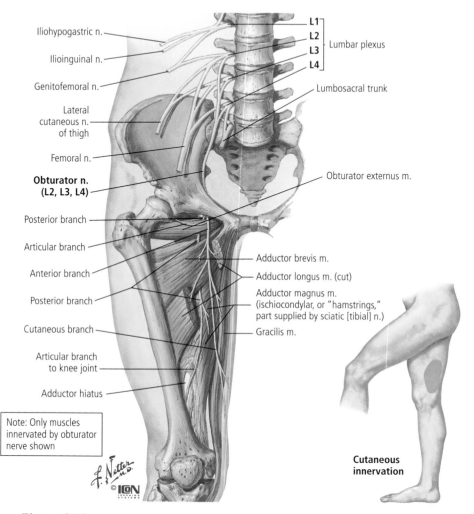

Figure 8-10

Nerves	Segmental Level	Sensory	Motor
Femoral	L2, L3, L4	Thigh via cutaneous nerves	Iliacus, sartorius, quadriceps femoris, articularis genu, pectineus
Obturator	L2, L3, L4	Medial thigh	Adductor longus, adductor brevis, adductor magnus (adductor part), gracilis, obturator externus
Saphenous	L2, L3, L4	Medial leg and foot	No motor
Tibial	L4, L5, S1, S2, S3	Posterior heel and plantar surface of foot	Semitendinosus, semimembranosus, biceps femoris, adductor magnus, gastrocnemius, soleus, plantaris, flexor hallucis longus, flexor digitorum longus, tibialis posterior
Common fibular	L4, L5, S1, S2	Lateral posterior leg	Biceps femoris

Nerves of Thigh and Knee (cont.)   **NERVES**

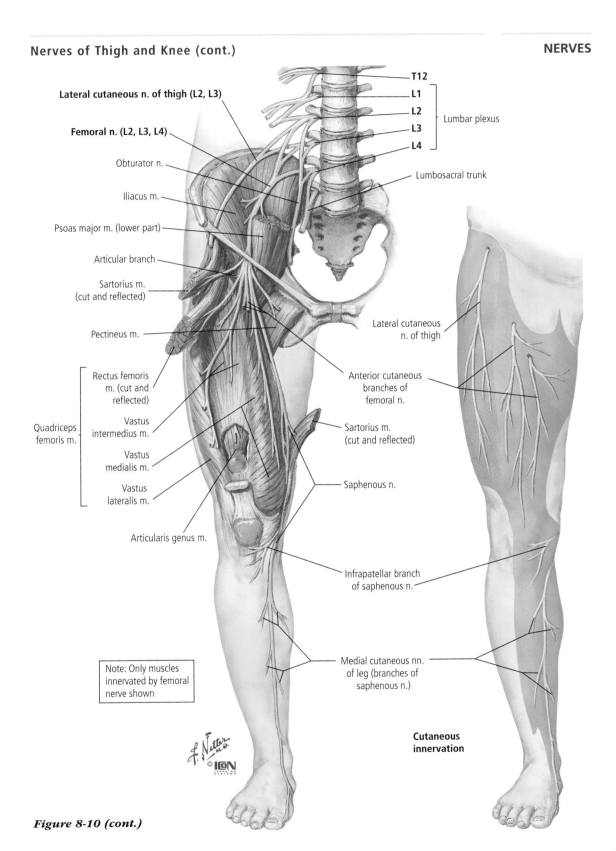

Lateral cutaneous n. of thigh (L2, L3)

Femoral n. (L2, L3, L4)

Obturator n.

Iliacus m.

Psoas major m. (lower part)

Articular branch

Sartorius m.
(cut and reflected)

Pectineus m.

Rectus femoris
m. (cut and
reflected)

Quadriceps
femoris m.

Vastus
intermedius m.

Vastus
medialis m.

Vastus
lateralis m.

Articularis genus m.

Note: Only muscles
innervated by femoral
nerve shown

T12

L1

L2

L3

L4

Lumbar plexus

Lumbosacral trunk

Lateral cutaneous
n. of thigh

Anterior cutaneous
branches of
femoral n.

Sartorius m.
(cut and reflected)

Saphenous n.

Infrapatellar branch
of saphenous n.

Medial cutaneous nn.
of leg (branches of
saphenous n.)

Cutaneous
innervation

Figure 8-10 (cont.)

NERVES   Nerves of Thigh and Knee (cont.)

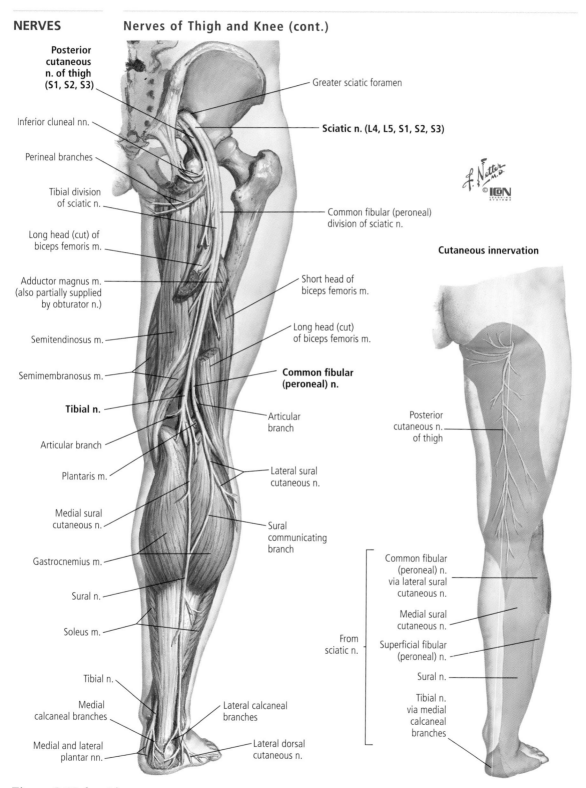

Posterior cutaneous n. of thigh (S1, S2, S3)

Inferior cluneal nn.

Perineal branches

Tibial division of sciatic n.

Long head (cut) of biceps femoris m.

Adductor magnus m. (also partially supplied by obturator n.)

Semitendinosus m.

Semimembranosus m.

Tibial n.

Articular branch

Plantaris m.

Medial sural cutaneous n.

Gastrocnemius m.

Sural n.

Soleus m.

Tibial n.

Medial calcaneal branches

Medial and lateral plantar nn.

Greater sciatic foramen

Sciatic n. (L4, L5, S1, S2, S3)

Common fibular (peroneal) division of sciatic n.

Short head of biceps femoris m.

Long head (cut) of biceps femoris m.

Common fibular (peroneal) n.

Articular branch

Lateral sural cutaneous n.

Sural communicating branch

Lateral calcaneal branches

Lateral dorsal cutaneous n.

Cutaneous innervation

Posterior cutaneous n. of thigh

From sciatic n.

Common fibular (peroneal) n. via lateral sural cutaneous n.

Medial sural cutaneous n.

Superficial fibular (peroneal) n.

Sural n.

Tibial n. via medial calcaneal branches

Figure 8-10 (cont.)

Initial Hypotheses Based on Patient Reports

Patient Reports	Initial Hypothesis
Patient reports a traumatic onset of knee pain that occurred during jumping, twisting, or changing direction with foot planted	Possible ligamentous injury[1, 2] (anterior cruciate) Possible patellar subluxation[2] Possible quadriceps rupture Possible meniscal tear
Patient reports traumatic injury that resulted in a posteriorly directed force to tibia with knee flexed	Possible PCL injury (posterior cruciate)[3]
Patient reports traumatic injury that resulted in a varus or valgus force exerted on the knee	Possible collateral ligament injury (fibular or tibial)[3]
Patient reports anterior pain with jumping and full knee flexion	Possible patellar tendonitis[2, 4] Possible patellofemoral pain syndrome[5, 6]
Patient reports swelling in knee with occasional locking and clicking	Possible meniscal tear[7] Possible loose body within knee joint
Patient reports pain with prolonged knee flexion, during squats, and while going up and down stairs	Possible patellofemoral pain syndrome[5, 6]
Patient reports pain and stiffness in the morning that diminishes after a few hours	Possible osteoarthritis (OA)[8, 9]

RELIABILITY OF THE CLINICAL EXAMINATION

Range-of-Motion Measurements

ROM Measurements	Instrumentation	Population	Reliability ICC			
Passive flexion and extension *Rothstein et al.*[10]	Three standard goniometers (metal, large plastic, and small plastic)	24 patients referred to PT	Intra-examiner			
				Flexion	Extension	
			Metal	.97	.96	
			Large plastic	.99	.91	
			Small plastic	.99	.97	
Passive flexion *Gogia et al.*[11]	1 large standard goniometer	30 asymptomatic subjects	Inter-examiner .99			
Passive flexion Passive extension *Watkins et al.*[12]	Standard goniometer	43 patients referred to PT when examination would normally include PROM measurements of knee	Intra-examiner		Inter-examiner	
			Flexion	.99	Flexion	.90
			Extension	.98	Extension	.86
Passive flexion Passive extension *Watkins et al.*[12]	Visual estimation		Inter-examiner			
			Flexion		.83	
			Extension		.82	
Active flexion Active extension *Clapper and Wolf*[13]	Standard goniometer	20 asymptomatic subjects	Intra-examiner			
			Flexion		.95	
			Extension		.85	
Active flexion *Brosseau et al.*[14]	Universal goniometer	60 healthy university students	Intra-examiner .86–.97 Inter-examiner .62–1.0			
Passive flexion Passive extension *Hayes et al.*[15]	Universal goniometer	79 patients with OA of knee	Intra-examiner			
			Flexion		.95–.96	
			Extension		.71–.86	
Passive flexion Passive extension *Fritz et al.*[16]	Standard goniometer	152 patients with unilateral knee dysfunction	Inter-examiner			
			Involved knee		Uninvolved knee	
			Flexion	.97	Flexion	.80
			Extension	.94	Extension	.72

ROM, range of motion; ICC, XXXX; PT, physical therapy; PROM, passive range of motion.

Range-of-Motion Measurements (cont.)

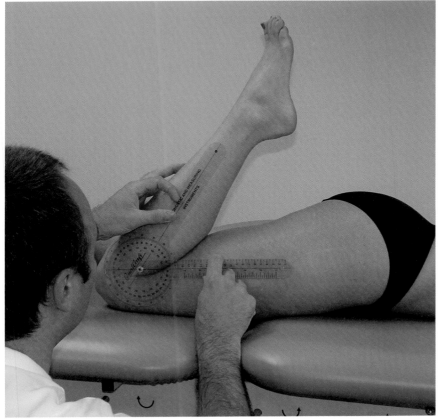

Figure 8-11: *Measurement of active knee flexion range of motion*

RELIABILITY OF THE CLINICAL EXAMINATION

Determining End-Feel of Knee

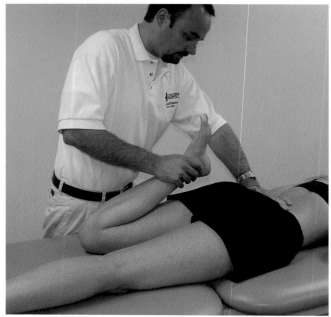

Figure 8-12: *Assessment of end-feel for knee flexion*

Test and Measure	Test Procedure	Population	Reliability Kappa Value (95% CI)			
Flexion end-feel Extension end-feel *Hayes et al.*[15]	End-feel is assessed at end of PROM and is categorized as capsular, tissue approximation, springy block, bony, spasm, or empty	79 patients with OA of knee	Intra-examiner			
			Flexion end-feel Extension end-feel		κ = .48 κ = .17	
Flexion end-feel Extension end-feel *Hayes et al.*[17]	End-feel is assessed at end of PROM and is graded on an 11-point scale with capsular at end of normal range, capsular early in range, capsular, tissue approximation, springy block, bony, spasm, or empty	40 patients with unilateral knee pain	Intra-examiner		Inter-examiner	
			Flexion end-feel	κ = .76 (.95, .97)	Flexion end-feel	κ= −.01 (−.36, .35)
			Extension end-feel	κ = 1 (1.0, 1.0)	Extension end-feel	κ = .43 (−.06, .92)
End-feel assessment during Lachman test *Cooperman et al.*[18]	Examiners asked to grade end-feel during Lachman test. End-feel graded as "hard" or "soft"	35 patients referred to PT clinics for rehabilitation of knee joint	Intra-examiner κ = .33			
End-feel of adduction stress applied to knee *McClure et al.*[19]	Examiner places knee in 0° and 30° of flexion and applies valgus force through knee. End-feel graded as soft or firm	50 patients referred to an outpatient orthopaedic clinic who would normally undergo valgus stress tests directed at knee	Inter-examiner 0° of flexion = .00 30° of flexion = .33			

CI, confidence interval.

Pain Resistance Sequence for Knee

Test and Measure	Test Procedure	Population	Reliability Kappa Value (95% CI)			
Pain resistance sequence: Passive flexion Passive extension Hayes et al.[15]	Pain sequence is assessed during PROM of knee. Pain is graded on a 4-point scale as no pain, pain that occurs after resistance is felt, pain that occurs at the same time resistance is felt, or pain that occurs before resistance is felt	79 patients with OA of knee	Intra-examiner			
			Passive flexion Passive extension		κ = .34 κ = .36	
Pain resistance sequence: Passive flexion Passive extension Hayes et al.[17]		40 patients with unilateral knee pain	Intra-examiner		Inter-examiner	
			Passive flexion	κ = .78 (.68, .87)	Passive flexion	κ = .51
			Passive extension	κ = .85 (.75, .95)	Passive extension	κ = .42
Pain resistance sequence: Passive flexion Fritz et al.[16]	Examiner passively flexes knee. Subject is directed to report when pain is above baseline levels. Examiner reports if pain occurs before, during, or after occurrence of PROM limitation	152 patients with unilateral knee dysfunction	Intra-examiner .28			
Assessment of pain during adduction stress applied to knee McClure et al.[19]	Examiner places knee in 0° and 30° of flexion and applies valgus force through knee. Pain responses recorded	50 patients referred to outpatient orthopaedic clinic who would normally undergo valgus stress tests directed at knee	Inter-examiner 0° of flexion = .40 30° of flexion = .33			

**RELIABILITY
OF THE
CLINICAL
EXAMINATION**

Detecting Cardinal Signs of Inflammation of Knee

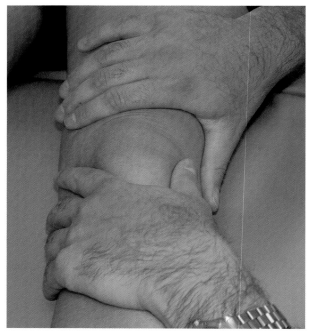

Figure 8-13: *Fluctuation test*

Test and Measure	Test Procedure	Population	Inter-examiner Reliability Kappa Values
Fluctuation test	Patient supine. Examiner places thumb and finger around patella while pushing any fluid from suprapatellar pouch with other hand. Positive if finger and thumb are pushed apart		κ = .37
Patellar tap test	Patient supine. Examiner presses suprapatellar pouch, then taps on patella. Patella remains in contact with femur if no swelling is present	152 patients with unilateral knee dysfunction	κ = .21
Palpation for warmth	Examiner palpates anterior aspect of knee. Results compared with uninvolved knee		κ = .66
Visual inspection for redness *Fritz et al.*[16]	Examiner visually inspects involved knee for redness and compares it with uninvolved side		κ = .21

Palpation in Patients With Osteoarthritis of Knee

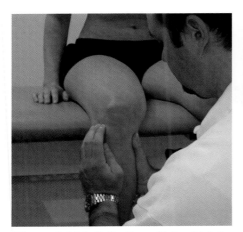

Figure 8-14A: *Palpation of lateral joint line*

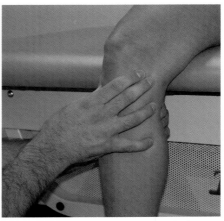

Figure 8-14B: *Palpation of medial joint line*

Physical Finding	Population	Reliability Kappa Values (95% CI)	
Tenderness at medial joint line	152 patients with OA of knee	Intra-examiner κ = .21 (.01, .41)	
Tenderness at lateral joint line Dervin et al.[20]		Inter-examiner κ = .25 (.07, .43)	
Medial tibiofemoral tenderness	6 subjects with OA of knee	Inter-examiner κ = .94	
Lateral tibiofemoral tenderness Cibere et al.[8]		Inter-examiner κ = .85	
Patellofemoral tenderness	49 patients presenting to outpatient rheumatology clinics for OA of knee	Intra-examiner κ = .61 (.43, .78)	Inter-examiner κ = .27 (.05, .48)
Medial tibiofemoral tenderness		κ = .60 (.47, .72)	κ = .35 (.24, .45)
Lateral tibiofemoral tenderness		κ = .60 (.44, .74)	κ = .29 (.14, .44)
Periarticular tenderness Jones et al.[9]		κ = .58 (.45, .73)	κ = .22 (.09, .36)

RELIABILITY OF THE CLINICAL EXAMINATION

Patients with Osteoarthritis of Knee

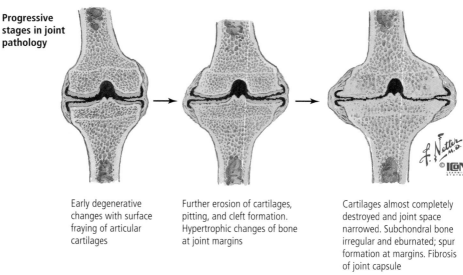

Progressive stages in joint pathology

Early degenerative changes with surface fraying of articular cartilages

Further erosion of cartilages, pitting, and cleft formation. Hypertrophic changes of bone at joint margins

Cartilages almost completely destroyed and joint space narrowed. Subchondral bone irregular and eburnated; spur formation at margins. Fibrosis of joint capsule

Figure 8-15: *Osteoarthritis of the knee*

History	Population	Reliability Kappa Values (95% CI)
Acute injury		κ = .21 (.03, .39)
Swelling		κ = .33 (.17, .49)
Giving way		κ = .12 (−.04, .28)
Locking		κ = .44 (.26, .62)
Generalized pain	152 patients with OA of knee	κ = −.03 (.15, .21)
Pain at rest		κ = .16 (.0, 32)
Pain on rising from chair		κ = .25 (.05, .45)
Pain on climbing stairs *Dervin et al.*[20]		κ - .21 (.06, .48)
Inactivity stiffness	49 patients presenting to outpatient rheumatology clinics for OA of knee	κ = .90 (.74, 1.0)
Pain on using stairs		κ = .86 (.70, 1.0)
Night pain *Jones et al.*[9]		κ = .81 (.66, .96)

Patients with Osteoarthritis of Knee (cont.)

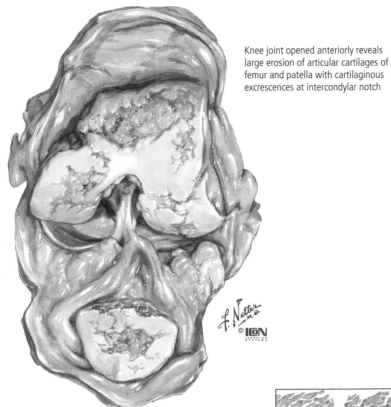

Knee joint opened anteriorly reveals large erosion of articular cartilages of femur and patella with cartilaginous excrescences at intercondylar notch

Section of articular cartilage shows fraying of surface and deep cleft. Hyaline cartilage abnormal with clumping of chondrocytes

Figure 8-15 (cont.): *Osteoarthritis of the knee*

Special Tests in Patients With Osteoarthritis of Knee

Test and Measure	Procedure	Determination of Positive Finding	Population	Inter-examiner Reliability Kappa Values (95% CI)
McMurray test	Knee is passively flexed, externally rotated, and axially loaded while brought into extension. Test is repeated in internal rotation.	Positive if a palpable or audible click or pain occurs during rotation	152 patients with knee OA	$\kappa = .16$ (−.01, .33)
Varus test	Not specified			$\kappa = 0$ (−.18, .18)
Valgus test				$\kappa = .05$ (−.13, 2.3)
Lachman test Dervin et al.[20]				$\kappa = −.08$ (−.12, .04)
Medial instability test	Not specified	Graded as normal or abnormal	6 subjects with knee OA	0 degrees of knee flexion $\kappa = .66$ 30 degrees of knee flexion $\kappa = .02$
Lateral instability test				0 degrees of knee flexion $\kappa = .88$ 30 degrees of knee flexion $\kappa = .34$
Anterior drawer test				$\kappa = .54$
Posterior drawer test Cibere et al.[8]				$\kappa = .82$

Testing Integrity of Anterior Cruciate Ligament Using Lachman Test

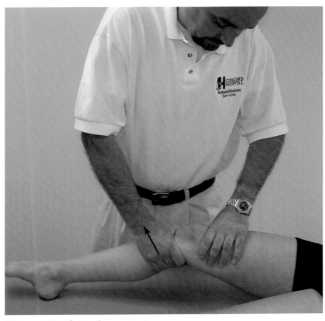

Figure 8-16: *Lachman test*

Test and Measure	Procedure	Determination of Positive Finding	Population	Reliability Kappa Values
Lachman test Cooperman et al.[18]	Examiners are instructed to perform Lachman test as they would in practice	Results are graded as positive or negative. Examiners also grade amount of anterior tibial translation as 0, 1+, 2+, or 3+. 0 represented no difference in tibial translation between unaffected and affected knees	35 patients referred to PT clinics for rehabilitation of knee joint	Intra-examiner for positive or negative findings κ = .51 Intra-examiner for grading of tibial translation ranged from κ = .44–.60 Inter-examiner for positive or negative findings κ = .19 Inter-examiner for grading of tibial translation κ = .02–.61

RELIABILITY OF THE CLINICAL EXAMINATION

Patellar Mediolateral Tilt

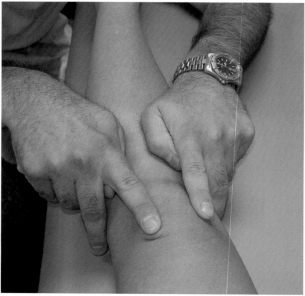

Figure 8-17: *Examination of mediolateral patellar tilt*

Test and Measure	Procedure	Determination of Positive Finding	Population	Reliability Kappa Values
Mediolateral tilt *Tomsich et al.*[21]	Examiner estimates patellar alignment while palpating medial and lateral aspects of patella	Patellar orientation graded according to an ordinal scale extending from −2 to +2, with −2 representing a lateral tilt, 0 no appreciable tilt, and +2 a medial tilt	27 asymptomatic subjects	Intra-examiner $\kappa = .57$ Inter-examiner $\kappa = .18$
Medial/lateral tilt *Fitzgerald et al.*[22]	Examiner palpates medial and lateral borders of patella with thumb and index finger	If digit palpating the medial border is higher than that palpating the lateral border, then the patella is considered laterally tilted. If digit palpating the lateral border is higher than that palpating the patella, then the patella is medially tilted	66 patients referred to PT who would normally undergo an evaluation of patellofemoral alignment	Inter-examiner $\kappa = .21$ Intra-examiner $\kappa = .28-.33$
Medial/lateral tilt *Watson et al.*[23]	Examiner attempts to palpate posterior surface of medial and lateral patellar borders	Scored 0, 1, or 2. 0 if examiner palpates posterior border on both medial and lateral sides. 1 if >50% of lateral border can be palpated but posterior surface cannot. 2 if <50% of lateral border can be palpated	56 subjects, 25 of whom had symptomatic knees	Inter-examiner $\kappa = .19$ Intra-examiner $\kappa = .44-.50$
Patellar tilt test *Watson et al.*[23]	Examiner lifts lateral edge of patella from lateral femoral epicondyle	Graded as having positive, neutral, or negative angle with respect to horizontal plane	99 knees, of which 26 were symptomatic	Inter-examiner $\kappa = .20-.35$

Patellar Mediolateral Orientation

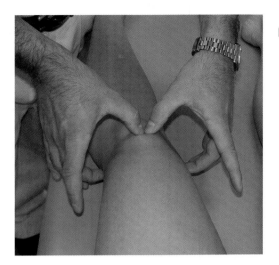

Figure 8-18: *Examination of mediolateral patellar orientation*

Test and Measure	Procedure	Determination of Positive Finding	Population	Reliability Kappa Value or ICC
Mediolateral position Tomsich et al.[24]	Examiner visually estimates patellar alignment while palpating sides of lateral epicondyles with index fingers, and patella midline with thumbs	Patellar orientation graded according to an ordinal scale extending from −2 to +2, with −2 representing a lateral displacement and +2 a medial displacement	27 asymptomatic subjects	Intra-examiner κ = .40 Inter-examiner κ = .03
Mediolateral orientation Herrington[25]	With knee supported in 20 degrees of flexion, the examiner identifies medial and lateral epicondyle of femur and midline of patella. Examiner then marks medial and lateral epicondyles and patellar midline with tape	Distances between patellar midline and medial and lateral condyles are measured	20 healthy physiotherapy students	Inter-examiner Medial distance: ICC = .91 Lateral distance: ICC = .94
Medial/lateral displacement Fitzgerald et al.[22]	Examiner palpates medial and lateral epicondyles with index fingers while simultaneously palpating midline of patella with thumbs	Distance between index fingers and thumbs should be the same. When distance to index finger palpating lateral epicondyle is less, patella is laterally displaced. When distance to index finger palpating medial epicondyle is less, patella is medially displaced	66 patients referred to PT who would normally undergo evaluation of patellofemoral alignment	Inter-examiner κ = .10
Medial/lateral glide Watson et al.[23]	Examiner uses a tape measure to record distance from medial and lateral femoral condyles to mid patella	Scored 0 or 1.0 if distance from medial epicondyle to mid patella equals distance from lateral epicondyle to mid patella. 1 if distance from medial epicondyle to mid patella is .5 cm greater than that from lateral condyle to mid patella	56 subjects, 25 of whom had symptomatic knees	Intra-examiner κ = .11–.35 Inter-examiner κ = .02

RELIABILITY OF THE CLINICAL EXAMINATION

Patellar Anterior/Posterior Tilt

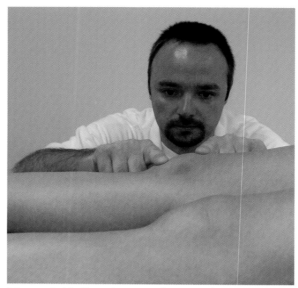

Figure 8-19: *Examination of anterior/posterior patellar tilt*

Test and Measure	Procedure	Determination of Positive Finding	Population	Reliability Kappa Values
Superoinferior tilt *Tomsich et al.*[24]	Examiner visually estimates patellar alignment while palpating superior and inferior patellar poles	Patellar orientation graded according to an ordinal scale extending from −2 to +2, with −2 representing inferior patellar pole below superior pole, and +2 representing inferior patellar pole above superior pole	27 asymptomatic subjects	Intra-examiner $\kappa = .50$ Inter-examiner $\kappa = .30$
Anterior tilt *Fitzgerald et al.*[22]	Examiner palpates inferior patellar pole	If examiner easily palpates inferior pole, no anterior tilt exists. If downward pressure on superior pole is required to palpate inferior pole, it is considered to have an anterior tilt	66 patients referred to PT who would normally undergo evaluation of patellofemoral alignment	Inter-examiner $\kappa = .24$
Anterior/posterior tilt component *Watson et al.*[23]	Examiner palpates inferior and superior patellar poles	Scored 0, 1, or 2. 0 if inferior patellar pole is as easily palpable as superior pole. 1 if inferior patellar pole is not as easily palpable as superior pole. 2 if inferior pole is not clearly palpable compared with superior pole	56 subjects, 25 of whom had symptomatic knees	Intra-examiner $\kappa = 0.03–0.23$ Inter-examiner $\kappa = .04$

Patellar Rotation

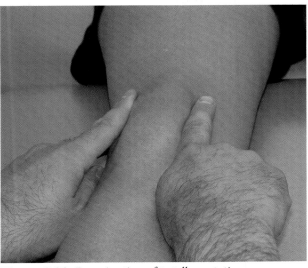

Figure 8-20: *Examination of patellar rotation*

Test and Measure	Procedure	Determination of Positive Finding	Population	Reliability Kappa Values
Rotation *Tomsich et al.*[24]	Examiner positions index fingers along longitudinal axes of patella and estimates acute angle formed	Graded according to ordinal scale extending from −2 to +2. −2 indicates that longitudinal axis of patella is more lateral than axis of femur. +2 indicates that patella is more medial than axis of femur	27 asymptomatic subjects	Intra-examiner $\kappa = .41$ Inter-examiner $\kappa = -.03$
Patellar rotation *Fitzgerald et al.*[22]		Longitudinal axis of patella should be in line with ASIS. If distal end of patella is medial, it is considered to be medially rotated. If distal end is lateral, it is considered to be laterally rotated	66 patients referred to PT who would normally undergo evaluation of patellofemoral alignment	Inter-examiner $\kappa = .36$
Patellar rotation component *Watson et al.*[23]	Examiner determines relationship between longitudinal axis of patella and femur	Scored as −1, 0, or +1. 0 when patellar long axis is parallel to long axis of femur. 1 when inferior patellar pole is lateral to axis of femur and classified as lateral patellar rotation. −1 when inferior pole is medial to axis of femur and classified as medial patellar rotation	56 subjects, 25 of whom had symptomatic knees	Intra-examiner $\kappa = -.06–.00$ Inter-examiner $\kappa = -.03$

**RELIABILITY
OF THE
CLINICAL
EXAMINATION**

Quadriceps Angle Measurements

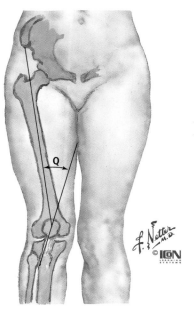

Q-angle formed by intersection of lines
from anterior superioriliac spine and from
tibial tuberosity through midpoint of
patella. Large Q-angle predisposes to
patellar subluxation

Figure 8-21: *Quadriceps angle*

Test and Measure	Procedure	Determination of Positive Finding	Population	Reliability ICC	
Q-angle *Tomsich et al.*[24]	Proximal arm of goniometer is aligned with ASIS, distal arm with tibial tubercle. Fulcrum is positioned over patellar midpoint		27 asymptomatic subjects	Intra-examiner .63 Inter-examiner .23	
Q-angle *Greene et al.*[26]	As above. Measure with knee fully extended and in 20° of flexion	Recorded to closest degree	50 asymptomatic knees	Full extension Inter-examiner	
				Right .14–.21	Left .08–.11
				20° of knee flexion Inter-examiner	
				Right .04–.08	Left .13–.16

A-Angle: The Relationship Between the Longitudinal Axis of the Patella and the Patellar Tendon

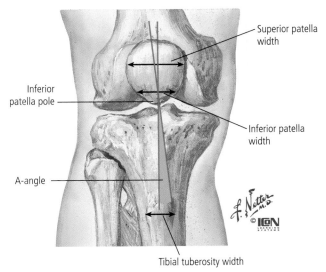

Superior patella width

Inferior patella pole

Inferior patella width

A-angle

Tibial tuberosity width

Figure 8-22: *A-angle*

Test and Measure	Procedure	Determination of Positive Finding	Population	Reliability ICC
A-angle Tomsich et al.[24]	Proximal and distal goniometer arms are aligned with middle of superior patellar pole and tibial tubercle. Fulcrum is positioned over midpoint of inferior patellar pole	Recorded in degrees	27 asymptomatic subjects	Intra-examiner .61 Inter-examiner .49
A-angle Ehrat et al.[27]	Superior patellar pole, superior patellar width, inferior patellar width, inferior patellar pole, and tibial tuberosity are identified. A-angle is then measured with a goniometer	Recorded to closest degree	36 asymptomatic subjects	Intra-examiner .20–.32 Inter-examiner −.01

Lateral Pull Test to Assess Patellar Alignment

Test and Measure	Procedure	Determination of Positive Finding	Population	Reliability Kappa Values
Lateral pull test *Watson et al.*[28]	Patient supine with knee extended. Examiner asks patient to perform isometric quadriceps contraction. Examiner observes patellar tracking during contraction	Positive if patella tracks more laterally than superiorly. Negative if superior displacement is equal to lateral displacement	99 knees, 26 of which were symptomatic	Intra-examiner $\kappa = .39–.47$ Inter-examiner $\kappa = .31$

Detecting Anterior Cruciate Ligament Ruptures

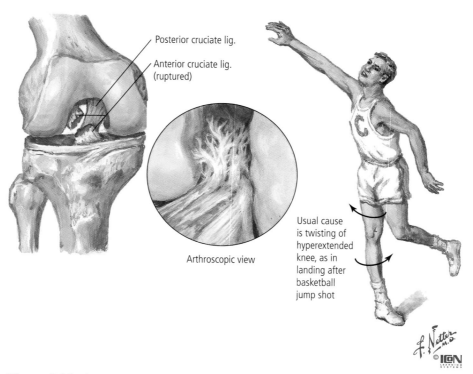

Posterior cruciate lig.

Anterior cruciate lig. (ruptured)

Arthroscopic view

Usual cause is twisting of hyperextended knee, as in landing after basketball jump shot

Figure 8-23: *Anterior cruciate ligament ruptures*

Detecting Anterior Cruciate Ligament Ruptures: The Lachman Test

See Figure 8-16.

Author	Test Procedure	Determination of Positive Finding	Population	Reference Standard	Sens	Spec	+LR	−LR
Katz et al.[29]	Patient supine. Knee joint is flexed between 10° and 20°, and femur is stabilized with one hand. Examiner uses other hand to attempt to translate tibia anteriorly	Lack of end point for tibial translation or subluxation is positive	85 patients presenting for arthroscopy to a community hospital	Arthroscopic visualization	.82	.97	27.3	.19
Kim and Kim[30]		Graded I, II, or III based on amount of anterior translation. Grade I = 5 mm, Grade II = 5–10 mm, Grade III = >1 cm	147 patients with chronic ACL injuries		.99	NR	NA	NA
Cooperman et al.[18]		Anterior tibial translation graded as 0, 1+, 2+, or 3+. 0 represents no difference between patient's knees. 1+ represents up to 5 mm of translation. 2+ represents 5–10 mm. 3+ represents >10 mm	32 patients referred to a PT clinic for evaluation of knee		.65	.42	1.12	.83
Liu et al.[31]			38 patients with arthroscopically proven ACL tears		.95 (.82, .99)	NR	NA	NA
Rubinstein et al.[32]		Increased posterior tibial displacement is positive for PCL injury	9 patients with ACL-deficient knees, 18 patients with PCL-deficient knees, and 12 subjects with normal knees	MRI confirmation	.96	1.0	NA	.04
Boeree and Ackroyd[33]	Not specified		203 patients visiting an orthopaedic clinic presenting with knee injuries	MRI	.63	.90	6.3	.41
Lee et al.[35]		Positive if anterior tibial subluxation is present	41 patients scheduled to undergo arthroscopic surgery	Arthroscopic visualization	.78	1.0	NA	.22

DIAGNOSTIC UTILITY OF THE CLINICAL EXAMINATION

Detecting Anterior Cruciate Ligament Ruptures: The Anterior Drawer Test

Test	Test Procedure	Determination of Positive Finding	Population	Reference Standard	Sens	Spec	+LR	−LR
Katz et al.[29]	Knee is flexed between 60° and 90° with foot on examination table. Examiner draws tibia anteriorly	Graded I, II, or III based on amount of anterior translation. Grade I = 5 mm, Grade II = 5–10 mm, Grade III = >1 cm	85 patients presenting for arthroscopy to a community hospital	Arthroscopic visualization	.41	.95	8.20	.62
Kim and Kim[30]			147 patients with chronic ACL injuries		.80	NR	NA	NA
Liu et al.[31]			38 patients with arthroscopically proven ACL tears		.61 (.54, .85)	NR	NA	NA
Rubinstein et al.[32]	Not specified	Increased anterior tibial displacement is positive for an ACL injury	9 patients with ACL-deficient knees, 18 patients with PCL-deficient knees, and 12 patients with normal knees	MRI confirmation	.76	.86	5.43	.28
Boeree and Ackroyd[33]			203 patients visiting an orthopaedic clinic presenting with knee injuries	MRI	.56	.92	7.0	.48
Braunstein[34]	Examiner places knee in 90° of flexion and glides tibial head anteriorly	Significant motion compared with opposite side is positive	100 consecutive knees scheduled to undergo arthroscopic surgery	Arthroscopic visualization	.91	1.0	NA	.09
Lee et al.[35]		Positive if there is anterior subluxation >5 mm	41 patients scheduled to undergo arthroscopic surgery		.78	1.0	NA	.22

LR, likelihood ratio; ACL, anterior cruciate ligament; MRI, magnetic resonance imaging; NR, not reported.

Detecting Anterior Cruciate Ligament Ruptures: The Anterior Drawer Test (cont.)

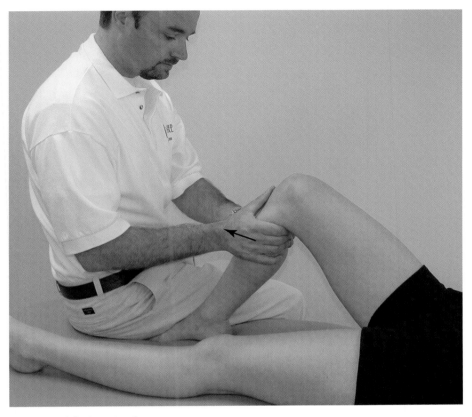

Figure 8-24: *Anterior drawer test*

DIAGNOSTIC UTILITY OF THE CLINICAL EXAMINATION

Detecting Anterior Cruciate Ligament Ruptures: Pivot Shift Test

Author	Test Procedure	Determination of Positive Finding	Population	Reference Standard	Sens	Spec	+LR	–LR
Katz et al.[29]		If lateral tibial plateau subluxes anteriorly, result is considered positive	85 patients presenting for arthroscopy to a community hospital	Arthroscopic visualization	.82	.98	41	.18
Kim and Kim[30]	Knee is placed in 10° to 20° of flexion, and tibia is rotated internally while examiner applies valgus force	Graded I, II, or III based on amount of anterior translation. Grade I = 5 mm, Grade II = 5–10 mm, Grade III = >1 cm	147 patients with chronic ACL injuries	Arthroscopic visualization	.90	NR	NA	NA
Liu et al.[31]			38 patients with arthroscopically proven ACL tears		.71 (.43, .76)	NR	NA	NA
Rubinstein et al.[32]	Not specified	Increased posterior tibial displacement is positive for PCL injury	9 patients with ACL-deficient knees, 18 patients with PCL-deficient knees, and 12 subjects with normal knees	MRI confirmation	.93	.89	8.45	.08
Boeree and Ackroyd[33]			203 patients visiting an orthopaedic clinic presenting with knee injuries	MRI	.30	.97	10	.72

Detecting Anterior Cruciate Ligament Ruptures: Pivot Shift Test (cont.)

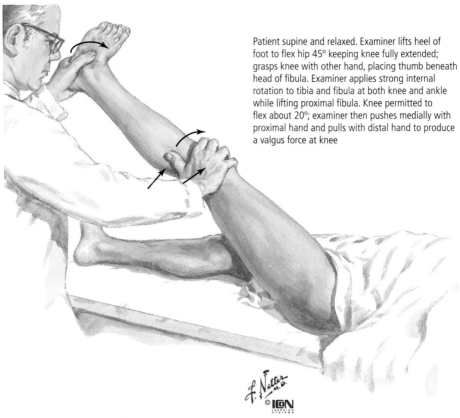

Patient supine and relaxed. Examiner lifts heel of foot to flex hip 45° keeping knee fully extended; grasps knee with other hand, placing thumb beneath head of fibula. Examiner applies strong internal rotation to tibia and fibula at both knee and ankle while lifting proximal fibula. Knee permitted to flex about 20°; examiner then pushes medially with proximal hand and pulls with distal hand to produce a valgus force at knee

Figure 8-25: *Pivot shift test*

Detecting Posterior Cruciate Ligament Ruptures: Miscellaneous Tests

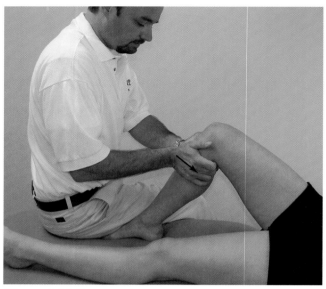

Figure 8-26: *Posterior drawer test*

Test	Test Procedure	Determination of Positive Finding	Population	Reference Standard	Sens	Spec	+LR	−LR
Posterior drawer test	NR				.90	.99	90	.10
Reverse Lachman	NR	Increased posterior tibial displacement is positive for PCL injury	9 patients with ACL-deficient knees, 18 patients with PCL-deficient knees, and 12 subjects with normal knees	MRI confirmation	.62	.89	5.64	.43
Reverse pivot shift	NR				.26	.59	.63	1.25
Posterior sagittal sign *Rubinstein et al.*[32]	NR				.79	1.0	NA	.21

Detecting Tibial Collateral Ligament Ruptures

DIAGNOSTIC UTILITY OF THE CLINICAL EXAMINATION

Usual cause is forceful impact on posterolateral aspect of knee with foot anchored, producing valgus stress on knee joint
Valgus stress may rupture tibial collateral and capsular ligaments

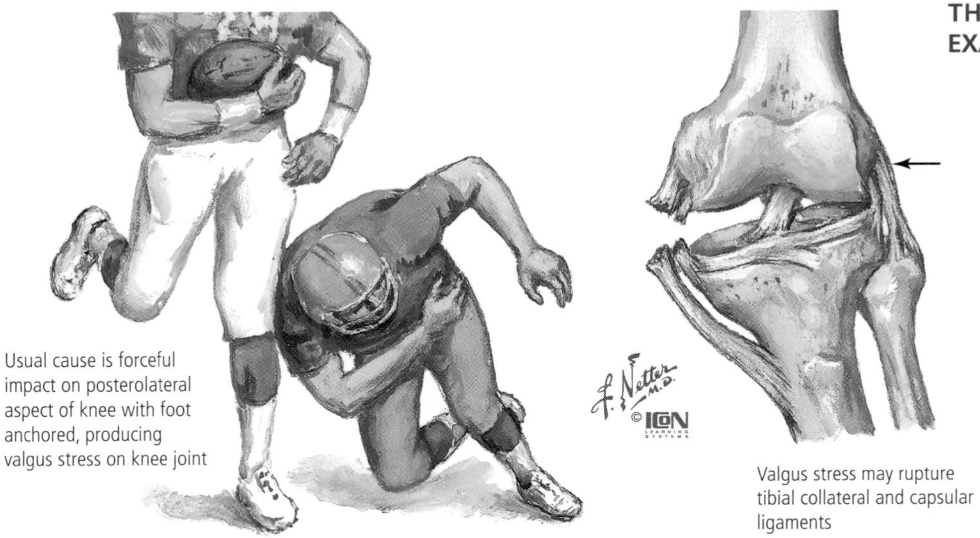

Figure 8-27: *Ruptured tibial collateral ligament*

Detecting FIbular Collateral Ligament Ruptures: Varus Stress Test

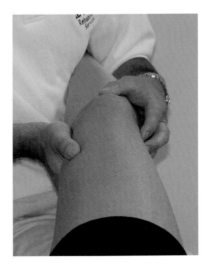

Figure 8-28: *Varus stress test*

Test	Test Procedure	Determination of Positive Findings	Population	Reference Standard	Sens	Spec	+LR	–LR
Varus stress test *Harilainen et al.*[36]	Patient supine. Examiner places patient's knee in 20° of flexion and applies a varus stress to knee	Positive if pain or laxity is present	4 patients with verified LCL tears	Arthroscopic visualization	.25	NR	NA	NA

LCL, lateral collateral ligament.

DIAGNOSTIC UTILITY OF THE CLINICAL EXAMINATION

Detecting Tibial Collateral Ligament Ruptures: Valgus Stress Test

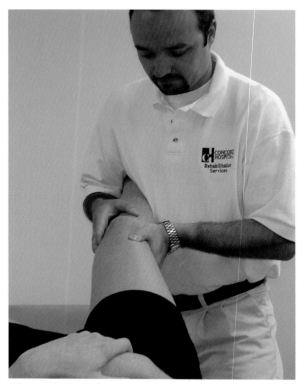

Figure 8-29: *Valgus stress test*

Test	Test Procedure	Determination of Positive Finding	Population	Reference Standard	Sens	Spec	+LR	−LR
Valgus stress test Harilainen [36]	Patient supine. Examiner places patient's knee in 20° of flexion and applies valgus stress to knee	Positive if pain or laxity is present	72 patients with verified MCL tears	Arthroscopic visualization	.86	NR	NA	NA
Valgus stress test Garvin et al. [37]	Nonstandardized physical examination	NR	Retrospective analysis of 23 patients who had undergone surgery	Surgical visualization	.96	NR	NA	NA

MCL, medial collateral ligament.

Detecting Meniscal Tears

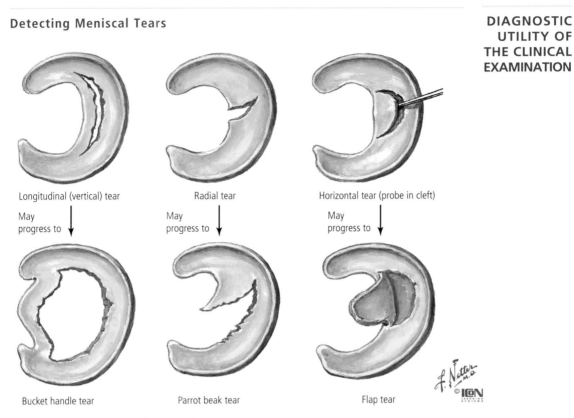

Longitudinal (vertical) tear

May
progress to ↓

Bucket handle tear

Radial tear

May
progress to ↓

Parrot beak tear

Horizontal tear (probe in cleft)

May
progress to ↓

Flap tear

Figure 8-30: *Types of meniscal tears*

DIAGNOSTIC UTILITY OF THE CLINICAL EXAMINATION

Detecting Meniscal Tears: The McMurray Test

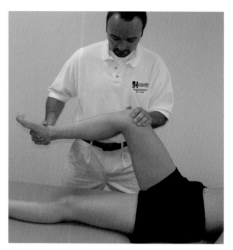

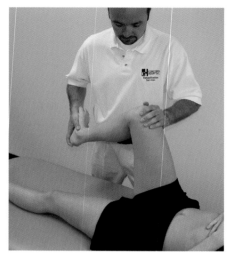

Figure 8-31A: *McMurray test with internal rotation of tibia*

Figure 8-31B: *McMurray test with external rotation of tibia*

Test	Test Procedure	Determination of Positive Findings	Population	Reference Standard	Sens	Spec	+LR	−LR
Evans et al.[38]	Examiner brings leg from extension into 90° of flexion while foot is held first in internal rotation, then in external rotation	A palpable "thud" or provocation of pain	104 knees awaiting arthroscopic surgery	Arthroscopic visualization	Medial thud			
					.16	.98	.8.0	.86
					Pain			
					.50	.94	8.33	.53
Fowler and Lubliner[39]			161 patients with knee pain undergoing arthroscopic procedure		.95	NR	NA	NA
Boeree and Ackroyd[33]			203 patients visiting an orthopaedic clinic who are presenting with knee injuries	MRI	Medial meniscus =			
					.29	.25	.39	2.84
					Lateral meniscus =			
					.25	.90	2.5	.83

Detecting Joint Line Tenderness

Test	Test Procedure	Determination of Positive Findings	Population	Reference Standard	Sens	Spec	+LR	−LR
Fowler and Lubliner [39]	Examiner palpates joint line	Positive if pain is reproduced. Graded as 1 for moderate pain and 2 for extreme pain	161 patients with knee pain undergoing arthroscopic procedure	Arthroscopic visualization	.85	.294	.1.2	.51
Eren [40]	Examiner palpates joint line with knee in 90° of flexion		104 male patients with suspected meniscal lesions scheduled to undergo arthroscopy		Medial joint line			
					.85	.67	2.61	.21
					Lateral joint line			
					.92	.97	30.67	.08
Shelbourne et al. [41]		Positive if pain is reproduced	173 patients scheduled to undergo ACL reconstruction	Surgical visualization	Medial joint line			
					.45	.35	.69	1.57
					Lateral joint line			
	Examiner palpates joint line				.58	.49	1.14	.86
Boeree and Ackroyd [83]			203 patients visiting an orthopaedic clinic who are presenting with knee injuries	MRI	Medial meniscus			
					.64	.70	2.13	.51
					Lateral meniscus			
					.28	.87	2.15	.83

Diagnosing a Meniscal Lesion: A Combination of Clinical Tests

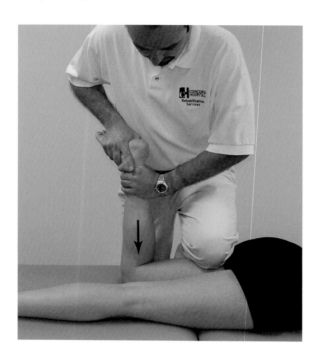

Figure 8-32: Apley grinding
test

Test	Test Procedure	Determination of Positive Finding	Population	Reference Standard	Sens	Spec	+LR	−LR
Tenderness to palpation of joint line	Examiner palpates joint line	Positive if palpation produces pain			If two tests were positive, then patient was considered to have meniscal lesion		NA	NA
Boehler test	Valgus or varus stress is applied to knee	Positive for lateral meniscus if valgus stress results in pain. Positive for medial meniscus if varus stress results in pain						
Steinmann test	Patient seated with knee in 90° of flexion. Examiner internally and externally rotates tibia	Positive if tibial rotation reproduces patient's pain	36 patients scheduled to undergo arthroscopic surgery	Arthroscopic visualization				
Apley grinding test	Patient prone with knee flexed to 90°. Examiner places downward pressure on foot, compressing knee, while internally and externally rotating tibia				.97	.87	7.46	.03
Payr test	Examiner flexes patient's knee to 90° and applies varus stress	Positive for medial meniscus tear if pain is elicited						
McMurray test Muellner et al.[7]	Knee is positioned in various degrees of flexion. Tibia is internally and externally rotated	A palpable "thud" or provocation of patient's pain						
Combined historical and physical examination Bonamo and Shulman[42]	Physical examination includes assessment of joint effusion, joint line tenderness, McMurray test, hyperflexion test, and squat test. Exact procedures for each test not defined	NR	100 consecutive patients who underwent arthroscopic surgery of knee	Arthroscopic visualization	.86	.83	5.06	.17

Managing Patients With Patellofemoral Pain Syndrome

Sutlive and colleagues[43] have identified predictor variables that identify persons with patellofemoral pain who are likely to improve with an off-the-shelf foot orthosis and modified activity. The study identified a number of predictor variables that are provided below.

Variable	Sens (95% CI)	Spec	+LR
2 or more degrees of forefoot valgus	.13 (.04, .24)	.97 (.90, 1.0)	4.0 (.7, 21.9)
78 degrees or less of great toe extension	.13 (.04, .24)	.97 (.90, 1.0)	4.0 (.7, 21.9)
3 mm or less of navicular drop	.47 (.32, .61)	.80 (.67, .93)	2.3 (1.3, 4.3)
5 degrees or less valgus, and any varus of relaxed calcaneal stance	.36 (.17, .55)	.81 (.71, .92)	1.9 (1.0, 3.6)
Tight hamstring muscles as measured by 90/90 straight-leg-raise test	.68 (.55, .80)	.56 (.37, .75)	1.5 (1.0, 2.3)
Reports of difficulty walking	.71 (.55, .86)	.48 (.33, .62)	1.4 (1.0, 1.8)

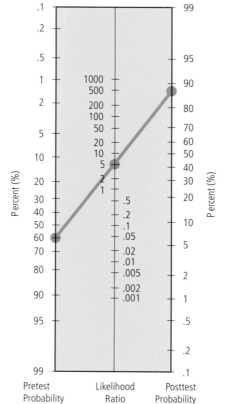

Figure 8-33: *Nomogram.* (Adapted with permission, Massachusetts Medical Society, Copyright © 2005.)

Considering a pretest probability of success of 60% (as determined in the Sutlive et al.[43] study), 2 or more degrees of forefoot valgus, or 78 or fewer degrees of great toe extension results in a posttest probability of 86%. This means that if a patient presented with one of the two aforementioned variables, the likelihood that a successful outcome would be achieved with off-the-shelf orthotics and activity modification would be 86%.

Identifying the Need to Order Radiographs After Acute Knee Trauma

Stiell and colleagues[45, 46] identified a clinical prediction rule to determine the need to order radiographs after knee trauma. If one of five variables identified were present, radiographs were required. The five variables included age ≥55 years, isolated patellar tenderness without other bone tenderness, tenderness of the fibular head, inability to bear weight immediately after injury, and inability to transfer weight onto each lower extremity (regardless of limping) in the emergency room. This rule has been validated in numerous studies in both adult[46-49] and pediatric[50, 51] populations. In the adult population, sensitivity has been shown to be 1.0, with specificity ranging from .49 to .56. Inter-examiner agreement between clinicians for identification of predictor variables exhibited a kappa value of .77, with a 95% confidence interval of .65 to .89.[46] In a group of children with a mean age of 11.8 years, Bulloch et al[51] determined a sensitivity of 1.0, with a 95% confidence interval of .95 to 1.0 and a specificity of .43, with a 95% confidence interval of .39 to .47.

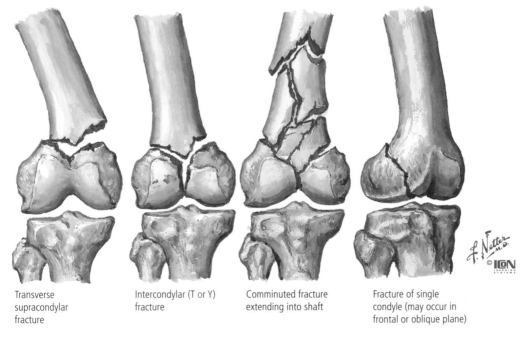

| Transverse supracondylar fracture | Intercondylar (T or Y) fracture | Comminuted fracture extending into shaft | Fracture of single condyle (may occur in frontal or oblique plane) |

Figure 8-34: *Types of fractures of the distal femur*

REFERENCES

1. Greenfield B, Tovin BJ. Knee. In: *Current Concepts in Orthopaedic Physical Therapy*. La Crosse: Orthopaedic Section, American Physical Therapy Association; 2001.
2. Hartley A. *Practical Joint Assessment*. St. Louis: Mosby; 1995.
3. DeHaven KE. Diagnosis of acute knee injuries with hemarthrosis. *Am J Sports Med*. 1980;8:9-14.
4. Cook J, Khan K, Kiss Z, Puram C, Griffiths L. Reproducibility and clinical utility of tendon palpation to detect patellar tendinopathy in young basketball players. *Br J Sports Med*. 2001;35:65-72.
5. Cleland JA, McRae M. Patellofemoral pain syndrome: a critical analysis of current concepts. *Phys Ther Rev*. 2002;7:153-161.
6. Grelsamer RP, McConnell J. *The Patella: A Team Approach*. Gaithersburg: Aspen Publishers; 1998.
7. Muellner T, Weinstabl R, Schabus R, Vecsei V, Kainberger F. The diagnosis of meniscal tears in athletes. A comparison of clinical and magnetic resonance imaging investigations. *Am J Sports Med*. 1997;25:7-12.
8. Cibere J, Bellamy N, Thorne A, et al. Reliability of the knee examination in osteoarthritis. *Arthritis Rheum*. 2004;50:458-468.
9. Jones A, Hopkinson N, Pattrick M, Berman P, Doherty M. Evaluation of a method for clinically assessing osteoarthritis of the knee. *Ann Rheum Dis*. 1992;51:243-245.
10. Rothstein JM, Miller PJ, Roettger R. Goniometric reliability in a clinical setting. Elbow and knee measurements. *Phys Ther*. 1983;63:1611-1615.
11. Gogia PP, Braatz JH, Rose S, Norton B. Reliability and validity of goniometric measurements of the knee. *Phys Ther*. 1987;67:192-195.
12. Watkins MA, Riddle DL, Lamb R, Personius W. Reliability of goniometric measurements and visual estimates of knee range of motion obtained in a clinical setting. *Phys Ther*. 1991;71:90-97.
13. Clapper MP, Wolf SL. Comparison of the reliability of the orthoranger and the standard goniometer for assessing active lower extremity range of motion. *Phys Ther*. 1988;68:215-218.
14. Brosseau L, Tousignant M, Budd J, et al. Intratester and intertester reliability and criterion validity of the parallelogram and universal goniometers for active knee flexion in healthy subjects. *Physiother Res Int*. 1997;2:150-166.
15. Hayes KW, Petersen C, Falconer J. An examination of Cyriax's passive motion tests with patients having osteoarthritis of the knee. *Phys Ther*. 1994;74:697-709.
16. Fritz JM, Delitto A, Erhard RE, Roman M. An examination of the selective tissue tension scheme, with evidence for the concept of a capsular of the knee. *Phys Ther*. 1998;78:1046-1061.
17. Hayes KW, Petersen CM. Reliability of assessing end-feel and pain and resistance sequence in subjects with painful shoulders and knees. *J Orthop Sports Phys Ther*. 2001;31:432-445.
18. Cooperman JM, Riddle DL, Rothstein J. Reliability and validity of judgments of the integrity of the anterior cruciate ligament of the knee using the Lachman test. *Phys Ther*. 1990;70:225-233.
19. McClure PW, Rothstein JM, Riddle D. Intertester reliability of clinical judgments of medial knee ligament integrity. *Phys Ther*. 1989;69:268-275.
20. Dervin GF, Stiell IG, Wells GA, Rody K, Grabowski J. Physicians' accuracy and interrater reliability for the diagnosis of unstable meniscal tears in patients having osteoarthritis of the knee. *Can J Surg*. 2001;44:267-274.
21. Mitchell J, McKay A. Comparison of left and right vertebral artery intracranial diameters. *Anat Rec*. 1995;242:350-354.

22. Fitzgerald GK, McClure PW. Reliability of measurements obtained with four tests for patellofemoral alignment. *Phys Ther.* 1995;75:84-92.

23. Watson CJ, Propps M, Galt W, Redding A, Dobbs D. Reliability of McConnell's classification of patellar orientation in symptomatic and asymptomatic subjects. *J Orthop Sports Phys Ther.* 1999;29:378-393.

24. Tomsich DA, Nitz AJ, Threlkeld AJ, Shapiro R. Patellofemoral alignment: reliability. *J Orthop Sports Phys Ther.* 1996;23:200-208.

25. Herrington LC. The inter-tester reliability of a clinical measurement used to determine the medial/lateral orientation of the patella. *Man Ther.* 2000;7:163-167.

26. Greene CC, Edwards TB, Wade MR, Carson EW. Reliability of the quadriceps angle measurement. *Am J Knee Surg.* 2001;14:97-103.

27. Ehrat M, Edwards J, Hastings D, Worrell T. Reliability of assessing patellar alignment: the A angle. *J Orthop Sports Phys Ther.* 1994;19:22-27.

28. Watson CJ, Leddy HM, Dynjan TD, Parham JL. Reliability of the lateral pull test and tilt test to assess patellar alignment in subjects with symptomatic knees: student raters. *J Orthop Sports Phys Ther.* 2001;31:368-374.

29. Katz JW, Fingeroth RJ. The diagnostic accuracy of ruptures of the anterior cruciate ligament comparing the Lachman test, the anterior drawer sign, and the pivot shift test in acute and chronic knee injuries. *Am J Sports Med.* 1986;14:88-91.

30. Kim SJ, Kim HK. Reliability of the anterior drawer test, the pivot shift test, and the Lachman test. *Clin Orthop.* 1995;317:237-242.

31. Liu SH, Osti L, Henry M, Bocchi L. The diagnosis of acute complete tears of the anterior cruciate ligament. *J Bone Joint Surg Br.* 1995;77:586-588.

32. Rubinstein RA Jr, Shelbourne KD, McCarroll JR, VanMeter CD, Rettig AC. The accuracy of the clinical examination in the setting of posterior cruciate ligament injuries. *Am J Sports Med.* 1994;22:550-557.

33. Boeree NR, Ackroyd CE. Assessment of the menisci and cruciate ligaments: an audit of clinical practice. *Injury.* 1991;22:291-294.

34. Braunstein EM. Anterior cruciate ligament injuries: a comparison of arthrographic and physical diagnosis. *Am J Roentgenol.* 1982;138:423-425.

35. Lee JK, Yao L, Phelps CT, Wirth CR, Czajka J, Lozman J. Anterior cruciate ligament tears: MR imaging compared with arthroscopy and clinical tests. *Radiology.* 1988;166:861-864.

36. Harilainen A. Evaluation of knee instability in acute ligamentous injuries. *Ann Chir Gynaecol.* 1987;76:269-273.

37. Garvin GJ, Munk P, Vellet A. Tears of the medial collateral ligament: magnetic resonance imaging findings and associated injuries. *Can Assoc Radiol J.* 1993;44:199-204.

38. Evans PJ, Bell GD, Frank C. Prospective evaluation of the McMurray test. *Am J Sports Med.* 1993;21:604-608.

39. Fowler PJ, Lubliner JA. The predictive value of 5 clinical signs in the evaluation of meniscal pathology. *Arthroscopy.* 1989;5:184-186.

40. Eren OT. The accuracy of joint line tenderness by physical examination in the diagnosis of meniscal tears. *Arthroscopy.* 2003;19:850-854.

41. Shelbourne KD, Martini DJ, McCarroll JR, VanMeter CD. Correlation of joint line tenderness and meniscal lesions in patients with acute anterior cruciate ligament tears. *Am J Sports Med.* 1995;23:166-169.

42. Bonamo JJ, Shulman G. Double contrast arthrography of the knee. A comparison to clinical diagnosis and arthroscopic finding. *Orthopedics.* 1988;11:1041-1046.

REFERENCES

43. Sutlive TG, Mitchell SD, Maxfield SN, et al. Identification of individuals with patellofemoral pain whose symptoms improved after a combined program of foot orthosis use and modified activity: a preliminary investigation. *Phys Ther.* 2004;84:49-61.

44. Petrone MR, Guinn J, Reddin A, Sutlive TG, Flynn TW, Garber MP. The accuracy of the Palpation Meter (PALM) for measuring pelvic crest height difference and leg length discrepancy. *J Orthop Sports Phys Ther.* 2003;33:319-325.

45. Stiell IG, Greenberg GH, Wells GA, et al. Derivation of a decision rule for the use of radiography in acute knee injuries. *Ann Emerg Med.* 1995;26:405-413.

46. Stiell IG, Wells GA, Hoag RH, et al. Implementation of the Ottawa Knee Rule for the use of radiography in acute knee injuries. *JAMA.* 1997;278:2075-2079.

47. Bachmann LM, Haberzeth S, Steurer J, ter Riet G. The accuracy of the Ottawa knee rule to rule out knee fractures: a systematic review. *Ann Intern Med.* 2004;140:121-124.

48. Ketelslegers E, Collard X, Vande Berg B, et al. Validation of the Ottawa Knee Rules in an emergency teaching center. *Eur Radiol.* 2002;12:1218-1220.

49. Emparanza JI, Aginaga JR, Estudio Multicentro en Urgencias de Osakidetza. Reglas de Ottawa (EMUORO) Group. Validation of the Ottawa Knee Rules. *Ann Emerg Med.* 2001;38:364-368.

50. Khine H, Dorfman DH, Avner JR. Applicability of Ottawa Knee Rule for knee injury in children. *Pediatr Emerg Care.* 2001;17:401-404.

51. Bulloch B, Neto G, Plint A, et al. Validation of the Ottowa Knee Rule in children: a multicenter study. *Ann Emerg Med.* 2003;42:48-55.

Foot and Ankle

Chapter 9

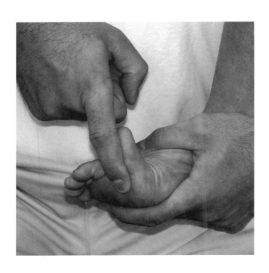

ANATOMY   Bones of Foot

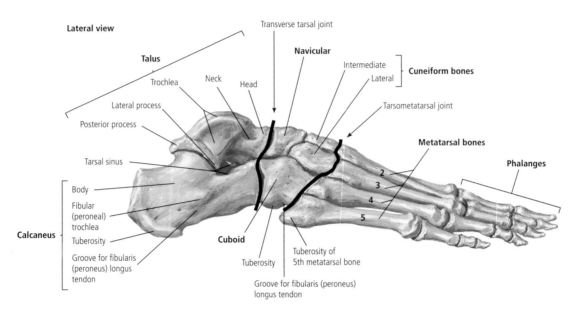

Lateral view

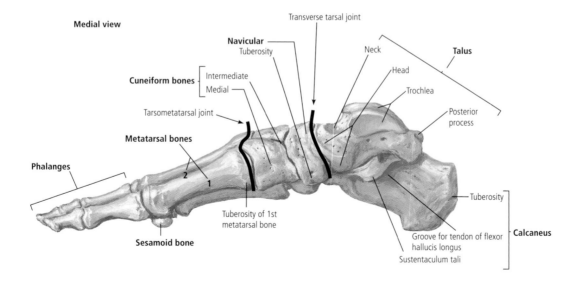

Medial view

Figure 9-1

Ankle

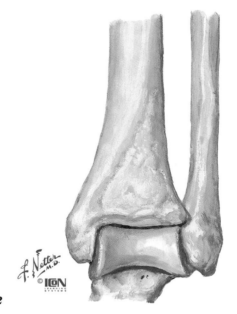

Figure 9-2

Joint	Type and Classification	Closed Packed Position	Capsular Pattern
Talocrural	Hinge synovial	Dorsiflexion	Plantarflexion slightly more limited than dorsiflexion
Distal tibiofibular	Syndesmosis	NA	NA

NA, not available.

Foot and Ankle

Joint	Type and Classification	Closed Packed Position	Capsular Pattern
Subtalar	Synovial: plane	Supination	Inversion greatly restricted; eversion not restricted
Talocalcaneonavicular	Synovial: plane	Supination	Supination more limited than pronation
Calcaneocuboid	Synovial: plane	Supination	
Transverse tarsal	Synovial: plane	Supination	
Tarsometatarsal	Synovial: plane	Supination	NA
MTP	Synovial: condyloid	Extension	Great toe: extension more limited than flexion MTP joints 2–5: variable
IP	Synovial: hinge	Extension	Extension more limited than flexion

MTP, metatarsophalangeal; IP, interphalangeal.

ARTHROLOGY Foot

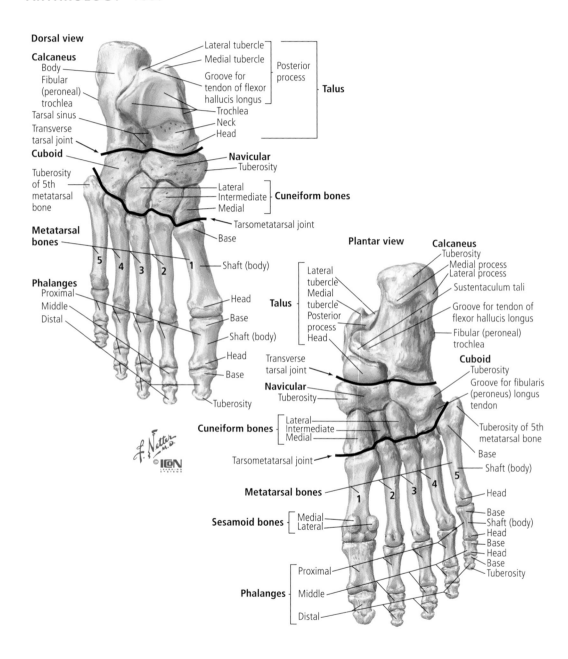

Dorsal view

Calcaneus
  Body
  Fibular (peroneal) trochlea
Tarsal sinus
Transverse tarsal joint
Cuboid
Tuberosity of 5th metatarsal bone
Metatarsal bones
  5 4 3 2 1
Phalanges
  Proximal
  Middle
  Distal

Lateral tubercle
Medial tubercle
Groove for tendon of flexor hallucis longus
Trochlea
Neck
Head
} Posterior process
} **Talus**

Navicular
  Tuberosity
Lateral
Intermediate
Medial
} **Cuneiform bones**
Tarsometatarsal joint
Base
Shaft (body)

Head
Base
Shaft (body)
Head
Base
Tuberosity

Talus

Plantar view

Lateral tubercle
Medial tubercle
Posterior process
Head

Transverse tarsal joint
Navicular
  Tuberosity
Cuneiform bones
  Lateral
  Intermediate
  Medial
Tarsometatarsal joint
Metatarsal bones
  1 2 3 4 5
Sesamoid bones
  Medial
  Lateral
Phalanges
  Proximal
  Middle
  Distal

Calcaneus
  Tuberosity
  Medial process
  Lateral process
  Sustentaculum tali
Groove for tendon of flexor hallucis longus
Fibular (peroneal) trochlea
Cuboid
  Tuberosity
  Groove for fibularis (peroneus) longus tendon
Tuberosity of 5th metatarsal bone
Base
Shaft (body)
Head
Base
Shaft (body)
Head
Base
Head
Base
Tuberosity

F. Netter M.D.
©ICON
LEARNING SYSTEMS

Figure 9-3

Posterior Ankle

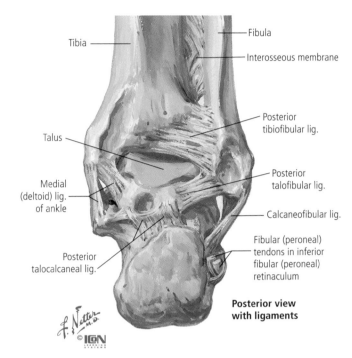

Tibia

Fibula

Interosseous membrane

Posterior tibiofibular lig.

Talus

Posterior talofibular lig.

Medial (deltoid) lig. of ankle

Calcaneofibular lig.

Posterior talocalcaneal lig.

Fibular (peroneal) tendons in inferior fibular (peroneal) retinaculum

Posterior view with ligaments

Figure 9-4

Ligaments	Attachments	Function
Posterior talocalcaneal	Superior body of calcaneus to posterior process of talus	Limit posterior separation of talus from calcaneus
Posterior tibiofibular	Distal posterior tibia to distal posterior fibula	Maintain distal tibiofibular joint
Posterior talofibular	Posterior talus to posterior lateral malleolus	Limit separation of fibula from talus
Interosseous membrane	Continuous connection between tibia and fibula	Reinforce approximation between tibia and fibula

LIGAMENTS   Lateral Ligaments of Ankle

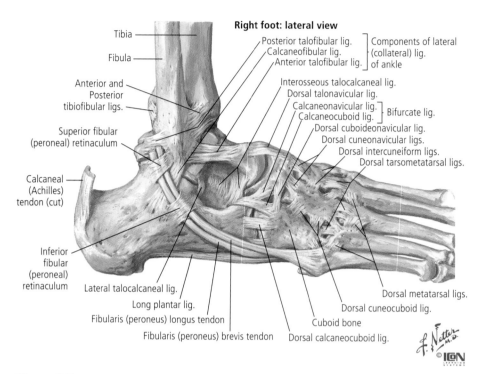

Right foot: lateral view

Tibia

Fibula

Anterior and Posterior tibiofibular ligs.

Superior fibular (peroneal) retinaculum

Calcaneal (Achilles) tendon (cut)

Inferior fibular (peroneal) retinaculum

Lateral talocalcaneal lig.

Long plantar lig.

Fibularis (peroneus) longus tendon

Fibularis (peroneus) brevis tendon

Posterior talofibular lig.
Calcaneofibular lig.
Anterior talofibular lig. ⎤ Components of lateral (collateral) lig. of ankle

Interosseous talocalcaneal lig.
Dorsal talonavicular lig.
Calcaneonavicular lig. ⎤ Bifurcate lig.
Calcaneocuboid lig. ⎦
Dorsal cuboideonavicular lig.
Dorsal cuneonavicular ligs.
Dorsal intercuneiform ligs.
Dorsal tarsometatarsal ligs.

Dorsal metatarsal ligs.
Dorsal cuneocuboid lig.
Cuboid bone
Dorsal calcaneocuboid lig.

Figure 9-5

Ligaments		Attachments	Function
Anterior tibiofibular		Anterior aspect of lateral malleolus to inferior border of medial tibia	Reinforce anterior tibiofibular joint
Lateral collateral	Posterior talofibular	Lateral malleolus talus to lateral	Limit ankle inversion
	Calcaneofibular	Lateral malleolus to lateral calcaneus talus	
	Anterior talofibular	Lateral malleolus to talus	
Interosseous talocalcaneal		Inferior aspect of talus to superior aspect of calcaneus	Limit separation of talus from calcaneus
Dorsal talonavicular		Dorsal aspect of talus to dorsal aspect of navicular	Limit separation of navaicular from talus
Bifurcate	Calcaneonavicular	Distal calcaneus to proximal navicular	Limit separation of navicular and cuboid calcaneus
	Calcaneocuboid	Distal calcaneus to proximal cuboid	
Dorsal cubonavicular		Lateral aspect of cuboid to dorsal aspect of navicular	Limit separation of navicular from cuboid
Dorsal cuneonavicular		Navicular to three cuneiforms	Limit separation of cuneiforms from navicular
Dorsal intercuneiform		Joining of three cuneiforms	Limit separation of cuneiforms
Dorsal tarsometatarsal		Dorsal tarsal bones to corresponding metatarsal bones	Reinforce tarsometatarsal joints

Medial Ligaments of Ankle

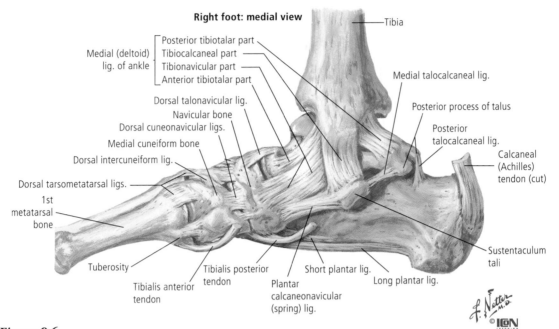

Right foot: medial view

Tibia

Medial (deltoid) lig. of ankle
- Posterior tibiotalar part
- Tibiocalcaneal part
- Tibionavicular part
- Anterior tibiotalar part

Medial talocalcaneal lig.

Dorsal talonavicular lig.

Navicular bone

Dorsal cuneonavicular ligs.

Medial cuneiform bone

Dorsal intercuneiform lig.

Dorsal tarsometatarsal ligs.

1st metatarsal bone

Posterior process of talus

Posterior talocalcaneal lig.

Calcaneal (Achilles) tendon (cut)

Sustentaculum tali

Tuberosity

Tibialis anterior tendon

Tibialis posterior tendon

Plantar calcaneonavicular (spring) lig.

Short plantar lig.

Long plantar lig.

Figure 9-6

Ligaments		Attachments	Function
Medial (deltoid)	Posterior tibiotalar	Medial malleolus to medial talus	Limit ankle eversion
	Tibiocalcaneal	Anterior distal medial malleolus to sustentaculum tali	
	Tibionavicular	Medial malleolus to proximal aspect of navicular	
	Anterior tibiotalar	Medial malleolus to talus	
Medial talocalcaneal		Sustentaculum tali to talus	Limit posterior separation of talus on calcaneus
Plantar calcaneonavicular (spring)		Sustentaculum tali to posteroinferior navicular	Maintain longitudinal arch of foot

LIGAMENTS

Plantar Ligaments of Foot

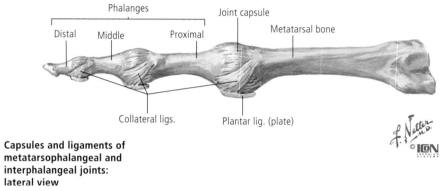

Capsules and ligaments of metatarsophalangeal and interphalangeal joints: lateral view
Figure 9-7

Ligaments	Attachments	Function
Long plantar	Plantar of calcaneus to cuboid	Support arches of foot
Plantar calcaneocuboid (short plantar)	Anteroinferior aspect of calcaneus to inferior aspect of cuboid	Support arches of foot
Plantar calcaneonavicular (spring)	Sustentaculum tali to posteroinferior aspect of talus	Support longitudinal arch of foot
Plantar cubonavicular	Inferior navicular to inferomedial cuboid	Limit separation of cuboid from navicular and support arch
Plantar tarsometatarsal	Connect metatarsals 1–5 to corresponding tarsal on plantar aspect	Limit separation of metatarsals from corresponding tarsal bones
Collateral	Distal aspect of proximal phalanx to proximal aspect of distal phalanx	Reinforce capsule of IP joints
Plantar plate	Thickening of plantar aspect of joint capsule	Reinforce plantar aspect of IP joint
Deep transverse metatarsal	MTP joints on plantar aspect	Limit separation of MTP joints

Plantar Ligaments of Foot (cont.)

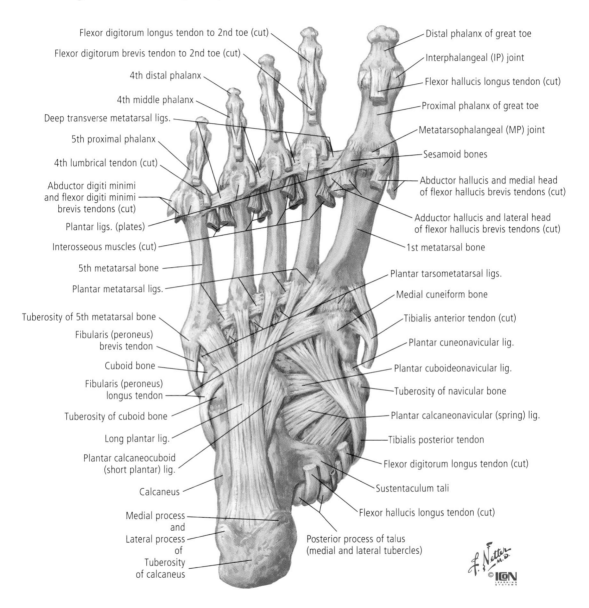

Flexor digitorum longus tendon to 2nd toe (cut)

Flexor digitorum brevis tendon to 2nd toe (cut)

4th distal phalanx

4th middle phalanx

Deep transverse metatarsal ligs.

5th proximal phalanx

4th lumbrical tendon (cut)

Abductor digiti minimi and flexor digiti minimi brevis tendons (cut)

Plantar ligs. (plates)

Interosseous muscles (cut)

5th metatarsal bone

Plantar metatarsal ligs.

Tuberosity of 5th metatarsal bone

Fibularis (peroneus) brevis tendon

Cuboid bone

Fibularis (peroneus) longus tendon

Tuberosity of cuboid bone

Long plantar lig.

Plantar calcaneocuboid (short plantar) lig.

Calcaneus

Medial process and Lateral process of Tuberosity of calcaneus

Distal phalanx of great toe

Interphalangeal (IP) joint

Flexor hallucis longus tendon (cut)

Proximal phalanx of great toe

Metatarsophalangeal (MP) joint

Sesamoid bones

Abductor hallucis and medial head of flexor hallucis brevis tendons (cut)

Adductor hallucis and lateral head of flexor hallucis brevis tendons (cut)

1st metatarsal bone

Plantar tarsometatarsal ligs.

Medial cuneiform bone

Tibialis anterior tendon (cut)

Plantar cuneonavicular lig.

Plantar cuboideonavicular lig.

Tuberosity of navicular bone

Plantar calcaneonavicular (spring) lig.

Tibialis posterior tendon

Flexor digitorum longus tendon (cut)

Sustentaculum tali

Flexor hallucis longus tendon (cut)

Posterior process of talus (medial and lateral tubercles)

Figure 9-7 (cont.)

MUSCLES   Lateral Muscles of Leg

Muscles	Proximal Attachments	Distal Attachments	Nerve and Segmental Level	Action
Gastrocnemius	Lateral head: lateral femoral condyle Medial head: popliteal surface of femur	Posterior aspect of calcaneus	Tibial nerve (S1, S2)	Plantarflex ankle and flex knee
Soleus	Posterior aspect of head of fibula, fibular soleal line, and medial aspect of tibia	Posterior aspect of calcaneus	(S1, S2)	Plantarflex ankle
Fibularis longus	Superolateral surface of fibula	Base of 1st metatarsal and medial cuneiform	Superficial fibular nerve (L5, S1, S2)	Evert foot and assist in plantarflexion
Fibularis brevis	Distal aspect of fibula	Tuberosity of base of 5th metatarsal	Superficial fibular nerve (L5, S1, S2)	Evert foot and assist in plantarflexion
Fibularis tertius	Anteroinferior aspect of fibula and interosseous membrane	Base of 5th metatarsal	Deep fibular nerve (L5, S1)	Dorsiflex ankle and evert foot
Extensor digitorum longus	Lateral condyle of tibia, medial surface of fibula	Middle and distal phalanges of digits 2–5	Deep fibular nerve (L5, S1)	Extend digits 2–5 and assist with ankle dorsiflexion
Extensor hallucis longus	Anterior fibula and interosseous membrane	Dorsal base of distal phalanx of great toe	Deep fibular nerve (L5, S1)	Extend great toe and assist with ankle dorsiflexion
Extensor digitorum brevis	Superolateral aspect of calcaneus, extensor retinaculum	Dorsal base of middle phalanx of digits 2–5	Deep fibular nerve (L5, S1)	Extend digits 2–4 at MTP joints
Tibialis anterior	Lateral condyle and anterior surface of tibia	Inferomedial aspect of medial cuneiform and base of 5th metatarsal	Deep fibular nerve (L4, L5)	Dorsiflex ankle and invert foot

Lateral Muscles of Leg (cont.)

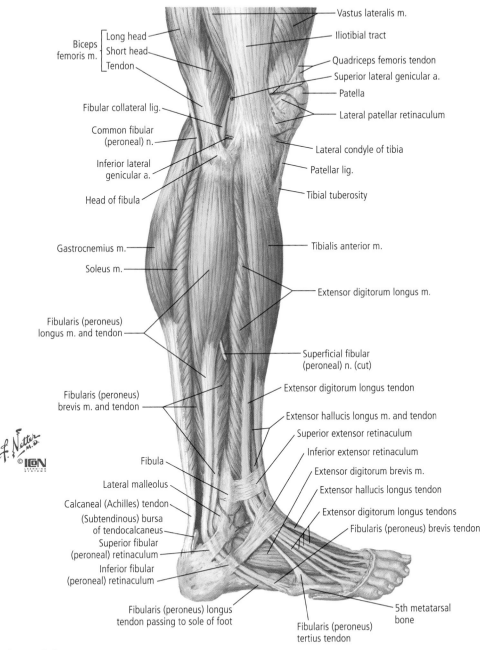

Vastus lateralis m.

Iliotibial tract

Quadriceps femoris tendon

Superior lateral genicular a.

Patella

Lateral patellar retinaculum

Lateral condyle of tibia

Patellar lig.

Tibial tuberosity

Tibialis anterior m.

Extensor digitorum longus m.

Superficial fibular (peroneal) n. (cut)

Extensor digitorum longus tendon

Extensor hallucis longus m. and tendon

Superior extensor retinaculum

Inferior extensor retinaculum

Extensor digitorum brevis m.

Extensor hallucis longus tendon

Extensor digitorum longus tendons

Fibularis (peroneus) brevis tendon

5th metatarsal bone

Fibularis (peroneus) tertius tendon

Biceps femoris m.
- Long head
- Short head
- Tendon

Fibular collateral lig.

Common fibular (peroneal) n.

Inferior lateral genicular a.

Head of fibula

Gastrocnemius m.

Soleus m.

Fibularis (peroneus) longus m. and tendon

Fibularis (peroneus) brevis m. and tendon

Fibula

Lateral malleolus

Calcaneal (Achilles) tendon

(Subtendinous) bursa of tendocalcaneus

Superior fibular (peroneal) retinaculum

Inferior fibular (peroneal) retinaculum

Fibularis (peroneus) longus tendon passing to sole of foot

Figure 9-8

MUSCLES   **Posterior Muscles of Leg**

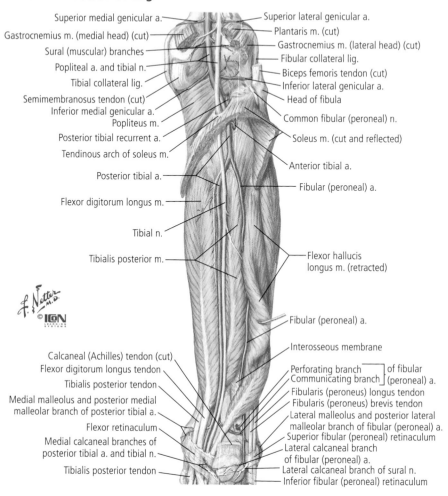

Figure 9-9

Muscles	Proximal Attachments	Distal Attachments	Nerve and Segmental Level	Action
Tibialis posterior	Interosseous membrane, posteroinferior aspect of tibia, and posterior fibula	Navicular tuberosity, cuneiform, cuboid, and bases of metatarsals 2–4	Tibial nerve (L4, L5)	Plantarflex ankle and invert foot
Flexor hallucis longus	Posteroinferior fibula and interosseous membrane	Base of distal phalanx of great toe	Tibial nerve (S2, S3)	Flex great toe and assist with ankle plantarflexion
Flexor digitorum longus	Posteroinferior tibia	Bases of distal phalanges 2–5	Tibial nerve (S2, S3)	Flex lateral four digits, plantarflex ankle, and support longitudinal arch of foot

Dorsum of Foot

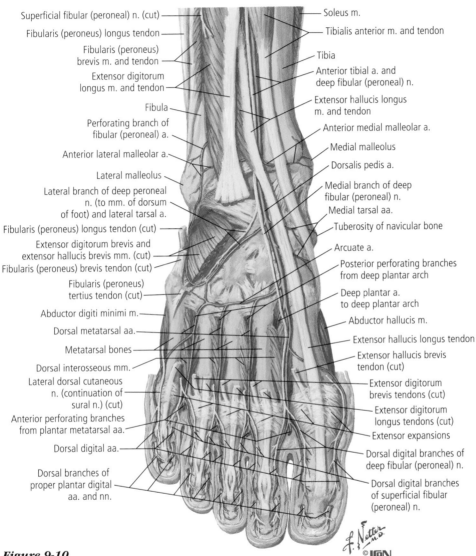

Superficial fibular (peroneal) n. (cut)
Fibularis (peroneus) longus tendon
Fibularis (peroneus) brevis m. and tendon
Extensor digitorum longus m. and tendon
Fibula
Perforating branch of fibular (peroneal) a.
Anterior lateral malleolar a.
Lateral malleolus
Lateral branch of deep peroneal n. (to mm. of dorsum of foot) and lateral tarsal a.
Fibularis (peroneus) longus tendon (cut)
Extensor digitorum brevis and extensor hallucis brevis mm. (cut)
Fibularis (peroneus) brevis tendon (cut)
Fibularis (peroneus) tertius tendon (cut)
Abductor digiti minimi m.
Dorsal metatarsal aa.
Metatarsal bones
Dorsal interosseous mm.
Lateral dorsal cutaneous n. (continuation of sural n.) (cut)
Anterior perforating branches from plantar metatarsal aa.
Dorsal digital aa.
Dorsal branches of proper plantar digital aa. and nn.

Soleus m.
Tibialis anterior m. and tendon
Tibia
Anterior tibial a. and deep fibular (peroneal) n.
Extensor hallucis longus m. and tendon
Anterior medial malleolar a.
Medial malleolus
Dorsalis pedis a.
Medial branch of deep fibular (peroneal) n.
Medial tarsal aa.
Tuberosity of navicular bone
Arcuate a.
Posterior perforating branches from deep plantar arch
Deep plantar a. to deep plantar arch
Abductor hallucis m.
Extensor hallucis longus tendon
Extensor hallucis brevis tendon (cut)
Extensor digitorum brevis tendons (cut)
Extensor digitorum longus tendons (cut)
Extensor expansions
Dorsal digital branches of deep fibular (peroneal) n.
Dorsal digital branches of superficial fibular (peroneal) n.

Figure 9-10

Muscles	Proximal Attachments	Distal Attachments	Nerve and Segmental Level	Action
Extensor digitorum brevis	Superolateral aspect of calcaneus and extensor retinaculum	Dorsal base of middle phalanx of digits 2–5	Deep fibular nerve (L5, S1)	Extend digits 2–4 at MTP joints
Extensor hallucis brevis	Superolateral aspect of calcaneus and extensor retinaculum	Dorsal base of proximal phalanx of great toe	Deep fibular nerve (L5, S1)	Extend great toe at MTP joints
Dorsal interossei	Sides of metatarsals 1–5	1st: medial aspect of proximal phalanx of 2nd digit; 2nd–4th: lateral aspect of digits 2–4	Lateral plantar nerve (S2, S3)	Abduct digits 2–4 and flex MTP joints

MUSCLES   Muscles of Sole of Foot, First Layer

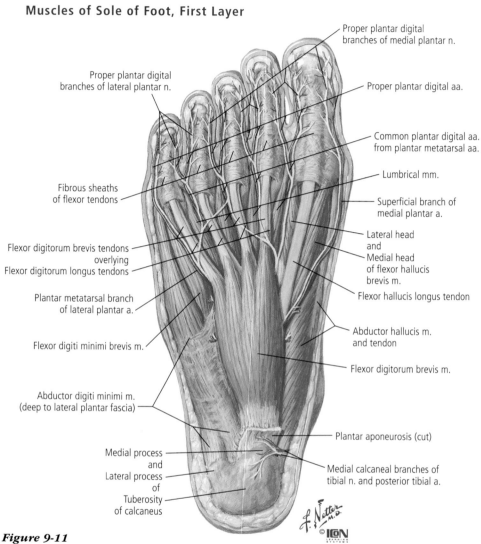

Figure 9-11

Muscles	Proximal Attachments	Distal Attachments	Nerve and Segmental Level	Action
First Layer				
Abductor hallucis longus	Medial calcaneal tuberosity, flexor retinaculum, and plantar aponeurosis	Base of proximal phalanx of 1st digit	Medial plantar nerve (S2, S3)	Abduct and flex great toe
Flexor digitorum brevis	Medial calcaneal tuberosity and plantar aponeurosis	Sides of middle phalanges of digits 2–5	Medial plantar nerve (S2, S3)	Flex digits 2–4
Abductor digiti minimi	Medial and lateral calcaneal tuberosities	Lateral aspect of base of proximal phalanx of 5th metatarsal	Lateral plantar nerve (S2, S3)	Abduct and flex 5th digit

Muscles of Sole of Foot, Second Layer

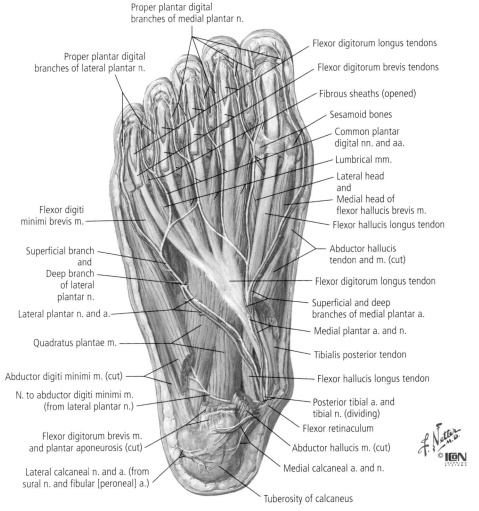

Proper plantar digital
branches of medial plantar n.

Proper plantar digital
branches of lateral plantar n.

Flexor digiti
minimi brevis m.

Superficial branch
and
Deep branch
of lateral
plantar n.

Lateral plantar n. and a.

Quadratus plantae m.

Abductor digiti minimi m. (cut)

N. to abductor digiti minimi m.
(from lateral plantar n.)

Flexor digitorum brevis m.
and plantar aponeurosis (cut)

Lateral calcaneal n. and a. (from
sural n. and fibular [peroneal] a.)

Flexor digitorum longus tendons

Flexor digitorum brevis tendons

Fibrous sheaths (opened)

Sesamoid bones

Common plantar
digital nn. and aa.

Lumbrical mm.

Lateral head
and
Medial head of
flexor hallucis brevis m.

Flexor hallucis longus tendon

Abductor hallucis
tendon and m. (cut)

Flexor digitorum longus tendon

Superficial and deep
branches of medial plantar a.

Medial plantar a. and n.

Tibialis posterior tendon

Flexor hallucis longus tendon

Posterior tibial a. and
tibial n. (dividing)

Flexor retinaculum

Abductor hallucis m. (cut)

Medial calcaneal a. and n.

Tuberosity of calcaneus

Figure 9-12

Muscles	Proximal Attachments	Distal Attachments	Nerve and Segmental Level	Action
Second Layer				
Lumbricals	Tendons of flexor digitorum longus	Medial aspect of expansion over lateral four digits	Lateral three: lateral plantar nerve (S2, S3) Medial one: medial plantar nerve (S2, S3)	Flex proximal phalanges and extend middle and distal phalanges of digits 2–5
Quadratus plantae	Medial and plantar aspects of calcaneus	Posterolateral aspect of tendon of flexor digitorum longus	Lateral plantar nerve (S2, S3)	Assist in flexing digits 2–5

MUSCLES

Muscles of Sole of Foot, Third Layer

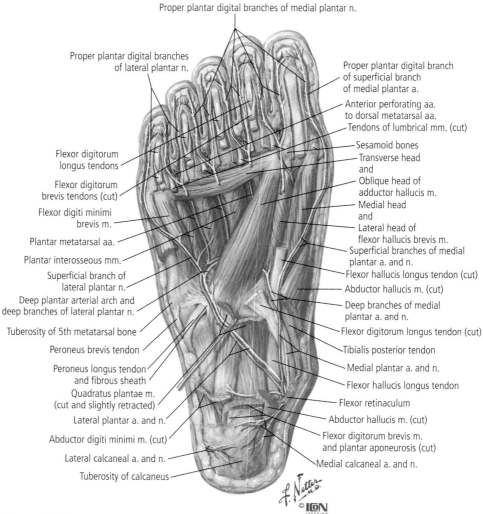

Proper plantar digital branches of medial plantar n.

Proper plantar digital branches of lateral plantar n.

Proper plantar digital branch of superficial branch of medial plantar a.

Anterior perforating aa. to dorsal metatarsal aa.

Tendons of lumbrical mm. (cut)

Sesamoid bones

Transverse head and

Oblique head of adductor hallucis m.

Medial head and

Lateral head of flexor hallucis brevis m.

Superficial branches of medial plantar a. and n.

Flexor hallucis longus tendon (cut)

Abductor hallucis m. (cut)

Deep branches of medial plantar a. and n.

Flexor digitorum longus tendon (cut)

Tibialis posterior tendon

Medial plantar a. and n.

Flexor hallucis longus tendon

Flexor retinaculum

Abductor hallucis m. (cut)

Flexor digitorum brevis m. and plantar aponeurosis (cut)

Medial calcaneal a. and n.

Flexor digitorum longus tendons

Flexor digitorum brevis tendons (cut)

Flexor digiti minimi brevis m.

Plantar metatarsal aa.

Plantar interosseous mm.

Superficial branch of lateral plantar n.

Deep plantar arterial arch and deep branches of lateral plantar n.

Tuberosity of 5th metatarsal bone

Peroneus brevis tendon

Peroneus longus tendon and fibrous sheath

Quadratus plantae m. (cut and slightly retracted)

Lateral plantar a. and n.

Abductor digiti minimi m. (cut)

Lateral calcaneal a. and n.

Tuberosity of calcaneus

Figure 9-13

Muscles		Proximal Attachments	Distal Attachments	Nerve and Segmental Level	Action
Third Layer					
Flexor digiti minimi brevis		Base of 5th metatarsal	Base of proximal phalanx of 5th toe	Superficial branch of lateral plantar nerve	Flex proximal phalanx of 5th digit
Adductor hallucis	Transverse head	Plantar ligaments of MTP joints	Lateral base of proximal phalanx of great toe	Deep branch of lateral plantar nerve (S2, S3)	Adduct great toe
	Oblique head	Bases of metatarsals 2–4			
Flexor hallucis brevis		Plantar cuboid and lateral cuneiforms	Sides of proximal phalanx of great toe	Medial plantar nerve (S2, S3)	Flex proximal phalanx of great toe

Interosseous Muscles of Sole of Foot

Dorsal view

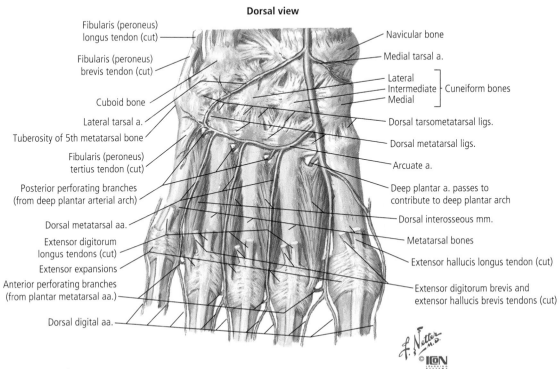

Fibularis (peroneus) longus tendon (cut)

Fibularis (peroneus) brevis tendon (cut)

Cuboid bone

Lateral tarsal a.

Tuberosity of 5th metatarsal bone

Fibularis (peroneus) tertius tendon (cut)

Posterior perforating branches (from deep plantar arterial arch)

Dorsal metatarsal aa.

Extensor digitorum longus tendons (cut)

Extensor expansions

Anterior perforating branches (from plantar metatarsal aa.)

Dorsal digital aa.

Navicular bone

Medial tarsal a.

Lateral
Intermediate] Cuneiform bones
Medial

Dorsal tarsometatarsal ligs.

Dorsal metatarsal ligs.

Arcuate a.

Deep plantar a. passes to contribute to deep plantar arch

Dorsal interosseous mm.

Metatarsal bones

Extensor hallucis longus tendon (cut)

Extensor digitorum brevis and extensor hallucis brevis tendons (cut)

Figure 9-14

Muscles	Proximal Attachments	Distal Attachments	Nerve and Segmental Level	Action
Deep Muscles				
Plantar interosseous	Bases of metatarsals 3–5	Medial base of proximal phalanges 3–5	Lateral plantar nerve (S2, S3)	Adduct digits 2–4 and flex MTP joints
Dorsal interossei	Sides of metatarsals 1–5	1st: medial aspect of proximal phalanx of 2nd digit 2nd–4th: lateral aspects of digits 2–4	Lateral plantar nerve (S2, S3)	Abduct digits 2–4 and flex MTP joints

MUSCLES   Interosseous Muscles of Sole of Foot (cont.)

Plantar view

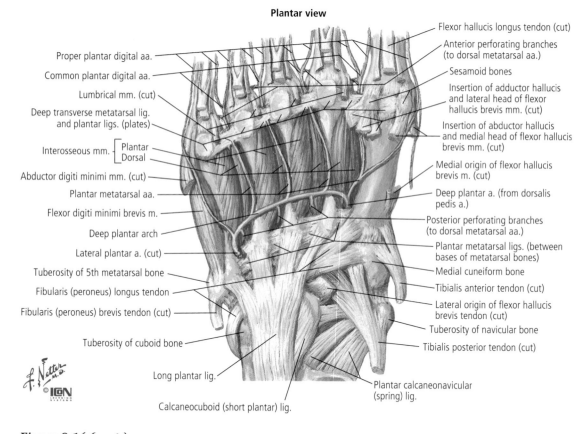

Proper plantar digital aa.

Common plantar digital aa.

Lumbrical mm. (cut)

Deep transverse metatarsal lig.
and plantar ligs. (plates)

Interosseous mm. { Plantar
Dorsal

Abductor digiti minimi mm. (cut)

Plantar metatarsal aa.

Flexor digiti minimi brevis m.

Deep plantar arch

Lateral plantar a. (cut)

Tuberosity of 5th metatarsal bone

Fibularis (peroneus) longus tendon

Fibularis (peroneus) brevis tendon (cut)

Tuberosity of cuboid bone

Long plantar lig.

Calcaneocuboid (short plantar) lig.

Flexor hallucis longus tendon (cut)

Anterior perforating branches
(to dorsal metatarsal aa.)

Sesamoid bones

Insertion of adductor hallucis
and lateral head of flexor
hallucis brevis mm. (cut)

Insertion of abductor hallucis
and medial head of flexor hallucis
brevis mm. (cut)

Medial origin of flexor hallucis
brevis m. (cut)

Deep plantar a. (from dorsalis
pedis a.)

Posterior perforating branches
(to dorsal metatarsal aa.)

Plantar metatarsal ligs. (between
bases of metatarsal bones)

Medial cuneiform bone

Tibialis anterior tendon (cut)

Lateral origin of flexor hallucis
brevis tendon (cut)

Tuberosity of navicular bone

Tibialis posterior tendon (cut)

Plantar calcaneonavicular
(spring) lig.

Figure 9-14 (cont.)

Tibial and Fibular Nerves

Nerves	Segmental Levels	Sensory	Motor
Sural	S1, S2	Posterior and lateral leg and lateral foot	No motor
Tibial	L4, L5, S1, S2, S3	Posterior heel and plantar surface of foot	Semitendinosus, semimembranosus, biceps femoris, adductor magnus, gastrocnemius, soleus, plantaris, flexor hallucis longus, flexor digitorum longus, tibialis posterior
Medial plantar	S2, S3	Medial 3½ digits	Flexor hallucis brevis, abductor hallucis, flexor digitorum brevis, lumbricales
Lateral plantar	S2, S3	Lateral 1½ digits	Adductor hallucis, abductor digiti minimi, quadratus plantae, lumbricales, flexor digiti minimi brevis, interossei
Saphenous	L2, L3, L4	Medial leg and foot	No motor
Deep fibular	L4, L5, S1	1st interdigital cleft	Tibialis anterior, extensor digitorum longus, extensor hallucis longus, fibularis tertius, extensor digitorum brevis, extensor hallucis brevis
Superficial fibular	L5, S1, S2	Distal anterior leg and dorsum of foot	Fibularis longus, fibularis brevis

NERVES   Tibial and Fibular Nerves (cont.)

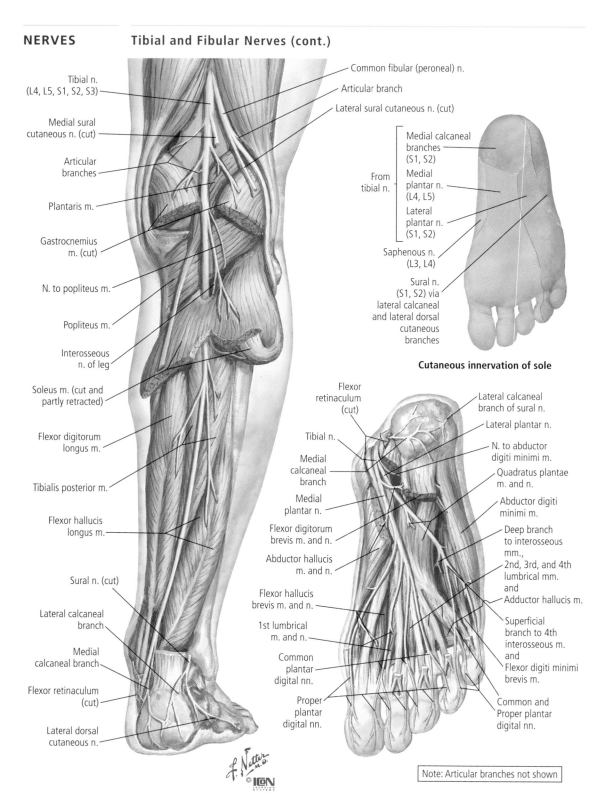

Tibial n.
(L4, L5, S1, S2, S3)

Medial sural
cutaneous n. (cut)

Articular
branches

Plantaris m.

Gastrocnemius
m. (cut)

N. to popliteus m.

Popliteus m.

Interosseous
n. of leg

Soleus m. (cut and
partly retracted)

Flexor digitorum
longus m.

Tibialis posterior m.

Flexor hallucis
longus m.

Sural n. (cut)

Lateral calcaneal
branch

Medial
calcaneal branch

Flexor retinaculum
(cut)

Lateral dorsal
cutaneous n.

Common fibular (peroneal) n.

Articular branch

Lateral sural cutaneous n. (cut)

Medial calcaneal
branches
(S1, S2)

From
tibial n.

Medial
plantar n.
(L4, L5)

Lateral
plantar n.
(S1, S2)

Saphenous n.
(L3, L4)

Sural n.
(S1, S2) via
lateral calcaneal
and lateral dorsal
cutaneous
branches

Cutaneous innervation of sole

Flexor
retinaculum
(cut)

Tibial n.

Medial
calcaneal
branch

Medial
plantar n.

Flexor digitorum
brevis m. and n.

Abductor hallucis
m. and n.

Flexor hallucis
brevis m. and n.

1st lumbrical
m. and n.

Common
plantar
digital nn.

Proper
plantar
digital nn.

Lateral calcaneal
branch of sural n.

Lateral plantar n.

N. to abductor
digiti minimi m.

Quadratus plantae
m. and n.

Abductor digiti
minimi m.

Deep branch
to interosseous
mm.,
2nd, 3rd, and 4th
lumbrical mm.
and
Adductor hallucis m.

Superficial
branch to 4th
interosseous m.
and
Flexor digiti minimi
brevis m.

Common and
Proper plantar
digital nn.

Note: Articular branches not shown

Figure 9-15

Tibial and Fibular Nerves (cont.)

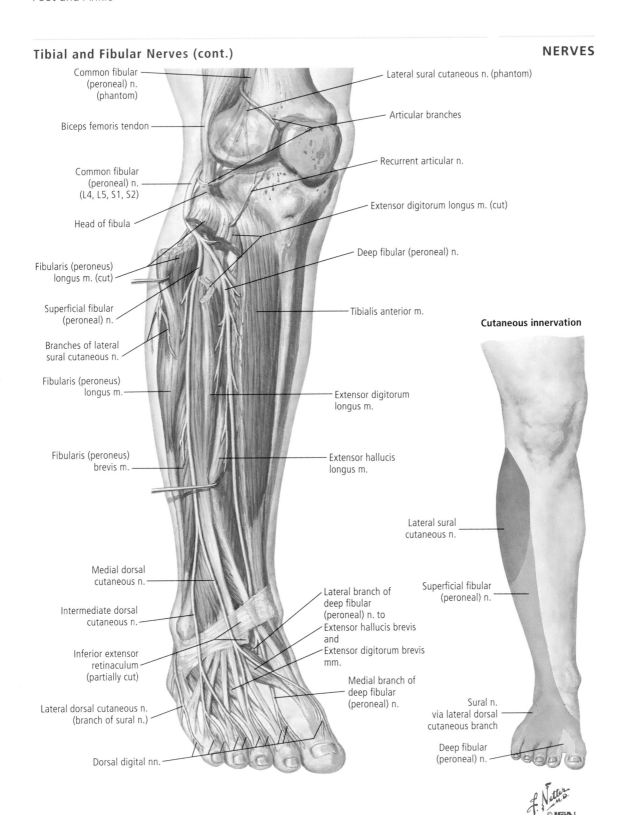

Common fibular (peroneal) n. (phantom)

Biceps femoris tendon

Common fibular (peroneal) n. (L4, L5, S1, S2)

Head of fibula

Fibularis (peroneus) longus m. (cut)

Superficial fibular (peroneal) n.

Branches of lateral sural cutaneous n.

Fibularis (peroneus) longus m.

Fibularis (peroneus) brevis m.

Medial dorsal cutaneous n.

Intermediate dorsal cutaneous n.

Inferior extensor retinaculum (partially cut)

Lateral dorsal cutaneous n. (branch of sural n.)

Dorsal digital nn.

Lateral sural cutaneous n. (phantom)

Articular branches

Recurrent articular n.

Extensor digitorum longus m. (cut)

Deep fibular (peroneal) n.

Tibialis anterior m.

Extensor digitorum longus m.

Extensor hallucis longus m.

Lateral branch of deep fibular (peroneal) n. to Extensor hallucis brevis and Extensor digitorum brevis mm.

Medial branch of deep fibular (peroneal) n.

Cutaneous innervation

Lateral sural cutaneous n.

Superficial fibular (peroneal) n.

Sural n. via lateral dorsal cutaneous branch

Deep fibular (peroneal) n.

Figure 9-15 (cont.)

EXAMINATION: Initial Hypotheses Based on Patient Reports
HISTORY

Patient Reports	Initial Hypothesis
Patient reports a traumatic incident resulting in forced inversion or eversion	Possible ankle sprain[1, 2] Possible fracture Possible fibular nerve involvement (if mechanism of injury is inversion)[3–5]
Patient reports trauma to ankle that included tibial rotation on a planted foot	Possible syndesmotic sprain[1]
Patient notes tenderness of anterior shin and may exhibit excessive pronation. Symptoms may be exacerbated by repetitive weight-bearing activities	Possible medial tibial stress syndrome[6]
Patient reports traumatic event resulting in inability to plantarflex ankle	Possible Achilles tendon rupture
Patient reports pain with stretch of calf muscles and during gait (toe push-off)	Possible Achilles tendonitis[7] Possible Sever disease[1]
Patient reports pain at heel with first few steps out of bed after prolonged periods of walking	Possible plantar fasciitis
Patient reports pain or paresthesias in plantar surface of foot	Possible tarsal tunnel syndrome[1] Possible sciatica Possible lumbar radiculopathy
Patient reports pain on plantar surface of foot between 3rd and 4th metatarsals. Might also state that pain is worse when walking with shoes compared with barefoot	Possible Morton neuroma[7] Possible metatarsalgia

Measurements of Relaxed Calcaneal Stance Position

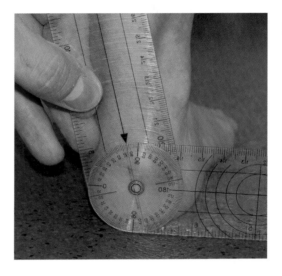

Figure 9-16: Measurement of relaxed calcaneal stance

Test Procedure	Instrumentation	Population	Reliability ICC (95% CI)	
			Intra-examiner	Inter-examiner
Relaxed calcaneal stance position Sobel et al.[16]	Standard goniometer	212 healthy subjects: 88 adults, 124 children	.61–.90	ICC not calculated; however, no significant difference between measurements obtained among examiners
Relaxed calcaneal stance Neutral calcaneal stance Van Gheluwe et al.[10]	Gravity goniometer	30 healthy subjects	Relaxed calcaneal stance .95–.97 Neutral calcaneal stance .87–.93	Relaxed calcaneal stance .61–.62 Neutral calcaneal stance .21–.31
Rearfoot angle Jonson and Gross[15]	Standard goniometer	63 healthy naval reserve officers	.88	.86

ICC, Intraclass Correlation Coefficient.

Goniometric Measurements

Test Procedure	Instrumentation	Population	Reliability ICC (95% CI)			
			Intra-examiner		**Inter-examiner**	
AROM Ankle dorsiflexion Ankle plantar flexion *Youdas et al.[8]*	Plastic goniometer	38 patients with orthopaedic disorders of ankle or knee	Ankle dorsiflexion Ankle plantarflexion	.89 .91	Ankle dorsiflexion Ankle plantar flexion	.28 .25
PROM Subtalar joint neutral Subtalar joint inversion Subtalar joint eversion Plantarflexion Dorsiflexion *Elveru et al.[9]*	Plastic goniometer	43 patients with orthopaedic or neurologic disorders in which measurements of foot and ankle would be appropriate in a clinical setting	Subtalar joint neutral Subtalar joint inversion Subtalar joint eversion Plantarflexion Dorsiflexion	.77 .62 .59 .86 .90	Subtalar joint neutral Subtalar joint inversion Subtalar joint eversion Plantarflexion Dorsiflexion	.25 .15 .12 .72 .50
PROM Pronation Supination Ankle dorsiflexion First ray plantarflexion First ray dorsiflexion *Van Gheluwe et al.[10]*	Inclinometer	30 healthy subjects	Pronation Supination Ankle dorsiflexion First ray plantarflexion First ray dorsiflexion	.89–.97 .90–.95 .86–.97 .72–.97 .90–.98	Pronation Supination Ankle dorsiflexion First ray plantarflexion First ray dorsiflexion	.46–.49 .28–.40 .26–.31 .91–.21 .14–.16
Weight-bearing lunge measurements of ankle dorsiflexion *Bennell et al.[11]*	Patients lunge forward until anterior knee touches wall. Inclinometer is used to record measurement between vertical and anterior tibia	13 healthy subjects	.98 (.93, .99)		.97 (.90, .99)	
Dorsiflexion in a modified lunge test *Menz et al.[12]*	A protractor is used to measure the angle formed by the horizontal and ‸ a line created between the fibular head and lateral malleolus as patient performs a lunge	31 subjects 76–87 years of age recruited from general population	Intra-examiner .87 (.74, .94)		NR	
Subtalar joint neutral: Open kinetic chain Closed kinetic chain *Picciano et al.[13]*	6 in universal goniometer	15 subjects with orthopaedic or neurologic condition of lower extremity	Open kinetic chain Closed kinetic chain	.06–.27 .14–.18	Open kinetic chain Closed kinetic chain	.0 .15
Open kinetic chain: Resting subtalar joint Subtar joint neutral *Sell et al.[14]*	Inclinometer	30 asymptomatic subjects	Resting subtalar joint Subtar joint neutral	.85 .85	Resting subtalar joint Subtar joint neutral	.68 .79
Passive dorsiflexion *Jonson and Gross[15]*	Standard goniometer	63 healthy naval reserve officers	Intra-examiner .74		Inter-examiner .65	

CI, confidence interval; AROM, active range of motion; PROM, passive range of motion.

Goniometric Measurements (cont.)

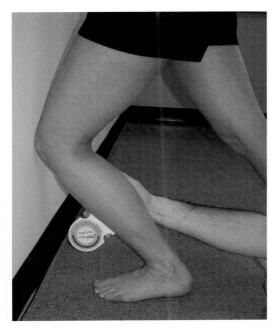

Figure 9-17: Weight-bearing lunge measurements of ankle dorsiflexion

Figure 9-18: Measurement of dorsiflexion with modified lunge test

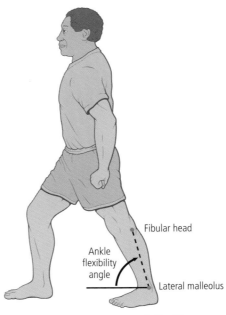

Fibular head

Ankle
flexibility
angle

Lateral malleolus

J. Perkins
MS, MFA
© ICON

Measurement of Navicular Height

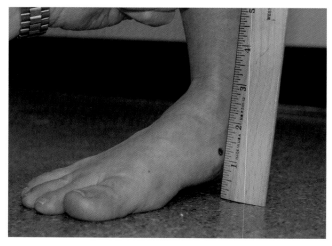

Figure 9-19: *Measurement of navicular height*

Test and Measure	Test Procedure	Population	Reliability ICC (95% CI)	
			Intra-examiner	Inter-examiner
Navicular height Menz et al.[12]	Navicular tuberosity is marked while patient is in weight-bearing position. Distance from ground to navicular tuberosity is measured	31 subjects 76–87 years of age recruited from general population	.64 (.38, .81)	NR
Navicular drop test Picciano et al.[13]	Navicular tuberosity is marked. Difference between navicular tuberosity height with foot resting on ground with weight bearing mostly on contralateral lower extremity while the examiner maintains subtalar joint neutral and during relaxed bilateral stance with full weight bearing is recorded.	15 subjects with orthopaedic or neurologic conditions of lower extremity	.61–.79`	.57
Navicular height technique Sell et al.[14]		30 asymptomatic subjects	.83	.73
Navicular drop test Vinicombe et al.[17]		20 symptomatic subjects	.33–.62	.31–.40
Navicular height Saltzman et al.[18]	Height of navicular tuberosity is calculated with a digital caliper	100 consecutive patients presenting to an orthopaedic foot and ankle clinic	.90	.74

Assessment of Medial Arch Height

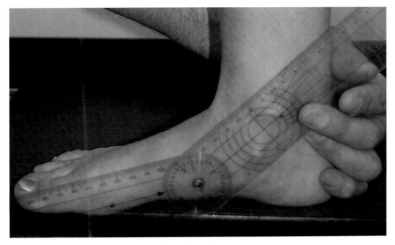

Figure 9-20: *Measurement of arch angle*

Test and Measure	Test Procedure	Population	Reliability ICC	
			Intra-examiner	Inter-examiner
Arch angle *Jonson and Gross*[15]	Patient in weight-bearing position. Examiner measures with standard goniometer angle formed by line connecting medial malleolus and navicular tuberosity and angle from tuberosity to medial aspect of first metatarsal head	63 healthy naval reserve officers	.90	.81
Arch height test *Saltzman et al.*[18]	Highest point of soft tissue margin along medial longitudinal arch was recoded with a digital caliper	100 consecutive patients presenting to an orthopaedic foot and ankle clinic	.91	.76
Visual assessment of arch height *Cowan et al.*[19]	Examiner makes a visual assessment of patient's arch height based on a 5-point scale ranging from 1 to 5. 1 = clearly flat-footed, and 5 = clearly high-arched	303 healthy army trainees	ICC values not calculated. Probability that two clinicians would agree that a foot presented was clearly flat was .57, and clearly high-arched was .17	

**RELIABILITY
OF THE
CLINICAL
EXAMINATION**

Measuring Forefoot Position

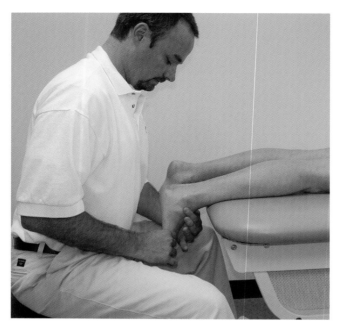

Figure 9-21: *Determination of forefoot varus/valgus*

Test and Measure	Test Procedure	Population	Reliability ICC			
			Intra-examiner		Inter-examiner	
Forefoot varus *Van Gheluwe et al.*[10]	Patient is prone with foot over edge of table. Examiner palpates medial and lateral talar head, then grasps 4th and 5th metatarsals and takes up slack in midtarsal joints. Subtalar neutral is position in which medial and lateral talar head is palpated equally *Root et al.*[20]	30 healthy subjects	.95–.99		.61	
Determination of forefoot varus/valgus: Goniometric Visual estimation *Somers et al.*[21]	Patient prone. Examiner places patient in subtalar neutral and places a dorsiflexion force through 4th and 5th metatarsal heads. Examiner takes goniometric measurements and makes visual estimation	10 asymptomatic subjects	Goniometric Visual estimation	.08–.78 .51–.76	Goniometric Visual estimation	.38–.42 .72–.81

Proprioceptive Measures

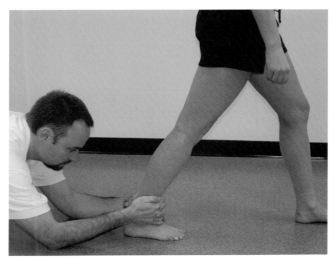

Figure 9-22: *Dorsiflexion-compression test*

Test	Procedure	Population	Test-Retest Reliability
Threshold for perception of passive movement	Examiner collects measurements with potentiometer	24 healthy adult subjects	.95
Active-to-active reproduction of joint position			.83
Reproduction of movement velocity			.79
Reproduction of torque *Deshpande et al.*[25]			Dorsiflexion .86 Plantarflexion .72

RELIABILITY OF THE CLINICAL EXAMINATION

Measuring Ankle Joint Swelling

Test and Measure	Test Procedure	Population	Reliability ICC	
			Intra-examiner	Inter-examiner
Figure-of-eight method *Tatro-Adams et al.*[22]	In open kinetic chain, examiner places tape measure midway between tibialis anterior tendon and lateral malleolus. Tape is then drawn medially and is placed just distal to navicular tuberosity. Tape is then pulled across arch and just proximal to base of 5th metatarsal. Tape is then pulled across anterior tibialis tendon and around ankle joint just distal to medial malleolus. Tape is finally pulled across Achilles tendon and is placed just distal to lateral malleolus and across start of tape	50 healthy subjects	.99	.99
Figure-of-eight method *Petersen et al.*[23]		29 persons with ankle swelling	.98	.98
Figure-of-eight method *Mawdsley et al.*[24]		15 healthy subjects	.99	NR
Water volumetrics *Petersen et al.*[23]	Water displacement is measured with patient's foot in a volumeter with toe tips touching front wall		.99	.99

Measuring Ankle Joint Swelling (cont.)

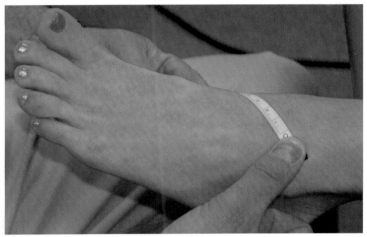

Figure 9-23A: *Start of figure-of-eight measurement*

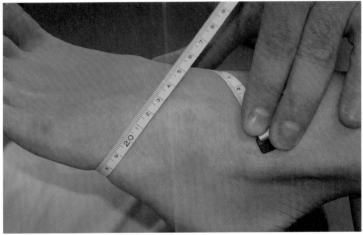

Figure 9-23B: *Figure-of-eight measurement, continued*

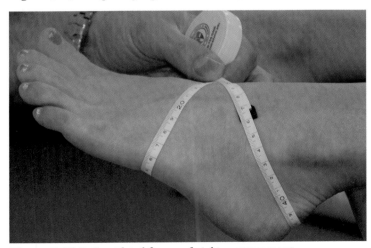

Figure 9-23C: *Completed figure-of-eight measurement*

Tests and Measures After Ankle Injury

Test	Test Procedure and Determination of Positive Finding	Population	Inter-examiner Reliability Kappa Values
Ability to bear weight	Calculated as tender or not. Swelling and ROM limitations dichotomized as "none-minimal" or "moderate-marked"	100 patients having sustained acute ankle trauma	$\kappa = .83$
Bone tenderness at base of 5th metatarsal			$\kappa = .78$
Bone tenderness at posterior edge of lateral malleolus			$\kappa = .75$
Bone tenderness at tip of medial malleolus			$\kappa = .66$
Bone tenderness at proximal fibula			$\kappa = -.01$
Combinations of bone tenderness			$\kappa = .76$
Soft tissue tenderness			$\kappa = .41$
Degree of swelling in area of anterior talofibular ligament			$\kappa = .18$
Ecchymosis			$\kappa = .39$
ROM restrictions present *Stiell et al.*[26]			$\kappa = .33$
Palpation test	Examiner palpates over anterior talofibular ligament. Positive if pain is reproduced	53 patients presenting for treatment of ankle injury	$\kappa = .36$
ER test	Patient sitting over edge of plinth. Passive ER stress is applied to foot and ankle. Positive if pain is reproduced over syndesmotic ligaments		$\kappa = .75$
Squeeze test	Patient sitting over edge of plinth. Examiner manually compresses fibula and tibia over calf midpoint. Positive if pain is reproduced over syndesmotic ligaments		$\kappa = .50$
Dorsiflexion-compression test *Alonso et al.*[27]	Patient is standing. Patient actively dorsiflexes ankle while weight bearing. Examiner applies manual compression around malleoli while in dorsiflexed position. Positive if significant increase in ankle dorsiflexion or reduction in pain with compression		$\kappa = .36$

ROM, range of motion; ER, external rotation.

Detecting Ligamentous Injuries: Tibiofibular Syndesmosis

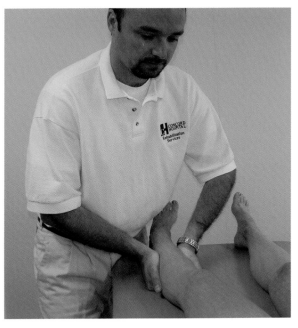

Figure 9-24: Squeeze test

Test	Test Procedure	Determination of Positive Finding	Population	Reference Standard	Sens (95% CI)	Spec (95% CI)	+LR (95% CI)	−LR (95% CI)
Cotton test	Patient is supine. Examiner assesses amount of talar translation from medial to lateral compared with uninjured side	Positive if pain is provoked or more movement is observed compared with uninjured side	12 persons, 3 with suspected syndesmotic rupture and 9 healthy	Arthroscopic visualization	Not reported. However, a relationship existed between confirmed diagnosis and squeeze (p=0.02), fibular translation (p=0.03), ER (p=0.03), and cotton tests (p=0.04)			
ER test	Patient is supine. Examiner places ER stress to involved ankle	Positive if pain is provoked at anterior or posterior syndesmotic ligaments or over interosseous membrane						
Squeeze test	Patient is supine. Fibula and tibia are compressed midway up calf	Positive if pain is provoked in area of syndesmosis						
Fibular translation test Beumer et al.[31]	Patient is supine. Examiner translates fibula anteriorly and posteriorly	Positive if pain is provoked or displacement of fibula is greater than on uninvolved side						

LR, likelihood ratio; MRI, magnetic resonance imaging.

DIAGNOSTIC UTILITY OF THE CLINICAL EXAMINATION

Detecting Ligamentous Injuries of Lateral Ankle

Test		Test Procedure	Determination of Finding	Population	Reference Standard	Sens (95% CI)	Spec (95% CI)	+LR (95% CI)	−LR (95% CI)
Anterior drawer test, pain on palpation, and formation of hematoma *van Dijk et al.*[28]	<48 hours after injury	Patient is supine. Examiner maintains ankle in 10° to 15° of plantarflexion while drawing heel gently forward	Test is positive for anterior talofibular ligament tear if talus rotates out of ankle mortise anteriorly	135 consecutive patients undergoing surgery for suspected lateral ankle ligament rupture	Surgical observation	.71	.33	1.06	.88
	5 days after injury					.96	.84	6.0	.05
Talar tilt test *Gaebler et al.*[29]		Patient's foot is inverted while under local anesthetic. Angle formed by a line drawn parallel to tibial plafond and superior talus surface is used to calculate degree of talar tilt	Amount of talar tilt is compared with uninvolved side and classified as <5°, 5° to 15°, or >15° of tilt	112 athletes with injuries to lateral ankle	MRI and surgical observation	Not calculated. However, talar tilt of ≥15 degrees always identified complete rupture of anterior tibial and calcaneotibular ligaments			
Anterior drawer		Patient is supine. Heel is drawn anterior. Amount of anterior translation is observed	Test is graded on a 4-point scale, 0–3. 0 represents no laxity. 3 represents gross laxity	12 volunteers with a history of unilateral ankle sprains	Stress fluoroscopy	Of nine patients considered to have excessive talar tilt on fluoroscopy, 78% exhibited laxity during anterior drawer and medial subtalar glide tests. 67% exhibited laxity with talar tilt test.			
Talar tilt		Patient is sidelying. Ankle is inverted. Amount of talar inversion is determined							
Medial subtalar glide *Hertel et al.*[30]		Examiner holds talus in subtalar neutral with one hand and glides calcaneus medially with other hand. Amount of medial calcaneus translation on talus is determined							

LR, likelihood ratio; MRI, magnetic resonance imaging.

Detecting Ligamentous Injuries of Lateral Ankle (cont.)

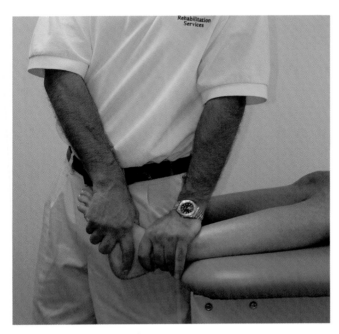

Figure 9-25: *Anterior drawer test*

DIAGNOSTIC UTILITY OF THE CLINICAL EXAMINATION

Detecting Anterolateral Ankle Impingement

Test	Test Procedure	Determination of Positive Finding	Population	Reference Standard	Sens (95% CI)	Spec (95% CI)	+LR (95% CI)	−LR (95% CI)
Impingement sign *Molloy et al.*[32]	Patient is seated. Examiner grasps calcaneus with one hand and uses other hand to grasp forefoot and bring it into plantarflexion. Examiner uses thumb to place pressure over anterolateral ankle. Foot is then brought from plantarflexion to dorsiflexion while thumb pressure is maintained	Positive if pain provoked with pressure from examiner's thumb is greater in dorsiflexion than in plantarflexion	73 patients with ankle pain	Arthroscopic visualization	.95	.88	7.91	.06
History and clinical examination *Liu et al.*[33]	Examiner records aggravating factors and reports loss of motion. Examination includes observation of swelling, passive forced ankle dorsiflexion and eversion, AROM, and double and single leg squats	Positive if five or more findings are positive: 1. Anterolateral ankle joint tenderness 2. Anterolateral ankle joint swelling 3. Pain with forced dorsiflexion and eversion 4. Pain with single leg squat 5. Pain with activities 6. Ankle instability	22 patients undergoing arthroscopic surgery for complaints of chronic ankle pain		.94	.75	3.76	.08

Detecting Anterolateral Ankle Impingement (cont.)

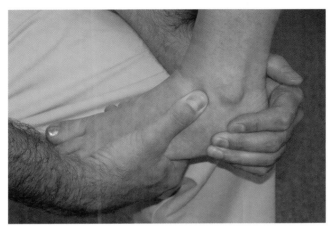

Figure 9-26A: *Impingement sign, plantarflexion*

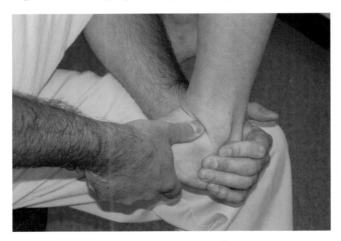

Figure 9-26B: *Impingement sign, dorsiflexion*

DIAGNOSTIC UTILITY OF THE CLINICAL EXAMINATION

Detecting Achilles Tendon Tears

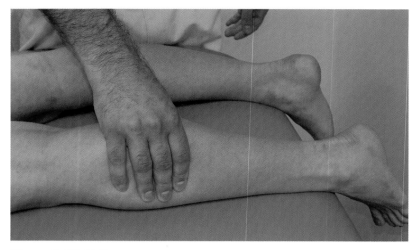

Figure 9-27: *Calf squeeze*

Test	Test Procedure	Determination of Positive Finding	Population	Reference Standard	Sens (95% CI)	Spec (95% CI)	+LR (95% CI)	−LR (95% CI)
Calf squeeze test	Patient is prone. Examiner gently squeezes calf	Positive if ankle remains still or minimal plantarflexion occurs	174 patients with complete Achilles tendon tears	Surgical observation	.96	NR	NA	NA
Copeland test	Patient is prone. Examiner places sphygmomanometer around middle of calf and inflates it to 100 mm Hg. Examiner then passively plantarflexes and dorsiflexes ankle	Positive if little or no pressure rise is noted on sphygmomanometer cuff			.78	NR	NA	NA
Gap test *Maffulli*[34]	Patient is prone. Examiner palpates course of Achilles tendon	Positive if gap in Achilles tendon is noted			.73	NR	NA	NA

NR, Not reported.

Detecting Plantar Fasciitis: Windlass Test

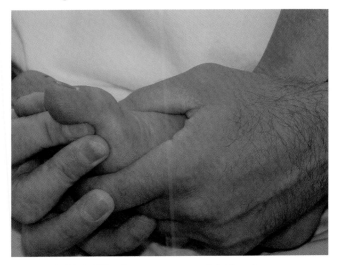

Figure 9-28A: *Windlass test, non–weight bearing*

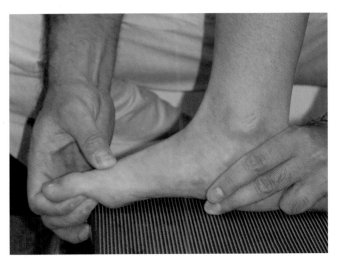

Figure 9-28B: *Windlass test, weight bearing*

De Garceau and colleagues[35] investigated the diagnostic utility of the Windlass test in detecting plantar fasciitis. The reference standard for plantar fasciitis was a detailed history and physical examination performed by a physician. Two methods of performing the Windlass test were used. In the first version, the patient's knee was flexed to 90° while in a non–weight-bearing position. The examiner stabilized the ankle and extended the MTP joint while allowing the IP joint to flex, thus preventing motion limitations due to a shortened hallucis longus muscle. The second method was performed with the patient standing on a step stool with toes over the stool's edge. Again, the MTP joint was extended while the IP joint was allowed to flex. In both methods, the test was considered positive if pain was reproduced at the end range of MTP extension. The sensitivity of the non–weight-bearing test was .14. The specificity was 1.0. The –LR was .86, and the +LR could not be calculated. The sensitivity of the weight-bearing test was .32. The specificity was 1.0. The –LR was .68, and the +LR could not be calculated.

DIAGNOSTIC UTILITY OF THE CLINICAL EXAMINATION

Accuracy of the Functional Hallux Limitus Test to Predict Abnormal Excessive Midtarsal Function During Gait

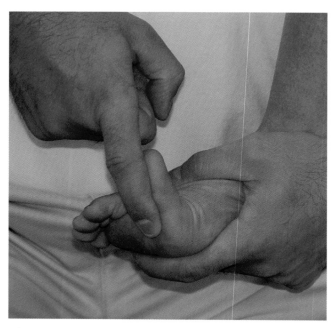

Figure 9-29: *Functional hallux limitus test*

Payne, Chuter, and Miller[36] investigated the accuracy of the functional hallux limitus test to identify abnormal midtarsal joint function during terminal stance. The authors identified abnormal midtarsal motion by observing whether the navicular moved in a plantar direction or adducted when the heel began to lift off the ground during gait. The test was performed with the patient in a non–weight-bearing position. The examiner used one hand to maintain the subtalar joint in a neutral position while maintaining the first ray in dorsiflexion. The other hand was used to dorsiflex the proximal phalanx of the hallux. The test was considered positive if the examiner noted immediate plantarflexion of the first metatarsal upon dorsiflexion of the proximal phalanx. The sensitivity of the test was .72. The specificity was .66. The +LR was 2.12, and the –LR was .42.

Ottawa Ankle Rules

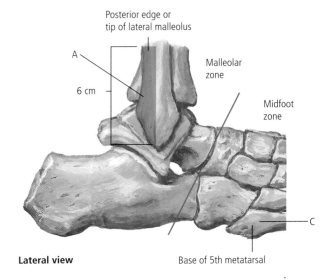

Posterior edge or
tip of lateral malleolus

A

6 cm

Malleolar
zone

Midfoot
zone

C

Lateral view

Base of 5th metatarsal

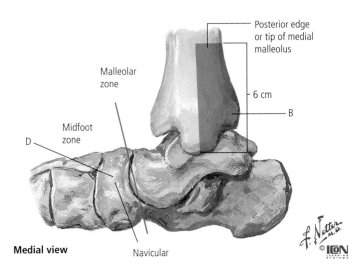

Posterior edge
or tip of medial
malleolus

Malleolar
zone

6 cm

B

Midfoot
zone

D

Medial view

Navicular

Figure 9-30

Stiell and colleagues[37] developed a clinical prediction rule, known as the Ottawa Ankle Rules, to determine the need to order radiographs after an acute ankle injury. The patient should be referred for radiographs if bone tenderness is exhibited at A or B or C or D, or if the patient cannot bear weight immediately after the injury or during the examination (four steps regardless of limping). The pooled sensitivity of 27 studies that investigated the utility of the Ottawa Ankle Rules was 97.6% (95% CI: 96.6, 98.9), and the –LR was .10 (95% CI: .06, .16).[38]

REFERENCES   1. Appling SA. Foot and ankle. In: *Current Concepts of Orthopeadic Physical Therapy*. La Crosse: Orthopaedic Section, American Physical Therapy Association; 2001.
   2. Hartley A. *Practical Joint Assessment*. St. Louis: Mosby; 1995.
   3. Hunt GC. Ankle sprain in a 14-year-old girl. In: Jones MA, Rivett DA, eds. *Clinical Reasoning for Manual Therapists*. Edinburgh: Butterworth Heinemann; 2004.
   4. Hunt GC, Sneed T, Hamann H, Chisam. Biomechanical and histilogical considerations for development of plantar fasciitis and evaluation of arch taping as a treatment option to control associated plantar heel pain: a single-subject design. *The Foot*. In press.
   5. Hunt GC. Injuries of peripheral nerves of the leg, foot and ankle: an often unrecognized consequence of ankle sprains. *The Foot*. 2003;13:14-18.
   6. Bennett JE, Reinking MF, Pluemer B, Pentel A, Seaton M, Killian C. Factors contributing to the development of medial tibial stress syndrome in high school runners. *J Orthop Sports Phys Ther*. 2001;31:504-510.
   7. Wooden MJ. Foot overuse syndromes of the foot and ankle. In: Wadsworth C, Kestel L, eds. *Orthopaedic Physical Therapy Home Study Course*. La Crosse: Orthopaedic Section, American Physical Therapy Association; 1995.
   8. Youdas JW, Bogard CL, Suman VJ. Reliability of goniometric measurements and visual estimates of ankle joint range of motion obtained in a clinical setting. *Arch Phys Med Rehabil*. 1993;74:1113-1118.
   9. Elveru RA, Rothstein JM, Lamb RL. Goniometric reliability in a clinical setting. *Phys Ther*. 1988;68:672-677.
  10. Van Gheluwe B, Kirby KA, Roosen P, Phillips R. Reliability and accuracy of biomechanical measurement of the lower extremities. *J Am Podiatr Med Assoc*. 2002;92:317-326.
  11. Bennell KL, Talbot RC, Wajswelner H, Techovanich W, Kelly DH, Hall AJ. Intra-rater and inter-rater reliability of a weight-bearing lunge measure of ankle dorsiflexion. *Aust J Physiother*. 1998;44:175-180.
  12. Menz HB, Tiedemann A, Kwan MM, Latt MD, Sherrington C, Lord SR. Reliability of clinical tests of foot and ankle characteristics in older people. *J Am Podiatr Med Assoc*. 2003;93:380-387.
  13. Picciano AM, Rowlands MS, Worrell T. Reliability of open and closed kinetic chain subtalar joint neutral positions and navicular drop test. *J Orthop Sports Phys Ther*. 1993;18:553-558.
  14. Sell KE, Verity TM, Worrell TW, Pease BJ, Wigglesworth J. Two measurement techniques for assessing subtalar joint position: a reliability study. *J Orthop Sports Phys Ther*. 1994;19:162-167.
  15. Jonson SR, Gross MT. Intraexaminer reliability, interexaminer reliability, and mean values for nine lower extremity skeletal measures in healthy naval shipmen. *J Orthop Sports Phys Ther*. 1997;25:253-263.
  16. Sobel E, Levitz SL, Caselli MA, et al. Reevaluation of the relaxed calcaneal stance position. Reliability and normal values in children and adults. *J Am Podiatr Med Assoc*. 1999;89:258-264.
  17. Vinicombe A, Raspovic A, Menz HB. Reliability of navicular displacement measurement as a clinical indicator of foot posture. *J Am Podiatr Med Assoc*. 2001;91:262-268.
  18. Saltzman CL, Nawoczenski DA, Talbot KD. Measurement of the medial longitudinal arch. *Arch Phys Med Rehabil*. 1995;76:45-49.

19. Cowan DN, Robinson JR, Jones BH, Polly DW Jr, Berrey BH. Consistency of visual assessments of arch height among clinicians. *Foot Ankle Int.* 1994;14:213-227.

20. Root ML, Orien WP, Weed JH. *Biomechanical Examination of the Foot.* Los Angeles: Clinical Biomechanics Corp; 1971.

21. Somers DL, Hanson JA, Kedzierski CM, Nestor KL, Quinlivan KY. The influence of experience on the reliability of goniometric and visual measurement of forefoot position. *J Orthop Sports Phys Ther.* 1997;25:192-202.

22. Tatro-Adams D, McGann SF, Carbone W. Reliability of figure-of-eight method of ankle measurement. *J Orthop Sports Phys Ther.* 1995;22:161-163.

23. Petersen EJ, Irish SM, Lyons CL, et al. Relaibility of water volumetry and the figure of eight method on subjects with ankle joint swelling. *J Orthop Sports Phys Ther.* 1999;29:609-615.

24. Mawdsley RH, Hoy DK, Erwin PM. Criterion-related validity of the figure-of-eight method of measuring ankle edema. *J Orthop Sports Phys Ther.* 2000;30:149-152.

25. Deshpande N, Connelly DM, Culham EG, Costigan PA. Reliability and validity of ankle proprioceptive measures. *Arch Phys Med Rehabil.* 2003;84:883-889.

26. Stiell IG, McKnight RD, Greenberg GH, Nair RC, McDowell I, Wallace GJ. Interobserver agreement in the examination of acute ankle injury patients. *Am J Emerg Med.* 1992;10:14-17.

27. Alonso A, Khoury L, Adams R. Clinical tests for ankle syndesmosis injury: reliability and prediction of return to function. *J Orthop Sports Phys Ther.* 1998;27:276-284.

28. van Dijk CN, Mol BW, Lim LS, Marti RK, Bossuyt PM. Diagnosis of a ligament rupture of the ankle joint. Physical examination, arthrography, stress radiography and sonography compared in 160 patients after inversion trauma. *Acta Orthop Scand.* 1996;67:566-570.

29. Gaebler C, Kukla C, Breitenseher MJ, et al. Diagnosis of lateral ankle ligament injuries. Comparison between talar tilt, MRI and operative findings in 112 athletes. *Acta Orthop Scand.* 1997;63:286-290.

30. Hertel J, Denegar CR, Monroe MM, Stokes WL. Talocrural and subtalar joint instability after lateral ankle sprain. *Med Sci Sports Exerc.* 1999;13:1501-1508.

31. Beumer A, Swierstra BA, Mulder PG. Clinical diagnosis of syndesmotic ankle instability: evaluation of stress tests behind the curtain. *Acta Orthop Scand.* 2002;73:667-669.

32. Molloy S, Solan MC, Bendall SP. Synovial impingement in the ankle: a new physical sign. *J Bone Joint Surg Br.* 2003;85:330-333.

33. Liu SH, Nuccion SL, Finerman G. Diagnosis of an anterolateral ankle impingement. *Am J Sports Med.* 1997;25:389-393.

34. Maffulli N. The clinical diagnosis of subcutaneous tears of the Achilles tendon. *Am J Sports Med.* 2004;26:266-270.

35. De Garceau D, Dean D, Requejo SM, Thordarson DB. The association between diagnosis of plantar fasciitis and windlass test results. *Foot Ankle Int.* 2003;24:251-255.

36. Payne C, Chuter V, Miller K. Sensitivity and specificity of the functional hallux limitus test to predict foot function. *J Am Podiatr Med Assoc.* 2002;92:269-271.

37. Stiell I, Greenberg G, McKnight R, et al. A study to develop clinical decision rules for the use of radiography in acute ankle injuries. *Ann Emerg Med.* 1992;21:384-390.

38. Bachmann LM, Kolb E, Koller MT, Steurer J, ter Riet G. Accuracy of Ottawa ankle rules to exclude fractures of the ankle and mid-foot: systematic review. *BMJ.* 2003;326:417.

Shoulder

Chapter 10

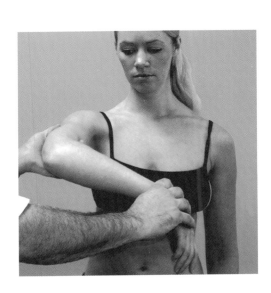

OSTEOLOGY   Humerus and Scapula

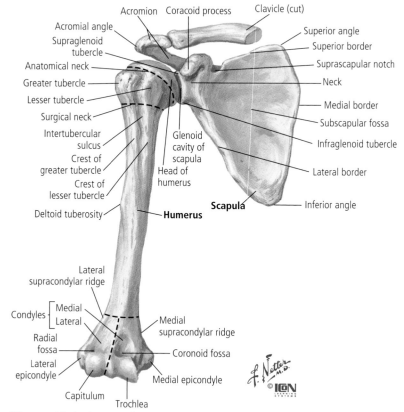

Figure 10-1: *Anterior humerus and scapula*

Superior and Inferior Clavicle

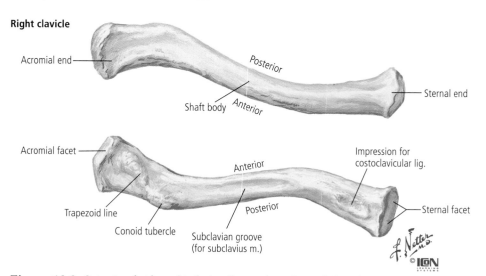

Figure 10-2: *Superior (top) and inferior (bottom) surface of clavicle*

Shoulder Joint

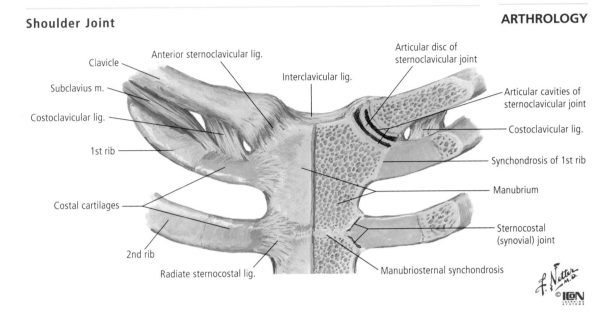

Clavicle

Anterior sternoclavicular lig.

Interclavicular lig.

Articular disc of sternoclavicular joint

Subclavius m.

Costoclavicular lig.

Articular cavities of sternoclavicular joint

Costoclavicular lig.

1st rib

Synchondrosis of 1st rib

Manubrium

Costal cartilages

Sternocostal (synovial) joint

2nd rib

Radiate sternocostal lig.

Manubriosternal synchondrosis

Figure 10-3: *Sternoclavicular joint*

Joint	Type and Classification	Closed Packed Position	Capsular Pattern
Glenohumeral	Spheroidal	Full abduction and ER	ER limited more than abduction, limited more than IR and flexion
Sternoclavicular	Saddle	Arm abducted to 90°	NR
AC	Plane synovial	Arm abducted to 90°	
Scapulothoracic	Not a true articulation	NA	NA

AC, acromioclavicular; ER, external rotation; NA, not applicable; IR, internal rotation; NR, not reported.

ARTHROLOGY   Shoulder Joint (cont.)

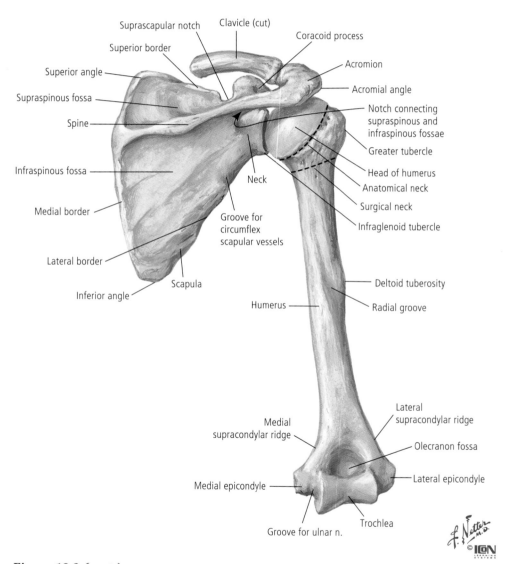

Figure 10-3 (cont.)

Scapulohumeral rhythm, which consists of integrated movements of the glenohumeral, scapulothoracic, AC, and sternoclavicular joints, occurs in sequential fashion to allow full functional motion of the shoulder complex. Scapulohumeral rhythm serves three functional purposes: it allows for greater overall shoulder range of motion (ROM), it maintains optimal contact between the humeral head and the glenoid fossa, and it assists with maintaining an optimal length-tension relationship of the glenohumeral muscles.[1] To complete 180° of abduction, the overall ratio of glenohumeral to scapulothoracic, AC, and sternoclavicular motion is 2:1.

Inman,[2] who was the first to explain scapulohumeral rhythm, described it as two phases that the shoulder complex completes to move through full abduction. The first phase (0° to 90°) entails the scapula setting against the thorax to provide initial stability as the humerus abducts to 30°.[1, 2] From 30° to 90° of abduction, the glenohumeral joint contributes another 30° of ROM while the scapula upwardly rotates 30°. This upward rotation results from clavicular elevation through the sternoclavicular and AC joints. The second phase (90° to 180°) entails 60° of glenohumeral abduction and 30° of upward rotation of the scapula. Rotation of the scapula is associated with 5° of elevation at the sternoclavicular joint and 25° of rotation at the acromioclavicluar joint.[2, 3]

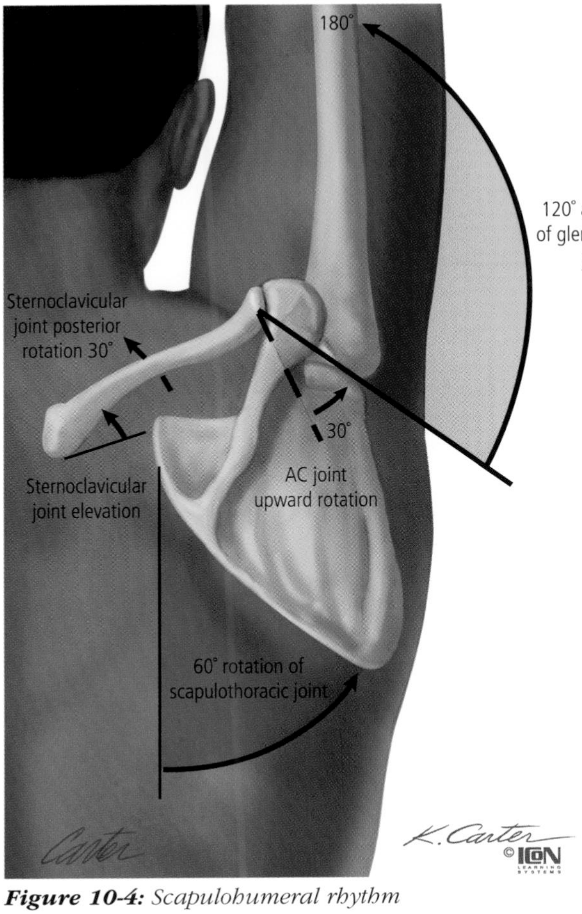

SCAPULO-HUMERAL RHYTHM

Figure 10-4: *Scapulohumeral rhythm*

LIGAMENTS   Shoulder Ligaments

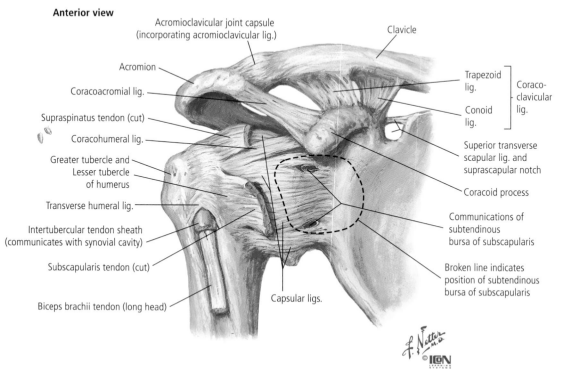

Anterior view

Acromioclavicular joint capsule
(incorporating acromioclavicular lig.)

Clavicle

Acromion

Coracoacromial lig.

Supraspinatus tendon (cut)

Coracohumeral lig.

Greater tubercle and
Lesser tubercle
of humerus

Transverse humeral lig.

Intertubercular tendon sheath
(communicates with synovial cavity)

Subscapularis tendon (cut)

Biceps brachii tendon (long head)

Trapezoid
lig.

Conoid
lig.

Coraco-
clavicular
lig.

Superior transverse
scapular lig. and
suprascapular notch

Coracoid process

Communications of
subtendinous
bursa of subscapularis

Broken line indicates
position of subtendinous
bursa of subscapularis

Capsular ligs.

Figure 10-5

Ligaments		Attachments	Function
Glenohumeral		Glenoid labrum to neck of humerus	Reinforce anterior glenohumeral joint capsule
Coracohumeral		Coracoid process to greater tubercle of humerus	Strengthen superior glenohumeral joint capsule
Coracoclavicular	Trapezoid	Superior aspect of coracoid process to inferior aspect of clavicle	Anchor clavicle to corocoid process
	Conoid	Corocoid process to conoid tubercle on inferior clavicle	
Acromioclavicular		Acromion to clavicle	Strengthen AC joint superiorly
Coracoacromial		Coracoid process to acromion	Prevent superior displacement of humeral head
Sternoclavicular		Clavicular notch of manubrium to medial base of clavicle anteriorly and posteriorly	Reinforce sternoclavicular joint anteriorly and posteriorly
Interclavicular		Medial end of one clavicle to medial end of another clavicle	Strengthen superior sternoclavicular joint capsule
Costoclavicular		Superior aspect of costal cartilage of 1st rib to inferior border of medial clavicle	Anchor medial end of clavicle to 1st rib

Shoulder Ligaments (cont.)

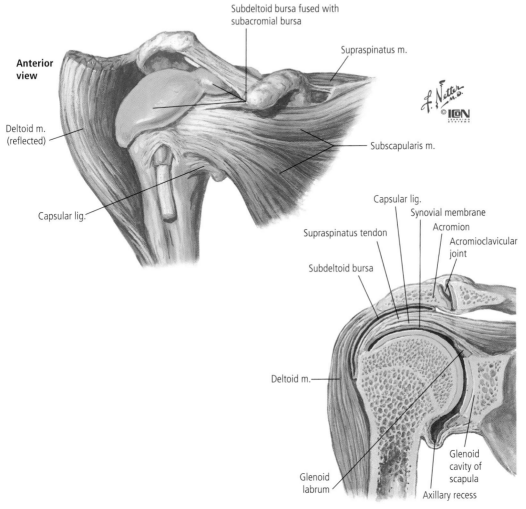

Subdeltoid bursa fused with subacromial bursa

Supraspinatus m.

Anterior view

Deltoid m. (reflected)

Subscapularis m.

Capsular lig.

Capsular lig.

Synovial membrane

Acromion

Acromioclavicular joint

Supraspinatus tendon

Subdeltoid bursa

Deltoid m.

Glenoid cavity of scapula

Glenoid labrum

Axillary recess

Coronal section through joint

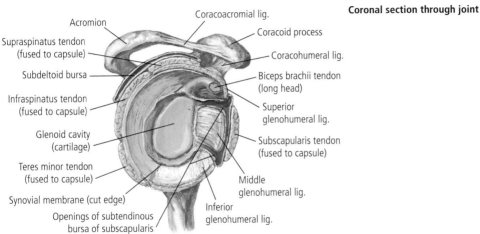

Acromion

Coracoacromial lig.

Supraspinatus tendon (fused to capsule)

Coracoid process

Coracohumeral lig.

Subdeltoid bursa

Biceps brachii tendon (long head)

Infraspinatus tendon (fused to capsule)

Superior glenohumeral lig.

Glenoid cavity (cartilage)

Subscapularis tendon (fused to capsule)

Teres minor tendon (fused to capsule)

Synovial membrane (cut edge)

Middle glenohumeral lig.

Openings of subtendinous bursa of subscapularis

Inferior glenohumeral lig.

Figure 10-5 (cont.)

MUSCLES   **Posterior Muscles of Shoulder**

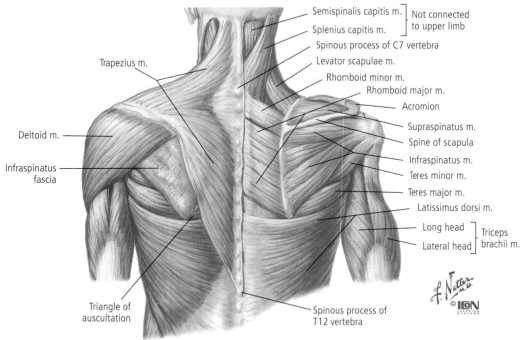

Figure 10-6

Muscles	Origin	Insertion	Nerve and Segmental Level	Action
Upper trapezius	Occipital protru-berance, nuchal line, ligamentum nuchae	Lateral clavicle and acromion	Cranial nerve XI and C2-C4	Rotate glenoid fossa upwardly, elevate scapula
Middle trapezius	Spinous process of T1-T5	Acromion and spine of scapula	Cranial nerve XI and C2-C4	Retract scapula
Lower trapezius	Spinous process of T6-T12	Apex of spine of scapula	Cranial nerve XI and C2-C4	Rotate glenoid fossa upwardly, depress scapula
Levator scapulae	Transverse processes of C1-C4	Superior medial scapula	Dorsal scapular (C3-C5)	Elevate and adduct scapula
Rhomboids	Ligamentum nuchae and spinous processes C7-T5	Medial scapular border	Dorsal scapular (C4-C5)	Retract scapula
Latissimus dorsi	Inferior thoracic vertebrae, thora-columbar fascia, iliac crest, and inferior ribs 3–4	Intertubercular groove of humerus	Thoracodorsal (C6-C8)	Internally rotate, adduct, and extend humerus
Serratus anterior	Ribs 1–8	Anterior medial scapula	Long thoracic (C5-C8)	Protract and upwardly rotate scapula

Anterior Muscles of Shoulder

Trapezius m.

Omohyoid m. and investing layer of deep cervical fascia

Acromion

Deltopectoral triangle

Sternocleidomastoid m.

Deltoid branch of thoracoacromial a.

Clavicle

Deltoid m.

Clavicular head

Cephalic v.

Sternocostal head

Pectoralis major m.

Abdominal part

Biceps brachii m. — Long head
Short head

Sternum

Triceps brachii m. (lateral head)

Latissimus dorsi m.

Serratus anterior m.

Anterior layer of rectus sheath

External oblique m.

6th costal cartilage

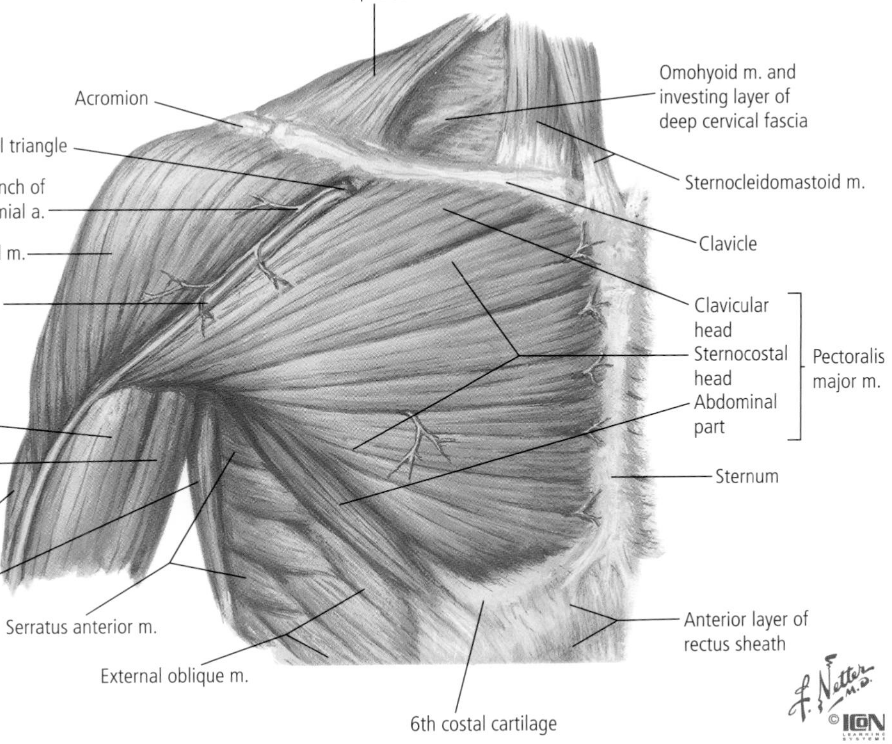

Figure 10-7

Muscles		Origin	Insertion	Nerve and Segmental Level	Action
Deltoid		Clavicle, acromion, spine of scapula	Deltoid tuberosity of humerus	Axillary (C5-C6)	Abduct arm
Pectoralis major	Clavicular head	Anterior medial clavicle	Intertubercular groove of humerus	Lateral and medial pectoral nerves (C5, C6, C7, C8, T1)	Adduct and internally rotate humerus
	Sternocostal head	Lateral border of sternum, superior six costal cartilages, and fascia of external oblique muscle			
Pectoralis minor		Just lateral to costal cartilage of ribs 3–5	Coracoid process	Medial pectoral nerve (C8, T1)	Stabilize scapula

MUSCLES

Muscles of Rotator Cuff

Superior view

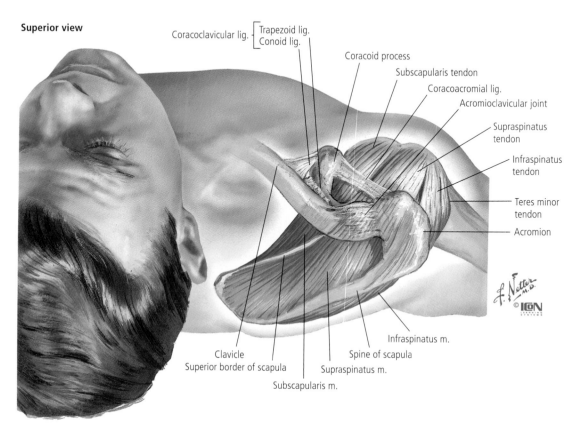

Coracoclavicular lig. ⎡ Trapezoid lig.
⎣ Conoid lig.

Coracoid process

Subscapularis tendon

Coracoacromial lig.

Acromioclavicular joint

Supraspinatus tendon

Infraspinatus tendon

Teres minor tendon

Acromion

Infraspinatus m.

Spine of scapula

Supraspinatus m.

Clavicle

Superior border of scapula

Subscapularis m.

Figure 10-8

Muscles	Origin	Insertion	Nerve and Segmental Level	Action
Supraspinatus	Supraspinous fossa of scapula	Greater tubercle of humerus	Suprascapular (C4-C6)	Assist deltoid in adduction of humerus
Infraspinatus	Infraspinatus fossa of scapula	Greater tubercle of humerus	Suprascapular (C5-C6)	Externally rotate humerus
Teres minor	Lateral border of scapula	Greater tubercle of humerus	Axillary (C5-C6)	Externally rotate humerus
Subscapularis	Subscapular fossa of scapula	Lesser tubercle of humerus	Upper and lower subscapular (C5-C6)	Internally rotate humerus
Teres major	Inferior angle of scapula	Intertubercular groove of humerus	Lower subscapular (C5-C6)	Internally rotate and adduct humerus

Muscles of Rotator Cuff (cont.)

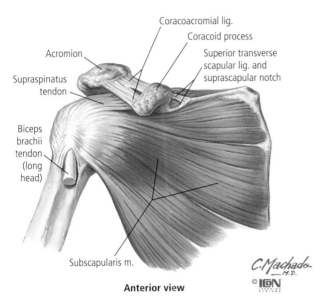

Coracoacromial lig.

Coracoid process

Acromion

Superior transverse scapular lig. and suprascapular notch

Supraspinatus tendon

Biceps brachii tendon (long head)

Subscapularis m.

Anterior view

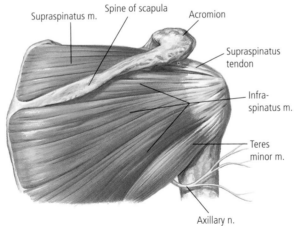

Spine of scapula

Supraspinatus m.

Acromion

Supraspinatus tendon

Infra-spinatus m.

Teres minor m.

Axillary n.

Posterior view

Figure 10-8 (cont.)

NERVES   Anterior Axilla

Nerves	Segmental Levels	Sensory	Motor
Radial	C5, C6, C7, C8, T1	Posterior aspect of forearm	Triceps brachii, anconeus, brachioradialis, extensor muscles of forearm
Ulnar	C7, C8, T1	Medial hand including medial half of 4th digit	Flexor carpi ulnaris, medial half of flexor digitorum profundus, and most small muscles in hand
Musculocutaneous	C5, C6, C7	Becomes lateral ante-brachial cutaneous nerve	Coracobrachialis, biceps brachii, brachialis
Axillary	C5, C6	Lateral shoulder	Teres minor, deltoid
Suprascapular	C4, C5, C6	No sensory	Supraspinatus, infraspinatus
Dorsal scapular	Ventral rami, C4, C5	No sensory	Rhomboids, levator scapulae
Lateral pectoral	C5, C6, C7	No sensory	Pectoralis major pectoralis minor
Medial pectoral	C8, T1	No sensory	Pectoralis minor
Long thoracic	Ventral rami, C5, C6, C7	No sensory	Serratus anterior
Upper subscapular	C5, C6	No sensory	Subscapularis
Lower subscapular	C5, C6	No sensory	Teres major, subscapularis
Medial cutaneous of arm	C8, T1	Medial arm	No motor

Anterior Axilla (cont.)

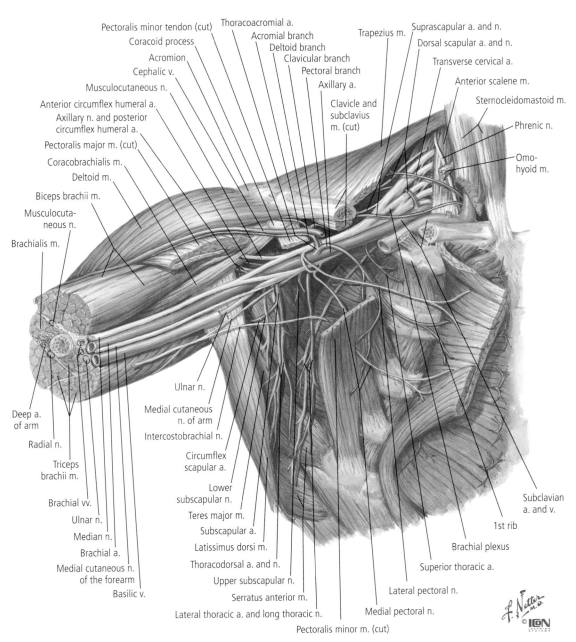

Pectoralis minor tendon (cut)
Coracoid process
Acromion
Cephalic v.
Musculocutaneous n.
Anterior circumflex humeral a.
Axillary n. and posterior circumflex humeral a.
Pectoralis major m. (cut)
Coracobrachialis m.
Deltoid m.
Biceps brachii m.
Musculocutaneous n.
Brachialis m.
Deep a. of arm
Radial n.
Triceps brachii m.
Brachial vv.
Ulnar n.
Median n.
Brachial a.
Medial cutaneous n. of the forearm
Basilic v.

Thoracoacromial a.
Acromial branch
Deltoid branch
Clavicular branch
Pectoral branch
Axillary a.
Clavicle and subclavius m. (cut)

Trapezius m.
Suprascapular a. and n.
Dorsal scapular a. and n.
Transverse cervical a.
Anterior scalene m.
Sternocleidomastoid m.
Phrenic n.
Omo-hyoid m.

Ulnar n.
Medial cutaneous n. of arm
Intercostobrachial n.
Circumflex scapular a.
Lower subscapular n.
Teres major m.
Subscapular a.
Latissimus dorsi m.
Thoracodorsal a. and n.
Upper subscapular n.
Lateral thoracic a. and long thoracic n.
Serratus anterior m.
Pectoralis minor m. (cut)
Medial pectoral n.
Lateral pectoral n.
Superior thoracic a.
Brachial plexus
1st rib
Subclavian a. and v.

Figure 10-9

**EXAMINATION:
HISTORY**

Initial Hypotheses Based on History

History	Initial Hypothesis
Patient reports of lateral/anterior shoulder pain with overhead activities or demonstration of a painful arc	Possible subacromial impingement[4, 5] Possible tendonitis[6] Possible bursitis[6]
Patient reports of instability, apprehension, and pain with activities most often when shoulder is abducted and externally rotated	Shoulder instability[4] Possible labral tear, if clicking is present[7, 8]
Decreased ROM and pain with resistance	Possible rotator cuff or long head of the bicep tendonitis[9]
Patient reports of pain and weakness with muscle loading, night pain. Age >60	Possible rotator cuff tear[6, 9]
Patient complaints of poorly located shoulder pain with occasional radiation into elbow. Pain is usually aggravated by movement and relieved by rest. Age >45. Females more often affected than males	Possible adhesive capsulitis[10]
Patient reports of a fall on the shoulder followed by pain over AC joint	Possible AC sprain[4]
Patient complaints of upper extremity heaviness or numbness with prolonged postures and when lying on involved side	Possible thoracic outlet syndrome[11, 12] Possible cervical radiculopathy[6, 13, 14]

Shoulder Range-of-Motion Measurements

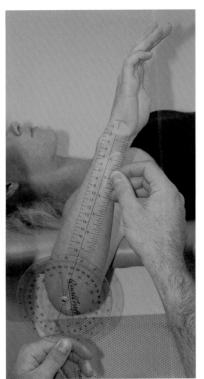

Figure 10-10A: *Measurements of internal rotation in 90° of abduction*

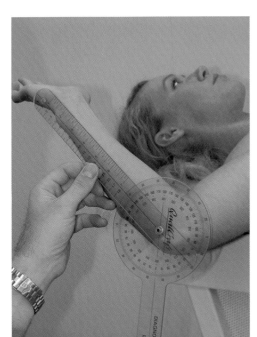

Figure 10-10B: *Measurements of external rotation in 90° of abduction*

Test Procedure	Instrumentation	Population	Reliability ICC (95% CI)	
			Intra-examiner	**Inter-examiner**
PROM Flexion Extension Abduction *Riddle et al.*[15]	Universal goniometer	100 patients referred to PT for shoulder impairments	Flexion .98 Extension .94 Abduction .98	Flexion .89 Extension.27 Abduction .87
AROM Flexion Abduction ER in neutral ER in abduction IR in abduction *Hoving et al.*[16]	Inclinometer	6 patients with shoulder pain and stiffness	Flexion .62 (.18, .83) Abduction .35 (.04, .65) ER in neutral .75 (.42, .89) ER in abduction .43 (.12, .80) IR in abduction .32 (.02, .67)	Flexion .65 (.32, .86) Abduction .51 (.22, .77) ER in neutral .29 (.02, .68) ER in abduction .11 (.02, .58) IR in abduction .06 (.01, .45)

ICC, Intraclass correlate coefficient; CI, confidence interval; PROM, passive range of motion; PT, physical therapy; AROM, active range of motion.

RELIABILITY OF THE CLINICAL EXAMINATION

Measuring Internal Rotation: Hand Behind Back Method

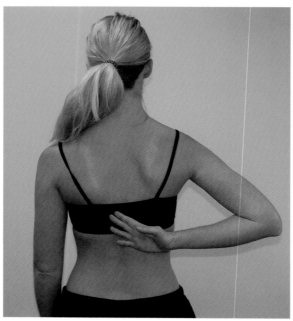

Figure 10-11: *Functional internal rotation of shoulder test*

Test and Measure	Test Procedure	Population	Reliability ICC (95% CI)	
			Intra-examiner	Inter-examiner
Hand behind back *Hoving et al.*[16]	Patient attempts to reach to highest level behind back while the examiner identifies vertebral level patient is able to reach	6 patients with pain and stiffness in the shoulder	.91 (.41, .97)	.80 (.19, .95)
Functional IR of shoulder *Edwards et al.*[17]		3 asymptomatic subjects	.44	.12–.27

Shoulder Assessment using Cyriax Schema

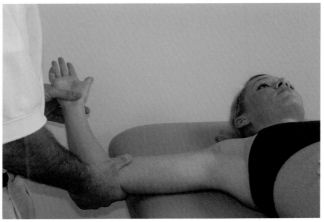

Figure 10-12: *Examination of end-feel for external rotation*

Test and Measure	Test Procedure	Population	Reliability Kappa Value	
			Intra-examiner	Inter-examiner
Cyriax examination *Pellecchia et al.[21]*	When using the Cyriax classification for shoulder diseases (including history and physical examination), examiner categorizes patient's diagnosis as arthritis, supraspinatus tendonitis, chronic subdeltoid bursitis, infraspinatus tendonitis, AC sprain, subscapularis tendonitis, biceps tendonitis, or suprascapular neuritis	19 patients with primary complaint of shoulder pain	NR	κ = .88
Examination of end-feel *Chesworth et al.[22]*	Examiner performs passive ER of shoulder and classifies as bone to bone, spasm, capsular (normal or abnormal), springy block, tissue approximation, or empty	36 patients with shoulder disease	κ = .48–.49	κ = .62–.76

RELIABILITY OF THE CLINICAL EXAMINATION

Detecting Scapular Asymmetry During Static and Dynamic Activity

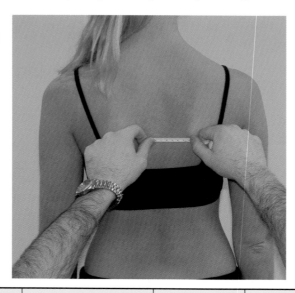

Figure 10-13A: *Lateral slide test position 1*

Test and Measure	Test Procedure	Population	Reliability ICC	
			Intra-examiner	**Inter-examiner**
Lateral scapular slide test Position 1	Patient is standing. Examiner records measurement between inferior angle of scapula and spinous process of thoracic vertebrae at same horizontal level in three positions. Position 1: with glenohumeral joint in neutral Position 2: with 45° of shoulder abduction and IR Position 3: with upper extremity in 90° of abduction and full IR A difference between sides >1 cm is considered scapular asymmetry	46 subjects with shoulder dysfunction and 26 subjects without shoulder dysfunction	With dysfunction .52 (.10, .74) Without dysfunction .75 (.56, .85)	With dysfunction .79 (.46, .91) Without dysfunction .67 (.25, .85)
Position 2			With dysfunction .66 (.36, .82) Without dysfunction .58 (.60, .86)	With dysfunction .45 (−.38, .78) Without dysfunction .43 (−.29, .75)
Position 3 Odom et al.[19]			With dysfunction .62 (.27, .79) Without dysfunction .80 (.65, .88)	With dysfunction .57 (−.23, .85) Without dysfunction .74 (.41, .88)
			Reliability Kappa	
Movement evaluation during abduction Kibler et al.[20]	Examiner classifies scapular movement during shoulder abduction into categories 1–4. Category 1 = inferior angle tilts dorsally compared with contralateral side Category 2 = medial border tilts dorsally compared with contralateral side Category 3 = shoulder shrug initiates movement Category 4 = scapulae move symmetrically	20 subjects with shoulder injuries and 6 asymptomatic subjects	$\kappa = .42$	NR

Detecting Scapular Asymmetry During Static and Dynamic Activity (cont.)

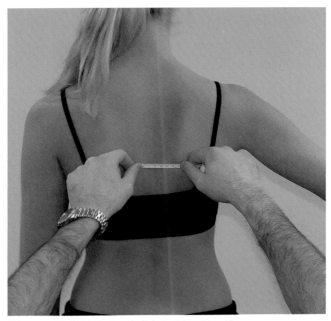

Figure 10-13B: *Lateral slide test position 2*

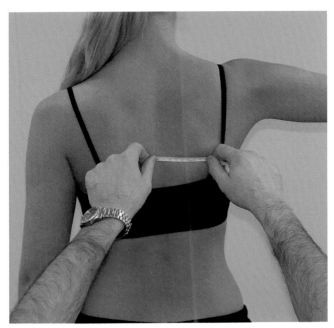

Figure 10-13C: *Lateral slide test position 3*

RELIABILITY OF THE CLINICAL EXAMINATION

Detecting Shoulder Instability

Test and Measure	Test Procedure	Population	Reliability Kappa Values and ICC	
Sulcus sign Levy et al.[24]	Patient supine. Examiner applies inferior distraction to shoulder. Amount of laxity is graded on a 0–3+ scale. 0 represents no laxity. 3+ represents maximum laxity	43 healthy college athletes	Inter-examiner $\kappa = .03–.06$	Intra-examiner $\kappa = .01–.20$
Palpation of subacromial space Boyd and Torrance[25]	Examiner palpates subacromial space and estimates distance as ¼, ½, ¾, or whole fingerbreadth	36 patients with shoulder subluxation	Intra-examiner ICC = .90–.94	Inter-examiner ICC = .77–.89
Load and shift test anterior	Test is performed with patient sitting and supine. For sitting patient, with glenohumeral joint in neutral, examiner stabilizes scapula with one hand and seats humeral head in glenoid fossa with the other hand. Examiner attempts to shift humeral head in anterior, posterior, and inferior directions. For supine patient, examiner grasps patient's elbow with one hand and the proximal humerus with the other hand. Arm is placed in 90° of abduction in the scapular plane. Examiner attempts to shift humeral head in anterior, posterior, and inferior directions. Amount of laxity is graded from 0 to 3. 0 indicates little or no movement. 3 indicates that humeral head can be dislocated off glenoid and remains so when pressure is released	13 patients with history indicating possible glenohumeral joint instability referred to an orthopaedic shoulder specialist	Inter-examiner reliability ICC 0° = .53 20° = .60 90° = .72	
Load and shift test posterior			Inter-examiner reliability ICC 0° = .68 20° = no variance observed 90° = .42	
Load and shift test inferior			Inter-examiner reliability ICC 0° = .79 20° = .79 90° = .65	
Sulcus sign	Patient sits, arms at sides. Examiner grasps patient's elbow and applies inferior force. If sulcus is identified, it is measured in centimeters		Inter-examiner reliability ICC .60	
Apprehension test	Patient is supine. The examiner positions arm in 90° of abduction and full ER. Examiner monitors for pain or apprehension		Pain = .31 Apprehension = .47 Pain and apprehension = .44	
Relocation test	Patient is supine with the arm abducted and in full ER. Examiner applies posterior force through humeral head. Positive if pain or apprehension is reduced with posteriorly applied force		Inter-examiner reliability ICC Pain = .31 Apprehension = .71 Pain and apprehension = .44	
Augmentation test	Patient is supine with arm in abduction and ER while examiner applies anterior force. Positive if pain or apprehension is provoked		Inter-examiner reliability ICC Pain = .09 Apprehension = .48 Pain and apprehension = .33	
Release test Tzannes et al.[26]	Patient is supine with arm in 90° of abduction and ER while examiner applies posterior force over humeral head. Examiner quickly releases posterior force. Positive if pain or apprehension is provoked		Inter-examiner reliability ICC Pain = .31 Apprehension = .63 Pain and apprehension = .45	

Detecting Shoulder Instability (cont.)

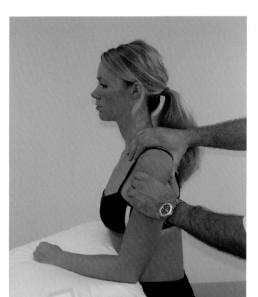

Figure 10-14: *Load and shift test anterior*

Measuring Proprioception During Internal and External Rotation

Test and Measure	Test Procedure	Population	Reliability ICC
Joint position sense *Dover and Powers[18]*	Patient is standing. Examiner measures full ER and IR of shoulder with inclinometer. Target angles are determined as 90% of IR and 90% of ER. With patient blindfolded, examiner guides patient's arm into target angle position and holds it for 3 sec. Patient's arm is returned to neutral. Patient is instructed to return arm to target angle. Examiner takes measurement with inclinometer	31 asymptomatic subjects	IR .98 ER .98

RELIABILITY OF THE CLINICAL EXAMINATION

Classifying Shoulder Disorders

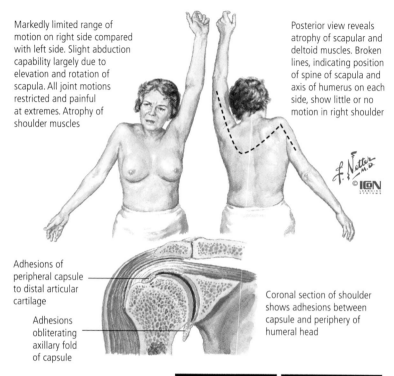

Markedly limited range of motion on right side compared with left side. Slight abduction capability largely due to elevation and rotation of scapula. All joint motions restricted and painful at extremes. Atrophy of shoulder muscles

Posterior view reveals atrophy of scapular and deltoid muscles. Broken lines, indicating position of spine of scapula and axis of humerus on each side, show little or no motion in right shoulder

Adhesions of peripheral capsule to distal articular cartilage

Adhesions obliterating axillary fold of capsule

Coronal section of shoulder shows adhesions between capsule and periphery of humeral head

Anteroposterior arthrogram of normal shoulder (left). Axillary fold and biceps brachii sheath visualized. Volume of capsule normal. Anteroposterior arthrogram of frozen shoulder (right). Joint capacity reduced. Axillary fold and biceps brachii sheath not evident

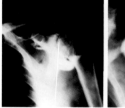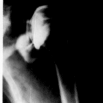

Figure 10-15: *Adhesive capsulitis of the shoulder*

Classification	Description of Procedure	Population	Inter-examiner Reliability Kappa Value
Capsular syndrome	Examiner obtains patient history. Physical examination consists of active, passive, and resistive movements. Determination of ROM, presence of painful arc or capsular pattern, and degree of muscle weakness are identified	201 patients with shoulder pain	κ = .63 (.50, .76)
Acute bursitis			κ = .50 (−.10, 1.0)
AC syndrome			κ = .24 (−.06, .53)
Subacromial syndrome			κ = .56 (.45, .68)
Rest group (does not fit any category above)			κ = .39 (.24, .54)
Mixed group (patient presents with two or more above classifications) de Winter et al[23]			κ = .14 (−.03, .30)

Shoulder Instability

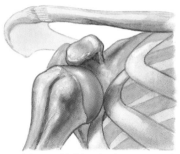

Subcoracoid dislocation (most common)

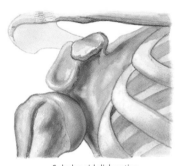

Subglenoid dislocation

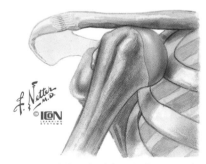

Subclavicular dislocation (uncommon).
Very rarely, humeral head penetrates
between ribs, producing intrathoracic
dislocation

Figure 10-16

Apprehension Test

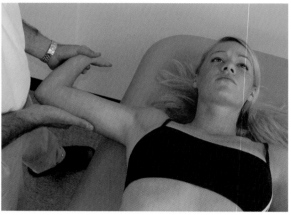

Figure 10-17

Test and Measure	Test Procedure	Determination of Positive Finding	Population	Reference Standard	Sens	Spec	+LR	−LR
Apprehension test Lo et al.[27]	Patient is supine with glenohumeral joint at edge of table, scapula supported by table. Shoulder is placed in 90° of abduction and elbow in 90° of flexion. Patient's shoulder is progressively externally rotated	Positive if patient reports pain or apprehension	46 patients with previously diagnosed shoulder disorder	Criteria for inclusion: 1. History of traumatic episode in abducted, ER position 2. Radiographic documentation of anterior glenohumeral dislocation 3. Reduction requiring physician assistance 4. Postreduction radiograph revealing concentric reduction 5. One or more recurrent episodes of instability 6. No history of surgery, instability of elbow or wrist, or shoulder disorder in extremity	.53	.99	53	.47

Sens, sensitivity; Spec, specificity; LR, likelihood ratio.

Relocation Test

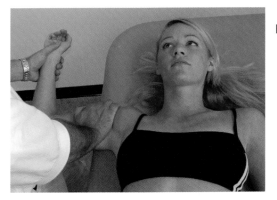

Figure 10-18

Test and Measure	Test Procedure	Determination of Positive Finding	Population	Reference Standard	Sens	Spec	+LR	−LR
Relocation test *Lo et al.*[27]	Patient supine with glenohumeral joint at edge of table. Examiner places shoulder in 90° of abduction and 90° of elbow flexion. Examiner then externally rotates shoulder and applies posterior force on head of humerus	Positive if patient's pain or apprehension diminishes with applied force	46 patients with previously diagnosed shoulder disorder	Criteria for inclusion: 1. History of traumatic episode in abducted, ER position 2. Radiographic documentation of anterior glenohumeral dislocation 3. Reduction requiring physician assistance 4. Postreduction radiograph revealing concentric reduction 5. One or more recurrent episodes of instability 6. No history of surgery, instability of elbow or wrist, or shoulder disorder in extremity	.46	.54	1.0	1.0
Relocation test with pain	Relocation test performed as above. After relocation test, examiner applies anteriorly directed force to proximal humerus		100 patients undergoing shoulder surgery	Surgical observation	.30	.58	.71	1.21
Relocation test with apprehension					.57	1.0	NA	.43
Anterior relocation test with pain					.54	.44	.96	1.05
Anterior relocation test with apprehension *Speer et al.*[28]					.68	1.0	NA	.32

NA, not available.

**DIAGNOSTIC
UTILITY OF
THE CLINICAL
EXAMINATION**

Anterior Release Test

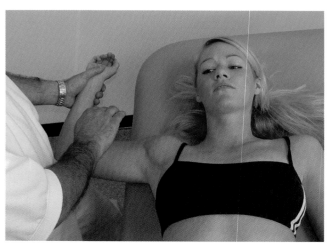

Figure 10-19

Test and Measure	Test Procedure	Determination of Positive Finding	Population	Reference Standard	Sens	Spec	+LR	−LR
Surprise Test *Lo et al.*[27]	Patient supine with shoulder in 90° of abduction and elbow in 90° of flexion. Patient's arm is ER while examiner applies posteriorly directed force. At end-range ER, examiner quickly releases posterior force to head of humerus	Positive if patient reports pain or apprehension when posterior force is removed	46 patients with a previously diagnosed shoulder disorder	Criteria for inclusion: 1. History of traumatic episode in abducted, ER position 2. Radiographic documentation of anterior glenohumeral dislocation 3. Reduction requiring physician assistance 4. Postreduction radiograph revealing concentric reduction 5. One or more recurrent episodes of instability 6. No history of surgery, instability of elbow or wrist, or shoulder disorder in extremity	.64	.99	64	.36
Anterior release test *Gross et al.*[29]			100 patients scheduled to undergo shoulder surgery	Surgical visualization	.92	.89	8.36	.09

Detecting Labral Tears: Anterior Slide Test

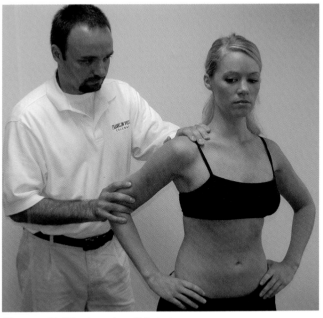

Figure 10-20: *Anterior slide test*

Test and Measure	Test Procedure	Determination of Positive Finding	Population	Reference Standard	Sens	Spec	+LR	−LR
Anterior slide test *Kibler*[35]	Patient is standing or sitting with hands on hips, thumbs facing posteriorly. The examiner stabilizes scapula with one hand and, with other hand on elbow, applies anteriorly and superiorly directed force through humerus. Patient is asked to push back against force	Positive if pain or click is elicited in anterior shoulder	126 athletes undergoing arthroscopic shoulder surgery and 100 asymptomatic athletes	Arthroscopic visualization	.78	.92	9.75	.24
Anterior slide test *McFarland et al.*[32]			426 patients who had undergone shoulder arthroscopy		.08	.84	.56	1.1

DIAGNOSTIC UTILITY OF THE CLINICAL EXAMINATION

Detecting Labral Tears: Crank Test

Test and Measure	Test Procedure	Determination of Positive Finding	Population	Reference Standard	Sens	Spec	+LR	−LR
Crank test *Stetson and Templin*[30]	Patient is supine while examiner elevates humerus 160° in scapular plane. Axial load is applied to humerus while shoulder is internally and externally rotated	Positive if pain is elicited	65 patients with symptoms of shoulder pain	Arthroscopic visualization	.46	.56	1.05	.96
Crank test *Mimori et al.*[31]			32 patients who had shoulder pain while throwing	Magnetic resonance arthrography	.83	1.0	NA	.17
Crank test *Liu et al.*[8]			62 patients scheduled to undergo arthroscopic shoulder surgery		.91	.93	13	.10
Compression rotation test *McFarland et al.*[32]	Patient is supine with arm abducted to 90° and elbow flexed to 90° while examiner applies axial force to humerus. Humerus is circumducted and rotated	Positive if pain or clicking is elicited	426 patients who had undergone shoulder arthroscopy	Arthroscopic visualization	.24	.76	1.0	1.0
Crank test *Guanche and Jones*[33]	Patient is supine. Examiner fully abducts humerus and internally and externally rotates arm while applying axial force through glenohumeral joint		62 shoulders undergoing arthroscopy		.40	.73	1.48	.82

Detecting Labral Tears: Crank Test (cont.)

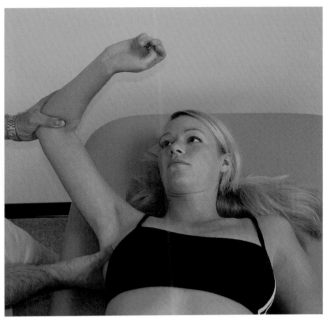

Figure 10-21: *The Crank test*

DIAGNOSTIC UTILITY OF THE CLINICAL EXAMINATION

Detecting Labral Tears: Active Compression Test

Test and Measure	Test Procedure	Determination of Positive Finding	Population	Reference Standard	Sens	Spec	+LR	−LR
Active compression test *O'Brien et al.*[34]	Standing patient is asked to flex arm to 90° with elbow in full extension. Patient then adducts arm 10° and internally rotates humerus. Examiner applies downward force to arm as patient resists. Patient then fully supinates arm and repeats procedure	Positive if pain or painful clicking in area of glenohumeral joint is elicited with first maneuver and reduced with second maneuver	318 patients with shoulder pain	Arthroscopic visualization	1.0	.98	50	0.0
Active compression test *McFarland et al.*[32]			426 patients who had undergone shoulder arthroscopy		.47	.55	1.04	.96
O'Brien test *Stetson and Templin*[30]	As above, except patient is seated		65 patients with symptoms of shoulder pain		.54	.31	.78	1.48
O'Brien test *Guanche and Jones*[33]	Seated patient adducts humerus 10° with thumb pointing down and elevates arm against resistance from examiner. Test is repeated with thumb pointing up	Positive if pain elicited is greater in thumb-down than in thumb-up position	62 shoulders undergoing arthroscopy		.63	.73	2.33	.51

Detecting Labral Tears: Active Compression Test (cont.)

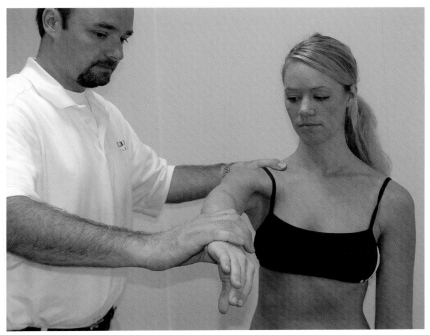

Figure 10-22A: Active compression test with internal rotation

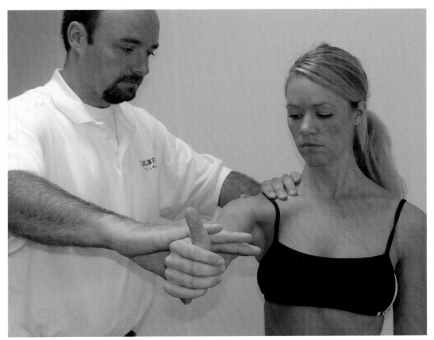

Figure 10-22B: Active compression test with external rotation

DIAGNOSTIC UTILITY OF THE CLINICAL EXAMINATION

Detecting Labral Tears: Miscellaneous Special Tests

Test and Measure	Test Procedure	Determination of Findings	Population	Reference Standard	Sens	Spec	+LR	−LR
Pain provocation test Mimori et al.[31]	Patient is sitting. Shoulder is abducted 90° to 100° and externally rotated by examiner. Performed with forearm pronation and supination	Positive if pain was provoked or more severe in pronated position	32 patients who had shoulder pain while throwing	Magnetic resonance arthrography	1.0	.9	10.0	0.0
Jobe relocation test	Patient is supine. Examiner abducts and externally rotates humerus. Examiner applies posterior pressure over humerus and releases it	Positive if pain is produced when force is released	62 shoulders scheduled to undergo arthroscopy	Arthroscopic visualization	.44	.87	3.38	.64
Anterior apprehension test	Patient is supine. Examiner passively abducts and externally rotates humerus	Positive if pain is produced with ER			.40	.87	3.08	.69
Bicipital groove tenderness	NR	NR			.44	.40	.73	1.40
Speed test	Patient is standing with arm in full elevation and forearm supination. Examiner applies resistance against elevation	Positive if pain is produced			.18	.87	1.38	.94
Yergason test Guanche and Jones[33]	Patient is standing with elbow at 90°. Patient supinates forearm against examiner's resistance. During procedure, examiner palpates long head of biceps tendon				.09	.93	1.29	.98

Detecting Labral Tears: Miscellaneous Special Tests (cont.)

Test and Measure	Test Procedure	Determination of Findings	Population	Reference Standard	Sens	Spec	+LR	−LR
Speed test*	As Speed test above	Positive if pain is produced	152 subjects with shoulder pain scheduled to undergo surgery	Surgical observation	.32	.75	1.28	.91
Yergason test* Holtby and Razmjou[36]	As Yergason test above				.43	.79	2.05	.72
SLAPrehension test Berg and Ciullo[7]	Patient is standing or seated and is asked to move humerus into horizontal adduction, IR, and elbow extension. Test is repeated with patient bringing humerus into ER	Positive if pain is produced with arm in IR to a greate extent than in ER	66 patients who had undergone arthroscopic shoulder surgery		.88	NR	NA	NA
Biceps load test Kim et al.[37]	Patient is supine with examiner grasping wrist and elbow. Arm is abducted to 90° with elbow flexed to 90° and forearm supinated. Examiner externally rotates arm until patient becomes apprehensive, at which time ER is stopped. Patient is asked to flex elbow against examiner's resistance	Positive if patient's apprehension remains or pain is produced	75 patients with unilateral recurrent anterior shoulder dislocations	Arthroscopic visualization	.90	.97	30	.10
Biceps load test II Kim et al.[38]	Patient is supine with examiner grasping wrist and elbow. Arm is elevated 120° and fully externally rotated with elbow held in 90° of flexion and forearm supinated. Examiner then resists elbow flexion by patient	Positive if resisted elbow flexion causes pain	127 patients experiencing shoulder pain scheduled to undergo arthroscopy		.90	.97	30	.10

*Positive tests are indicative of biceps tendon disease, labral tear, or both.

**DIAGNOSTIC
UTILITY OF
THE CLINICAL
EXAMINATION**

Detecting Labral Tears: Miscellaneous Special Tests (cont.)

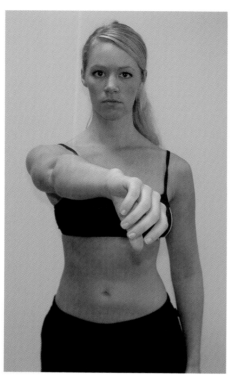

Figure 10-23A: *SLAPrebension test with internal rotation*

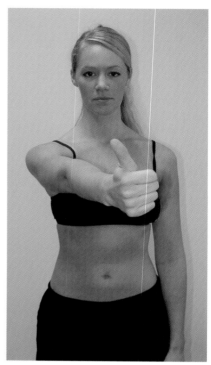

Figure 10-23B: *SLAPrebension test with external rotation*

Predicting Glenoid Labral Tears: Combination of Tests

Test and Measure	Test Procedure	Determination of Findings	Patient Population	Reference Standard	Sens	Spec	+LR	−LR
Crank test	Patient is supine while examiner elevates humerus 160° in scapular plane. Axial loads is applied to humerus while shoulder is internally and externally rotated	Positive if click is heard or apprehension is	54 patients with shoulder pain	Arthroscopic visualization	.90	.85	6	.12
Apprehension test	Patient is supine or seated with arm in 90° of abduction and ER. Examiner applies anteriorly directed load on humeral head	Positive if patient exhibits apprehension						
Relocation test	Patient is supine with the arm in 90° of abduction and ER. Examiner applies Examiner applies posteriorly directed load on humeral head	Positive if apprehension is eliminated						
Load and shift test	Patient is seated or supine. Examiner places arm in 20° of abduction and flexion. Examiner stabilizes scapular with one hand. With other hand, examiner loads humeral head into glenoid fossa and performs anterior and posterior translation	Positive if amount of translation is excessive compared with contralateral side						
Inferior sulcus sign *Liu et al*[39]	Not described	Not described						
Jobe relocation and O'Brien	Jobe relocation test: Patient is supine. Examiner abducts and externally rotates humerus. Examiner applies posterior pressure over humerus and releases it. Positive if pain is produced when force is released		62 shoulders scheduled to undergo arthroscopy		.41	.91	4.56	.65
Jobe relocation and anterior apprehension	Anterior apprehension test: Patient is supine. Examiner passively abducts and externally rotates humerus. Positive if pain is produced with ER				.38	.93	5.43	.67
O'Brien and anterior apprehension	O'Brien test: Seated patient adducts humerus 10° with thumb pointing down and elevates arm against resistance from examiner. Test is reported with thumb pointing up. Positive if pain elicited is greater in thumb-down than in thumb-up position				.38	.82	2.11	.76
Jobe and O'Brien and apprehension *Guanche and Jones*[33]					.34	.91	3.78	.73

DIAGNOSTIC UTILITY OF THE CLINICAL EXAMINATION

Detecting Subacromial Impingement: Hawkins and Kennedy Test

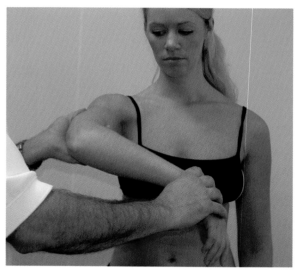

Figure 10-24: Hawkins and Kennedy test

Test and Measure	Test Procedure	Determination of Positive Findings	Patient Population	Reference Standard	Sens	Spec	+LR	−LR
Hawkins test *Calis et al.*[40]	Patient's arm is passively flexed to 90° and forcefully moved into IR		125 painful shoulders	Subacromial injection	.92	.25	1.23	.32
Hawkins sign* *MacDonald et al.*[41]		Positive if pain occurs with IR	85 patients scheduled to undergo shoulder arthroscopy	Arthroscopic visualization	.92	.44	1.64	.18
Hawkins and Kennedy test *Leroux et al.*[42]	Patient is standing. Examiner elevates patient's arm to 90° with elbow in 90° of flexion and forcefully internally rotates arm		55 patients scheduled to undergo shoulder surgery	Surgical observation	.87	NR	NA	NA

*Indicative of subacromial bursitis.

Detecting Subacromial Impingement: Neer Test

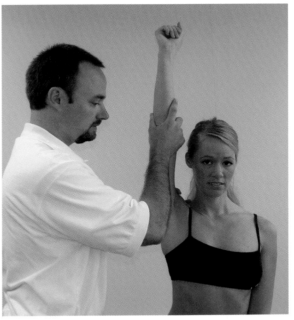

Figure 10-25: *Neer test*

Test and Measure	Test Procedure	Determination of Positive Findings	Population	Reference Standard	Sens	Spec	+LR	−LR
Neer test *Calis et al.*[40]	Examiner stabilizes scapula with one hand and forces patient's arm into maximal elevation with the other		125 painful shoulders	Subacromial injection	.89	.31	1.29	.35
Neer sign *MacDonald et al.*[41]	Examiner passively elevates shoulder with maximal IR while stabilizing scapula	Positive if pain is produced	85 patients scheduled to undergo shoulder arthroscopy	Arthroscopic visualization	.75	.48	1.44	.52
Neer and Welsh test *Leroux et al.*[42]	Patient is seated. Examiner stands behind patient, stabilizing scapula with one hand, and forcefully elevates humerus with the other		55 patients scheduled to undergo shoulder surgery	Surgical observation	.89	NR	NA	NA

DIAGNOSTIC UTILITY OF THE CLINICAL EXAMINATION

Detection of Subacromial Impingement: Miscellaneous Special Tests

Test and Measure	Test Procedure	Determination of Positive Findings	Population	Reference Standard	Sens	Spec	+LR	−LR
Yocum test *Leroux et al.*[42]	Patient is seated or standing and is asked to place hand of involved shoulder on contralateral shoulder and raise elbow	Positive if pain is elicited	55 patients scheduled to undergo shoulder surgery	Surgical observation	.78	NR	NA	NA
Horizontal adduction test	Examiner forces patient's arm into horizontal adduction while elbow is flexed				.82	.28	1.14	.64
Painful arc test	Patient is instructed to perform straight plane abduction throughout full ROM	Positive if pain occurs between 60° and 100° of abduction			.33	.81	1.74	.83
Drop arm test	Patient is instructed to abduct shoulder to 90°, then lower it slowly to neutral position	Positive if patient is unable to do this secondary to pain			.08	.97	2.67	.95
Yergason test	Patient's elbow is flexed to 90° with forearm in pronation. Patient is then instructed to actively supinate forearm against resistance	Positive if pain is produced in area of bicipital groove	125 painful shoulders	Subacromial injection	.37	.86	2.64	.73
Speed test *Calis et al.*[40]	Patient elevates humerus to 60° with elbow flexion and forearm supination. Patient holds this position while examiner applies resistance against elevation	Positive if pain is elicited			.69	.56	1.57	.55

Detection of Subacromial Impingement: Miscellaneous Special Tests (cont.)

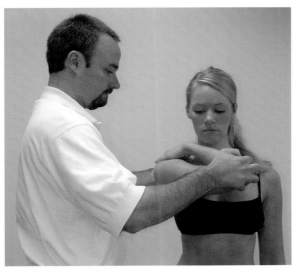

Figure 10-26: *Horizontal adduction test*

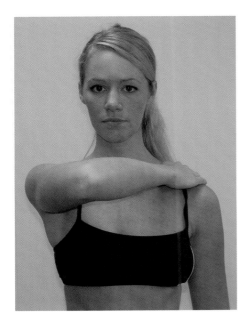

Figure 10-27: *Yocum test*

DIAGNOSTIC UTILITY OF THE CLINICAL EXAMINATION

Detecting Subacromial Impingement: Internal Rotation Resistance Strength Test

Zaslav[43] investigated the ability of the internal rotation resistance strength (IRRS) test to delineate intra-articular disease from impingement syndrome in a group of 115 patients who underwent arthroscopic shoulder surgery. The IRRS test is performed with the patient standing. The examiner positions the patient's arm in 90° of abduction and 80° of ER. The examiner applies resistance against ER, then IR in the same position. The test is considered positive for intra-articular disease if the patient exhibits greater weakness in IR when compared with ER. If the patient demonstrated greater weakness with ER, they were considered positive for impingement syndrome. The IRRS test demonstrated a sensitivity of .88, a specificity of .96, a +LR of 8.2, and a –LR of .13.

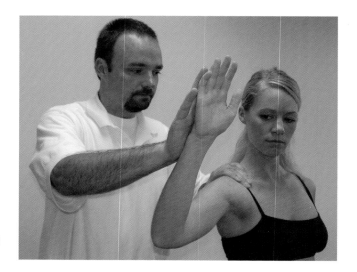

Figure 10-28A: Internal rotation resistance strength test, resistance against external rotation

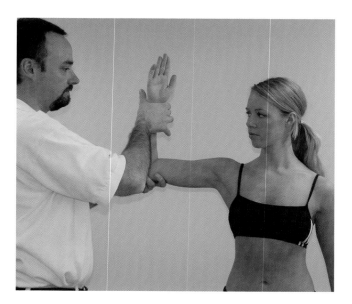

Figure 10-28B: Internal rotation resistance strength test, resistance against internal rotation

Detecting Subacromial Impingement: Combination of Tests

Calis et al.[40] calculated the diagnostic usefulness of combinations of the following tests for detecting subacromial impingement: Neer test, Hawkins test, horizontal adduction test, painful arc test, drop arm test, Yergason test, and Speed test. Each test is performed as described on pages 400 to 403.

Number of Positive Tests	Sens	Spec	+LR	−LR
All seven positive	.04	.97	1.33	.99
At least six positive	.30	.89	2.73	.79
At least five positive	.38	.86	2.71	.72
At least four positive	.70	.67	2.12	.45
At least three positive	.84	.44	1.5	.36

Detecting Rotator Cuff Tears: Historical Examination

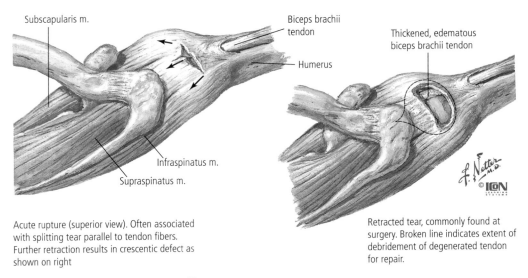

Acute rupture (superior view). Often associated with splitting tear parallel to tendon fibers. Further retraction results in crescentic defect as shown on right

Retracted tear, commonly found at surgery. Broken line indicates extent of debridement of degenerated tendon for repair.

Figure 10-29: *Superior rotator cuff tear*

Patient Reports	Sens	Spec	+LR	−LR
History of trauma	.36	.73	1.33	.88
Night pain Litaker et al.[9]	.88	.20	1.10	.60

Supraspinatus Tear

Test or Measure		Test Procedure	Determination of Finding	Population	Reference Standard	Sens (95% CI)	Spec (95% CI)	+LR (95% CI)	−LR (95% CI)
Full can test	Pain	Patient is standing with arms elevated to shoulder level in scapular plane, thumbs pointing up. Patient is asked to resist downward force applied by examiner	Muscle strength is graded on a 0 to 5 scale. 0 indicates no muscle contraction. 5 indicates full resistance. Presence or absence of pain is recorded	136 patients with shoulder symptoms	Magnetic resonance imaging (MRI)	.66	.64	1.83	.53
	Muscle weakness					.77	.74	2.96	.31
	Pain, muscle weakness, or both					.86	.57	2.0	.25
Empty can test *Itoi et al.[45]*	Pain	Patient is standing with arms elevated to shoulder level in scapular plane, thumbs pointing down. Patient is asked to resist downward force applied by examiner				.63	.55	1.40	.67
	Muscle weakness					.77	.68	2.41	.34
	Pain, muscle weakness, or both					.89	.50	1.78	.22
Weakness with elevation test *Litaker et al.[9]*			Positive if weakness is present	448 patients undergoing arthrography	Arthrographic confirmation of complete or partial rotator cuff tear	.64	.65	1.83	.55
Supraspinatus test *Holtby and Razmjou[46]*	Tendonitis or partial-thickness tear*	Patient is standing, shoulders abducted to 90° in scapular plane and IR of humerus.	Examiner records weakness or pain	50 patients with shoulder pain scheduled to undergo	Surgical observation	.62 (.49, .75)	.54 (.40, .68)	1.35	.70
	Full-thickness tear†					.41 (.27, .55)	.70 (.57, .83)	1.37	.84
	Large or massive full-thickness tear†	Examiner applies isometric resistance. Strength of involved side is compared with uninvolved side				.88 (.79, .97)	.70 (.58, .82)	2.93	.17
ER lag sign *Hertel et al.[47]*		Patient is seated. Examiner passively flexes elbow to 90° and elevates shoulder to 20° in scapular plane. Examiner then places shoulder in near maximal rotation (5° from full). Patient is asked to maintain position of ER when examiner releases arm. Tests integrity of supraspinatus and infraspinatus tendons	Positive if patient is unable to maintain ER	74 patients scheduled to undergo arthroscopic shoulder surgery	Arthroscopic visualization	.70	1.0	NA	.30

*Tendonitis defined as inflammation or fraying of supraspinatus tendon. Partial thickness defined as partial tear of supraspinatus tendon.
†Full-thickness tear categorized as small, moderate, large, or massive. Small indicates tear <1 cm, moderate indicates tear 1–3 cm that includes infraspinatus, large indicates tear 3–5 cm that includes infraspinatus and teres minor, and massive indicates tear >5 cm that includes infraspinatus, teres minor, and subscapularis.

Supraspinatus Tear (cont.)

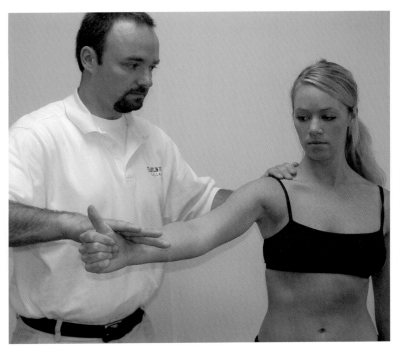

Figure 10-30: *Full can*

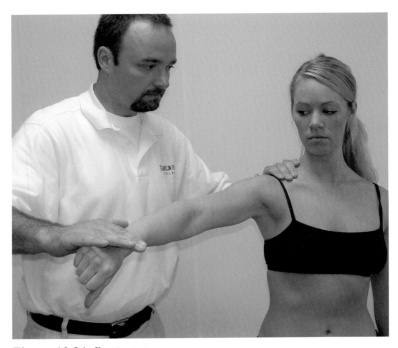

Figure 10-31: *Empty can*

DIAGNOSTIC UTILITY OF THE CLINICAL EXAMINATION

Identifying Impairments Associated With Rotator Cuff Injury

Test and Measure	Test Procedure and Determination of Positive Findings	Population	Reference Standard	Sens (95% CI)	Spec	+LR	−LR
Passive elevation less than 170°	Patient supine while examiner maximally elevates shoulder	448 patients undergoing arthrography	Arthrographic confirmation of complete or partial rotator cuff tear	.30	.78	1.36	.90
Passive ER less than 70°	Patient supine with arm at side. Examiner externally rotates arm			.19	.84	1.19	.96
Arc of pain sign	Patient standing while examiner passively abducts arm to 170°. Patient is then instructed to slowly lower arm to the side. Positive if patient reports pain at 120° to 70° of abduction			.98	.10	1.09	.20
Atrophy of the supraspinatus muscle	Examiner determines atrophy through visual inspection			.56	.73	2.07	.60
Atrophy of the infraspinatus muscle Litaker et al.[9]				.56	.73	2.07	.60
Strength testing of supraspinatus and infraspinatus combined with palpation Lyons and Tomlinson[44]	Isometric strength of supraspinatus is tested at 20° of abduction. Isometric strength of infraspinatus is tested by assessing resistance of IR while arm is in neutral position and elbow is at 90°. Examiner palpates rotator cuff while passively rotating arm internally and externally	42 patients scheduled to undergo shoulder surgery	Arthroscopic visualization	.91 (.76, .98)	.75	3.64	.12

Infraspinatus or Teres Minor Tears

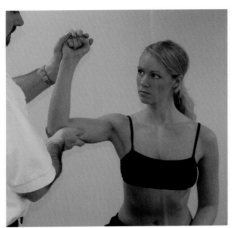

Figure 10-32A: *Hornblower's sign*

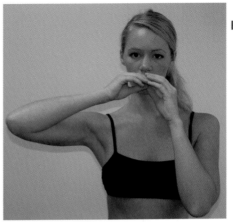

Figure 10-32B: *Patient with a positive hornblower's sign often has difficulty raising the hand to the mouth without abducting the shoulder.*

Test and Measure	Test Procedure	Determination of Positive Finding	Population	Reference Standard	Sens	Spec	+LR	−LR
Hornblower's signs (teres minor)	Patient is seated. Examiner places patient's arm in 90° of scaption and asks the patient to externally rotate against resistance	Positive if patient is unable to externally rotate shoulder	54 patients who had undergone shoulder surgery to repair rotator cuff	Stage of fatty degeneration of muscle as determined by computed tomography (CT) scan	1.0	.93	14.29	0.0
Dropping sign (infraspinatus) Walch et al.[48]	Patient is seated. Examiner places patient's shoulder in 0° of abduction and 45° of ER with elbow flexed to 90°. Patient is instructed to hold position when examiner releases forearm	Positive if patient is unable to hold position and arm returns to 0° of ER			1.0	1.0	NA	0.0
Drop sign (infraspinatus) Hertel et al.[47]	Patient is seated. Examiner elevates patient's arm to 90° of elevation in scapular plane with full ER and 90° of elbow flexion. Patient is instructed to maintain position when examiner releases arm	Positive if a lag or drop of arm occurs when arm is released	74 patients scheduled to undergo arthroscopic shoulder surgery	Arthroscopic visualization	.36*	1.00*	NA	.64

*Positive test is indicative of supraspinatus and infraspinatus tears.

Subscapularis Tears

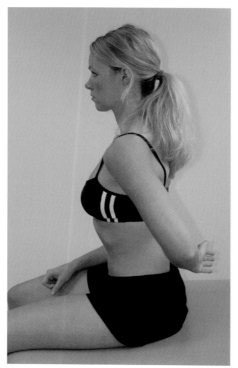

Figure 10-33A: *Internal rotation lag sign, negative test*

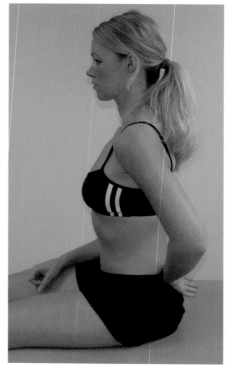

Figure 10-33B: *Internal rotation lag sign, positive test*

Test and Measure	Test Procedure	Determination of Positive Findings	Population	Reference Standard	Sens	Spec	+LR	−LR
IR lag sign *Hertel et al.*[47]	Patient is seated. Examiner brings shoulder to maximum IR by placing patient's forearm behind the back. While maintaining elbow in 90° of flexion, examiner extends shoulder 20°. Patient is instructed to maintain position when examiner releases arm	Positive if lag or drop of arm occurs when arm is released	74 patients scheduled to undergo arthroscopic shoulder surgery	Arthroscopic visualization	.97	.96	24.3	.03

Detecting Biceps Tendon Lesions: Speed Test

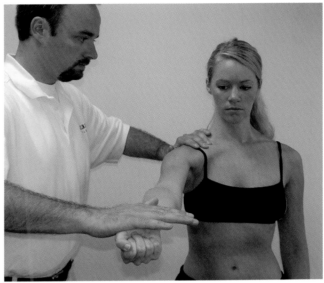

Figure 10-34: *Speed test*

Test and Measure	Test Procedure	Determination of Positive Findings	Population	Reference Standard	Sens	Spec	+LR	−LR
Speed test Bennett[51]	Patient is standing with arm flexed to 90°, elbow extended, and forearm fully supinated. Patient is asked to resist downward force applied by examiner	Positive if patient experiences pain in proximal shoulder during application of force	46 patients with shoulder pain	Arthroscopic visualization	.90	.14	1.0	.71
Gilcrest palm-up test Leroux et al.[42]	Patient is asked to elevate arm with elbow extended and forearm supinated against resistance applied by examiner	Positive if patient feels pain at anterior aspect of arm along course of biceps brachii	55 patients scheduled to undergo shoulder surgery	Surgical observation	.63	.35	.97	1.06

DIAGNOSTIC UTILITY OF THE CLINICAL EXAMINATION

Rotator Cuff Tears (Unspecified Muscles)

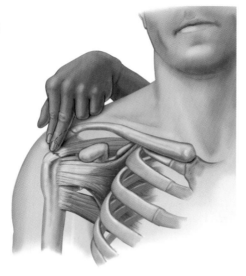

Figure 10-35: *Rent test*

Test and Measure	Test Procedure	Determination of Positive Findings	Population	Reference Standard	Sens	Spec	+LR	−LR
Neer sign	Examiner stabilizes scapula with one hand and forces patient's arm into maximal elevation with other hand	Positive if pain is produced	85 patients scheduled to undergo shoulder arthroscopy	Arthroscopic visualization	.83	.51	1.69	.33
Hawkins sign	Patient's arm is passively flexed to 90° and forcefully moved into IR	Positive if pain occurs with IR			.88	.43	1.54	.28
Both Hawkins and Neer *MacDonald et al.*[41]					.83	.56	1.89	.30
Impingement sign *Litaker et al.*[9]	As Neer sign above	Positive if pain is reproduced	448 patients undergoing arthrography	Arthrographic confirmation of complete or partial rotator cuff tear	.97	.09	1.07	.33
Rent test *Wolf and Agrawal*[49]	Patient is seated with arm by side. Examiner palpates anterior margin of acromion through deltoid. Examiner then passively extends patient's arm and internally and externally rotates to palpate rotator cuff tendons	Positive if examiner palpates eminence or rent	109 patients undergoing arthroscopic shoulder surgery	Arthroscopic visualization	.96	.97	32.0	.04

Rotator Cuff Tears (Unspecified Muscles) (cont.)

Murrell and Walton[50] identified predictor variables from the patient history and physical examination that could be used to determine the likelihood of a rotator cuff tear. Variables associated with rotator cuff tears were identified as age, supraspinatus weakness, weakness in ER, and impingement. The table below describes the relationship between the number of variables present and the associated posttest probability of rotator cuff tear.

Number of Positive Diagnostic Features	Age Group (y)	Posttest Probability (95% CI)
All three	Any	.98 (.89, 1.0)
Any two	<60	.64 (.47, .79)
Any two	>60	.98 (.89, 1.0)
Any one	<40	.12 (.25, .31)
Any one	40–69	.45 (.36, .55)
Any one	≥70	.76 (.56, .90)
None	Any	.05 (.02, .11)

DIAGNOSTIC UTILITY OF THE CLINICAL EXAMINATION

Detecting Acromioclavicular Lesions

A common mechanism of injury for acromioclavicular tears is a fall on the tip of the shoulder.

Test and Measure	Test Procedure	Determination of Positive Findings	Patient Population	Reference Standard	Sens	Spec	+LR	−LR
Active compression test O'Brien et al.[34]	Patient is standing. Examiner asks patient to flex arm to 90° with elbow in full extension. Patient then adducts arm 10° and internally rotates humerus. Examiner applies downward force to arm as patient resists. Patient fully supinates arm and repeats procedure	Positive if pain is localized to AC joint	318 patients with shoulder pain	Radiographic confirmation	1.0	.97	33.3	0.0
O'Brien sign			1013 patients with pain between mid clavicle and deltoid	AC joint infiltration test: Patients were injected with lidocaine in AC joint. Those who experienced at least a 50% reduction in symptoms within 10 minutes were considered to have AC disease	.16	.90	1.6	.93
Paxinos test	Patient is sitting with arm by side. With one hand, examiner places thumb over posterolateral aspect of acromion and index finger superior to midportion of clavicle. Examiner then applies compressive force	Positive if pain is reported in area of AC joint			.79	.50	1.58	.42
Palpation of the AC joint Walton et al.[53]	NR	NR			.96	.10	1.07	.40
Cross-body adduction stress test	Examiner flexes shoulder to 90° and adducts it across body				.77	.79	3.67	.29
AC-resisted extension test	Patient is standing with arm flexed to 90°, elbow bent to 90°. Patient is asked to extend arm against examiner's resistance	Positive if pain is reproduced at AC joint	315 patients undergoing shoulder surgery	Arthroscopic visualization	.72	.85	4.80	.33
Active compression test Chronopoulos et al.[54]	Patient is standing. Examiner asks patient to flex arm to 90° with elbow in full extension. Patient then adducts arm 10° and internally rotates humerus. Examiner applies downward force to arm as patient resists. Patient fully supinates arm and repeats procedure				.41	.95	8.20	.62

Detecting Acromioclavicular Lesions (cont.)

Test and Measure	Test Procedure	Determination of Positive Findings	Patient Population	Reference Standard	Sens	Spec	+LR	−LR
Neer impingement sign	NR	NR	315 patients undergoing shoulder surgery	Arthroscopic visualization	.57	.41	.97	1.05
Hawkins impingement sign					.47	.45	.85	1.18
Painful arc sign					.50	.47	.94	1.06
Drop arm sign					.35	.72	1.25	.90
Speed test *Chronopoulos et al[54]*					.24	.71	.83	1.07

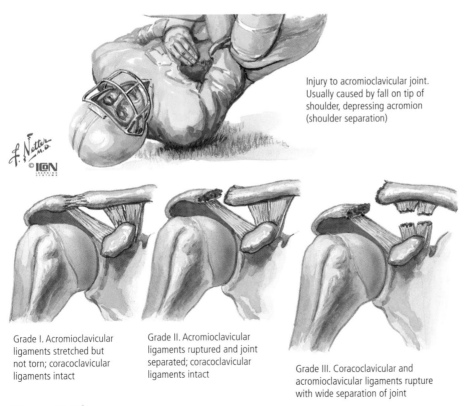

Injury to acromioclavicular joint. Usually caused by fall on tip of shoulder, depressing acromion (shoulder separation)

Grade I. Acromioclavicular ligaments stretched but not torn; coracoclavicular ligaments intact

Grade II. Acromioclavicular ligaments ruptured and joint separated; coracoclavicular ligaments intact

Grade III. Coracoclavicular and acromioclavicular ligaments rupture with wide separation of joint

Figure 10-36

**DIAGNOSTIC
UTILITY OF
THE CLINICAL
EXAMINATION**

Classifying Shoulder Disorders: Special Tests

Naredo et al.[52] investigated the diagnostic utility of the physical examination in identifying specific disorders as confirmed by ultrasonographic findings in 31 consecutive patients referred to a rheumatology clinic with shoulder pain. The following special tests were used to classify the shoulder disorder.

Pathology	Test and Measure	Test Procedure	Determination of Positive Findings		Sens	Spec	+LR	−LR
Impingement	Neer test	Patient is standing. Examiner stabilizes scapula with one hand while forcefully elevating patient's arm with other hand	Positive if pain is reproduced		.65	.73	2.41	.48
	Hawkins test	Patient is standing. Examiner elevates patient's arm to 90° with elbow flexed to 90°. Examiner then forcefully internally rotates arm						
	Yocum test	Patient places involved hand on contralateral shoulder and is asked to raise elbow without elevating shoulder						
Tendon disease of infraspinatus and teres minor	Pattes	Examiner supports patient's elbow in 90° of elevation in scapular plane. Patient is asked to rotate arm laterally against examiner's resistance	Positive for tendonitis if pain is produced. If patient is unable to resist force, test is considered positive for tendon rupture	Lesion	.71	.90	7.1	.32
				Tendonitis	.57	.71	1.97	.61
				Tear	.36	.95	7.2	.67
Tendon disease of supraspinatus	Jobes	Patient places both arms in 90° of elevation with IR of shoulder. Patient then resists downward force applied by examiner		Lesion	.79	.50	1.58	.42
				Tendonitis	.72	.38	1.16	.74
				Tear	.19	1.0	NA	.81
Tendon disease of subscapularis	Gerber lift-off test	Patient is standing with hand against back at waist level. Examiner pulls patient's arm 5° to 10° away from back while maintaining elbow flexion. Patient is asked to maintain position when examiner releases arm	Positive for complete tendon rupture if patient cannot hold position	Lesion	.50	.84	3.13	.60
				Tendonitis	.50	.88	4.17	.57
				Tear	.50	.95	10	.53
Tendon disease of biceps brachii *Naredo et al.*[52]	Yergason test	With patient's arm at side, patient is asked to perform elbow flexion with medial rotation of arm against resistance	Positive if biceps tendon slips out of bicipital groove or if patient's pain is reproduced	Tendonitis	.74	.58	1.76	.45
	Palm-up test	Patient is asked to elevate arm with palm facing upward	Positive if movement recreates patient's pain along course of biceps brachii					

*Lesion indicates involvement of any tendon as determined by ultrasonographic findings.

Classifying Shoulder Disorders: Special Tests (cont.)

Chronopoulos et al.[54] investigated the diagnostic utility of three combined special tests for identifying AC lesions. The tests investigated were the cross-body adduction stress test, the AC resisted-extension test, and the active compression test. Results demonstrated that if two of the tests were positive, the sensitivity was .81, and the specificity was .89. The +LR was 7.36, and the –LR was .21. If all three tests were positive, the sensitivity was determined to be .25, with a specificity of .97, a +LR of 36.4, and a –LR of .77

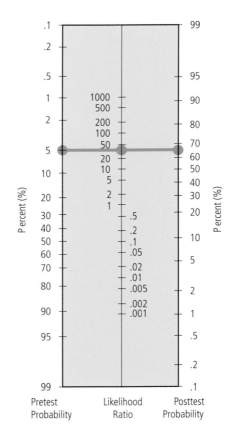

Figure 10-37: *Nomogram representing a dramatic change from the pretest (6%) to the posttest probability (70%) if the cross-body adduction stress test, the AC resisted-extension test, and the active compression test were all found to be positive (+LR 36.4).* (Nomogram adapted with permission, Massachusetts Medical Society, Copyright © 2005.)

REFERENCES

1. Norkin CC, Levangie PK. The shoulder complex. *Joint Structure and Function: A Comprehensive Analysis.* 2nd ed. Philadelphia: F.A. Davis Company; 1992:240-261.

2. Inman VT, Saunders JB, Abbott LC. Observations on the function of the shoulder joint. *Clin Orthop.* 1996;330:3-12.

3. Neumann DA. Shoulder complex. In: *Kinesiology of Musculoskeletal System: Foundations for Physical Rehabilitation.* St. Louis: Mosby; 2002:189-248.

4. Brody LT. Shoulder. In: *Current Concepts of Orthopaedic Physical Therapy.* La Crosse: Orthopaedic Section, American Physical Therapy Association; 2001.

5. Michener LA, Walsworth MK, Burnet EN. Effectiveness of rehabilitation for patients with subacromial impingement syndrome: a systematic review. *J Hand Ther.* 2004;17:152-164.

6. Hartley A. *Practical Joint Assessment.* St. Louis: Mosby; 1995.

7. Berg EE, Ciullo JV. A clinical test for superior glenoid labral or 'SLAP' lesions. *Clin J Sport Med.* 1998;8:121-123.

8. Liu SH, Henry MH, Nuccion SL. A prospective evaluation of a new physical examination in predicting glenoid labral tears. *Am J Sports Med.* 1996;24:721-725.

9. Litaker D, Pioro M, El Bilbeisi H, Brems J. Returning to the bedside: using the history and physical examination to identify rotator cuff tears. *J Am Geriatr Soc.* 2000;48:1633-1637.

10. Cleland J, Durall CJ. Physical therapy for adhesive capsulitis. *Physiotherapy.* 2002;88:450-457.

11. Rayan GM, Jensen C. Thoracic outlet syndrome: provocative examination maneuvers in a typical population. *J Shoulder Elbow Surg.* 1995;4:113-117.

12. Winsor T, Brow R. Costoclavicular syndrome: its diagnosis and treatment. *JAMA.* 2004;196:109-111.

13. Wainner RS, Gill H. Diagnosis and nonoperative management of cervical radiculopathy. *J Orthop Sports Phys Ther.* 2000;30:728-744.

14. Wainner RS, Fritz JM, Irrgang JJ, Boninger ML, Delitto A, Allison A. Reliability and diagnostic accuracy of the clinical examination and patient self-report measures for cervical radiculopathy. *Spine.* 2003;28:52-62.

15. Riddle D, Rothstein J, Lamb R. Goniometric reliability in a clinical setting: shoulder measurements. *Phys Ther.* 1987;67:668-673.

16. Hoving JL, Buchbinder R, Green S, et al. How reliably do rheumatologists measure shoulder movement? *Ann Rheum Dis.* 2002;61:612-616.

17. Edwards TB, Bostick RD, Greene CC, Baratta RV, Drez D. Interobserver and intraobserver reliability of the measurement of shoulder internal rotation by vertebral level. *J Shoulder Elbow Surg.* 2002;11:40-42.

18. Dover G, Powers ME. Reliability of joint position sense and force-reproduction measures during internal and external rotation of the shoulder. *J Athl Train.* 2003;38:304-310.

19. Odom CJ, Taylor AB, Hurd CE, Denegar CR. Measurement of scapular asymmetry and assessment of shoulder dysfunction using the Lateral Scapular Slide Test: a reliability and validity study. *Phys Ther.* 2001;81:799-809.

20. Kibler WB, Uhl TL, Maddux JW, Brooks PV, Zeller B, McMullen J. Qualitative clinical evaluation of scapular dysfunction: a reliability study. *J Shoulder Elbow Surg.* 2002;11:550-556.

21. Pellecchia GL, Paolino J, Connell J. Intertester reliability of the Cyriax evaluation in assessing patients with shoulder pain. *J Orthop Sports Phys Ther.* 1996;23:34-38.

22. Chesworth BM, MacDermid JC, Roth JH, Patterson SD. Movement diagram and "end-feel" reliability when measuring passive lateral rotation of the shoulder in patients with shoulder pathology. *Phys Ther*. 1998;78:593-601.

23. de Winter AF, Jans MP, Scholten RJ, Deville W, van Schaardenburg D, Bouter LM. Diagnostic classification of shoulder disorders: interobserver agreement and determinants of disagreement. *Ann Rheum Dis*. 1999;58:272-277.

24. Levy AS, Lintner S, Kenter K, Speer KP. Intra- and interobserver reproducibility of the shoulder laxity examination. *Am J Sports Med*. 1999;27:460-463.

25. Boyd EA, Torrance GM. Clinical measures of shoulder subluxation: their reliability. *Can J Public Health*. 1992;83:S24-S28.

26. Tzannes A, Paxinos A, Callanan M, Murrell GA. An assessment of the interexaminer reliability of tests for shoulder instability. *J Shoulder Elbow Surg*. 2004;13:18-23.

27. Lo IK, Nonweiler B, Woolfrey M, Litchfield R, Kirkley A. An evaluation of the apprehension, relocation, and surprise tests for anterior shoulder instability. *Am J Sports Med*. 2004;32:301-307.

28. Speer KP, Hannafin JA, Altchek DW, Warren RF. An evaluation of the shoulder relocation test. *Am J Sports Med*. 1994;22:177-183.

29. Gross ML, Distefano MC. Anterior release test. A new test for occult shoulder instability. *Clin Orthop*. 1997;339:105-108.

30. Stetson WB, Templin K. The crank test, the O'Brien test, and routine magnetic imaging scans in the diagnosis of labral tears. *Am J Sports Med*. 2002;30:806-809.

31. Mimori K, Muneta T, Nakagawa T, Shinomiya K. A new pain provocation test for superior labral tears of the shoulder. *Am J Sports Med*. 1999;27:137-142.

32. McFarland EG, Kim TK, Savino RM. Clinical assessment of three common tests for superior labral anterior-posterior lesions. *Am J Sports Med*. 2002;30:810-815.

33. Guanche CA, Jones DC. Clinical testing for tears of the glenoid labrum. *Arthroscopy*. 2003;19:517-523.

34. O'Brien SJ, Pagnani MJ, Fealy S, McGlynn SR, Wilson JB. The active compression test: a new and effective test for diagnosing labral tears and acromioclavicular joint abnormality. *Am J Sports Med*. 1998;26:610-613.

35. Kibler WB. Specificity and sensitivity of the anterior slide test in throwing athletes with superior glenoid labral tears. *Arthroscopy*. 1995;11:296-300.

36. Holtby R, Razmjou H. Accuracy of the Speed's and Yergason's tests in detecting biceps pathology and SLAP lesions: comparison with arthroscopic findings. *Arthroscopy*. 2004;20:231-236.

37. Kim SH, Ha KI, Han KY. Biceps load test: a clinical test for superior labrum anterior and posterior lesions in shoulders with recurrent anterior dislocations. *Am J Sports Med*. 1999;27:300-303.

38. Kim SH, Ha KI, Ahn JH, Kim SH, Choi HJ. Biceps load test II: a clinical test for SLAP lesions of the shoulder. *Arthroscopy*. 2001;17:160-164.

39. Liu SH, Henry MH, Nuccion S, Shapiro MS, Dorey F. Diagnosis of glenoid labral tears. A comparison between magnetic resonance imaging and clinical examinations. *Am J Sports Med*. 1996;24:149-154.

40. Calis M, Akgun K, Birtane M, Karacan I, Calis H, Tuzun F. Diagnostic values of clinical diagnostic tests in subacromial impingement syndrome. *Ann Rheum Dis*. 2000;59:44-47.

41. MacDonald P, Clark P, Sutherland K. An analysis of the diagnostic accuracy of the

REFERENCES

Hawkins and Neer subacromial impingement signs. *J Shoulder Elbow Surg.* 2000;9:299-301.

42. Leroux JL, Thomas E, Bonnel F, Blotman F. Diagnostic value of clinical tests for shoulder impingement syndrome. *Rev Rhum Engl Ed.* 1995;62:423-428.

43. Zaslav KR. Internal rotation resistance strength test: a new diagnostic test to differentiate intra-articular pathology from outlet (Neer) impingement syndrome in the shoulder. *J Shoulder Elbow Surg.* 2001;10:23-27.

44. Lyons A, Tomlinson J. Clinical diagnosis of tears of the rotator cuff. *J Bone Joint Surg.* 1992;74B:414-415.

45. Itoi E, Kido T, Sano A, Urayama M, Sato K. Which is more useful, the "full can test" or the "empty can test" in detecting the torn supraspinatus tendon? *Am J Sports Med.* 1999;27:65-68.

46. Holtby R, Razmjou H. Validity of the supraspinatus test as a single clinical test in diagnosing patients with rotator cuff pathology. *J Orthop Sports Phys Ther.* 2004;34:194-200.

47. Hertel R, Ballmer FT, Lombert SM, Gerber C. Lag signs in the diagnosis of rotator cuff rupture. *J Shoulder Elbow Surg.* 1996;5:307-313.

48. Walch G, Boulahia A, Calderone S, Robinson AH. The 'dropping' and 'hornblower's' signs in evaluation of rotator cuff tears. *J Bone Joint Surg.* 1998;80:624-628.

49. Wolf EM, Agrawal V. Transdeltoid palpation (the rent test) in the diagnosis of rotator cuff tears. *J Shoulder Elbow Surg.* 2001;10:470-473.

50. Murrell GA, Walton JR. Diagnosis of rotator cuff tears. *Lancet.* 2001;357:769-770.

51. Bennett WF. Specificity of the Speed's test: arthroscopic technique for evaluating the biceps tendon at the level of the bicipital groove. *Arthroscopy.* 1998;14:789-796.

52. Naredo E, Aguado P, De Miguel E, et al. Painful shoulder: comparison of physical examination and ultrasonographic findings. *Ann Rheum Dis.* 2001;61:132-136.

53. Walton J, Mahajan S, Paxinos A, et al. Diagnostic values of tests for acromioclavicular joint pain. *J Bone Joint Surg Am.* 2004;86A:807-812.

54. Chronopoulos E, Kim TK, Park HB, Ashenbrenner D, McFarland EG. Diagnostic value of physical tests for isolated chronic acromioclavicular lesions. *Am J Sports Med.* 2004;32:655-661.

Elbow and Forearm

Chapter 11

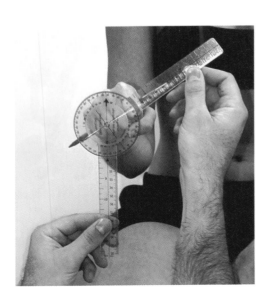

ANATOMY   Elbow

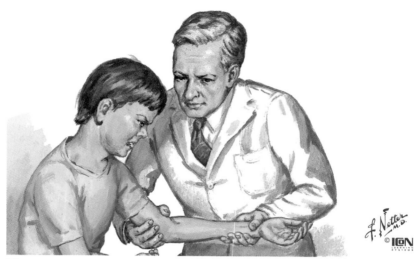

Figure 11-1

Bones of Elbow

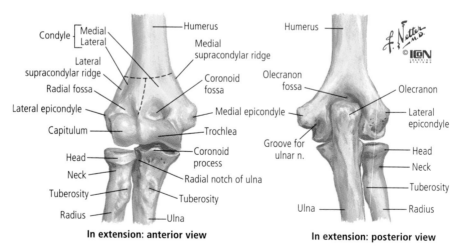

Condyle [Medial / Lateral]

Humerus

Medial supracondylar ridge

Lateral supracondylar ridge

Radial fossa

Coronoid fossa

Lateral epicondyle

Capitulum

Trochlea

Head

Coronoid process

Neck

Radial notch of ulna

Tuberosity

Tuberosity

Radius

Ulna

Medial epicondyle

In extension: anterior view

Humerus

Olecranon fossa

Olecranon

Medial epicondyle

Lateral epicondyle

Groove for ulnar n.

Head

Neck

Tuberosity

Ulna

Radius

In extension: posterior view

Figure 11-2: *Bones of right elbow*

Bones of Elbow (cont.)

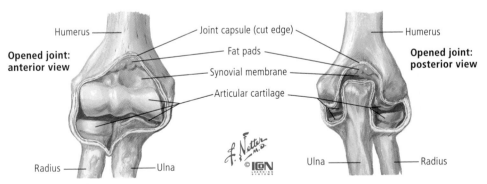

Humerus — Radius — Humerus

In extension: lateral view   **In extension: medial view**

Humerus
Lateral epicondyle
Capitulum
Head
Neck
Tuberosity

Radius

Radial notch
Coronoid process — of ulna
Trochlear notch
Olecranon
Ulna

In 90° flexion: lateral view

Humerus
Medial epicondyle
Capitulum
Trochlea
Head
Neck
Tuberosity

Tuberosity
Coronoid process
Trochlear notch
Olecranon

In 90° flexion: medial view

Figure 11-2 (cont.)

Anterior and Posterior Opened Elbow Joint

Humerus — Joint capsule (cut edge) — Humerus

Opened joint: anterior view

Fat pads
Synovial membrane
Articular cartilage

Opened joint: posterior view

Radius — Ulna   Ulna — Radius

Figure 11-3

Joint	Type and Classification	Closed Packed Position	Capsular Pattern
Humeroulnar	Synovial: hinge	Elbow extension	Flexion is limited more than extension
Humeroradial	Synovial: condyloid	0° of flexion, 5° of supination	Flexion is limited more than extension
Proximal radioulnar	Synovial: trochoid	5° of supination	Pronation = supination
Distal radioulnar	Synovial: trochoid	5° of supination	Pronation = supination

LIGAMENTS   Ligaments of Elbow

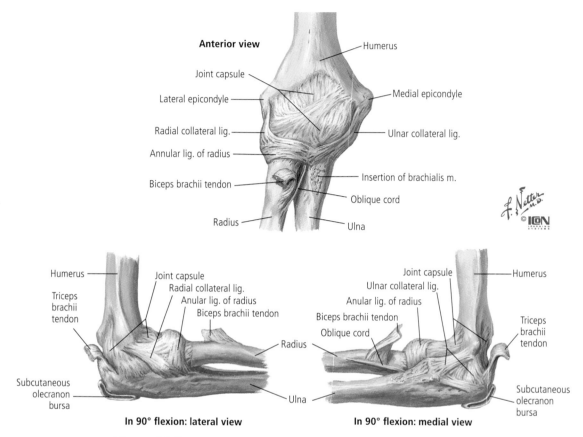

Anterior view

Humerus

Joint capsule

Lateral epicondyle

Medial epicondyle

Radial collateral lig.

Ulnar collateral lig.

Annular lig. of radius

Biceps brachii tendon

Insertion of brachialis m.

Oblique cord

Radius

Ulna

Humerus

Joint capsule

Joint capsule

Humerus

Triceps brachii tendon

Radial collateral lig.

Ulnar collateral lig.

Anular lig. of radius

Anular lig. of radius

Biceps brachii tendon

Biceps brachii tendon

Triceps brachii tendon

Radius

Oblique cord

Subcutaneous olecranon bursa

Ulna

Subcutaneous olecranon bursa

In 90° flexion: lateral view

In 90° flexion: medial view

Figure 11-4

Ligaments	Attachments	Function
Radial collateral	Lateral epicondyle of humerus to annular ligament of radius	Resist varus stress
Annular ligament of radius	Coronoid process of ulna, around radial head to lateral border of radial notch of ulna	Hold head of radius in radial notch of ulna, and allow forearm supination and pronation
Ulnar collateral	Medial epicondyle of humerus to coronoid process and olecranon of ulna	Resist valgus stress

Ligaments of Forearm

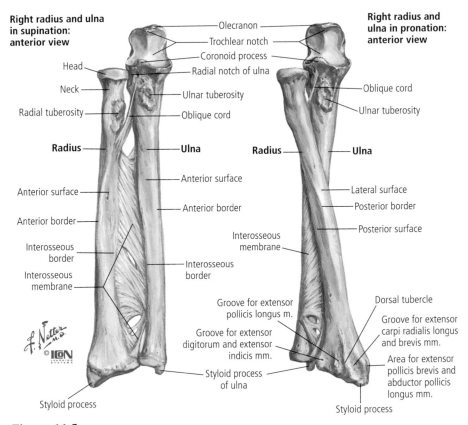

Right radius and ulna in supination: anterior view

- Head
- Neck
- Radial tuberosity
- **Radius**
- Anterior surface
- Anterior border
- Interosseous border
- Interosseous membrane

- Olecranon
- Trochlear notch
- Coronoid process
- Radial notch of ulna
- Ulnar tuberosity
- Oblique cord
- **Ulna**
- Anterior surface
- Anterior border
- Interosseous border
- Groove for extensor pollicis longus m.
- Groove for extensor digitorum and extensor indicis mm.
- Styloid process of ulna

- Styloid process

Right radius and ulna in pronation: anterior view

- Oblique cord
- Ulnar tuberosity
- **Radius** — **Ulna**
- Lateral surface
- Posterior border
- Posterior surface
- Interosseous membrane
- Dorsal tubercle
- Groove for extensor carpi radialis longus and brevis mm.
- Area for extensor pollicis brevis and abductor pollicis longus mm.
- Styloid process

Figure 11-5

Ligaments	Attachments	Function
Oblique cord	Tuberosity of ulna to just distal to tuberosity of radius	Transfer forces from radius to ulna, and reinforce proximity of ulna to radius
Interosseous membrane	Lateral border of ulna to medial border of radius	Transfer force from radius to ulna, and reinforce proximity of ulna to radius

MUSCLES

Anterior and Posterior Muscles of Arm

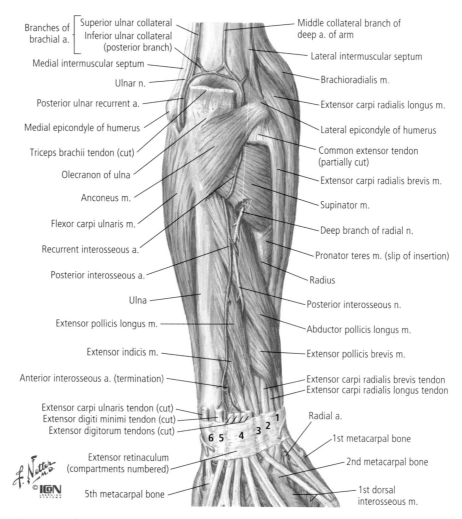

Branches of brachial a. — Superior ulnar collateral
Inferior ulnar collateral (posterior branch)

Medial intermuscular septum

Ulnar n.

Posterior ulnar recurrent a.

Medial epicondyle of humerus

Triceps brachii tendon (cut)

Olecranon of ulna

Anconeus m.

Flexor carpi ulnaris m.

Recurrent interosseous a.

Posterior interosseous a.

Ulna

Extensor pollicis longus m.

Extensor indicis m.

Anterior interosseous a. (termination)

Extensor carpi ulnaris tendon (cut)
Extensor digiti minimi tendon (cut)
Extensor digitorum tendons (cut)

Extensor retinaculum (compartments numbered)

5th metacarpal bone

Middle collateral branch of deep a. of arm

Lateral intermuscular septum

Brachioradialis m.

Extensor carpi radialis longus m.

Lateral epicondyle of humerus

Common extensor tendon (partially cut)

Extensor carpi radialis brevis m.

Supinator m.

Deep branch of radial n.

Pronator teres m. (slip of insertion)

Radius

Posterior interosseous n.

Abductor pollicis longus m.

Extensor pollicis brevis m.

Extensor carpi radialis brevis tendon
Extensor carpi radialis longus tendon

Radial a.

1st metacarpal bone

2nd metacarpal bone

1st dorsal interosseous m.

Figure 11-6

Muscle		Proximal Attachment	Distal Attachment	Nerve and Segmental Level	Action
Triceps brachii	Long head	Infraglenoid tubercle of scapula	Olecranon process of ulna	Radial nerve (C6, C7, C8)	Extend elbow
	Lateral head	Superior to radial groove of humerus			
	Medial head	Inferior to radial groove of humerus			
Anconeus		Lateral epicondyle of humerus	Superoposterior aspect of ulna	Radial nerve (C7, C8, T1)	Assist in elbow extension, stabilize elbow joint

Anterior and Posterior Muscles of Arm (cont.)

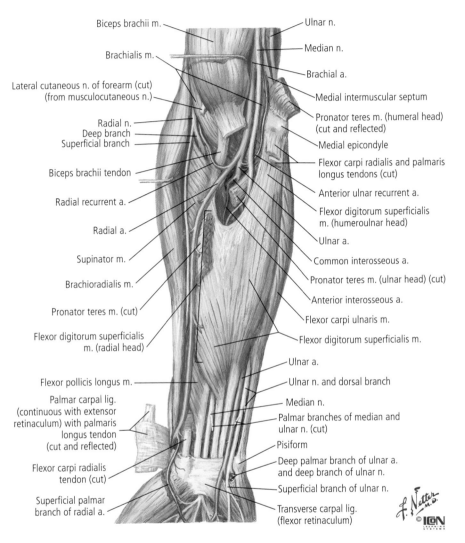

Biceps brachii m.

Brachialis m.

Lateral cutaneous n. of forearm (cut)
(from musculocutaneous n.)

Radial n.
Deep branch
Superficial branch

Biceps brachii tendon

Radial recurrent a.

Radial a.

Supinator m.

Brachioradialis m.

Pronator teres m. (cut)

Flexor digitorum superficialis
m. (radial head)

Flexor pollicis longus m.

Palmar carpal lig.
(continuous with extensor
retinaculum) with palmaris
longus tendon
(cut and reflected)

Flexor carpi radialis
tendon (cut)

Superficial palmar
branch of radial a.

Ulnar n.

Median n.

Brachial a.

Medial intermuscular septum

Pronator teres m. (humeral head)
(cut and reflected)

Medial epicondyle

Flexor carpi radialis and palmaris
longus tendons (cut)

Anterior ulnar recurrent a.

Flexor digitorum superficialis
m. (humeroulnar head)

Ulnar a.

Common interosseous a.

Pronator teres m. (ulnar head) (cut)

Anterior interosseous a.

Flexor carpi ulnaris m.

Flexor digitorum superficialis m.

Ulnar a.

Ulnar n. and dorsal branch

Median n.

Palmar branches of median and
ulnar n. (cut)

Pisiform

Deep palmar branch of ulnar a.
and deep branch of ulnar n.

Superficial branch of ulnar n.

Transverse carpal lig.
(flexor retinaculum)

F. Netter M.D.

Figure 11-6 (cont.)

Muscle		Proximal Attachment	Distal Attachment	Nerve and Segmental Level	Action
Biceps brachii	Short head	Coronoid process of scapula	Radial tuberosity and fascia of forearm	Musculocutaneous nerve (C5, C6)	Supinate forearm and flex elbow
	Long head	Supraglenoid tubercle of scapula			
Brachialis		Distal aspect of humerus	Coronoid process and tuberosity of ulna	Musculocutaneous nerve (C5, C6)	Flex elbow

MUSCLES   **Supinators/Pronators of the Forearm**

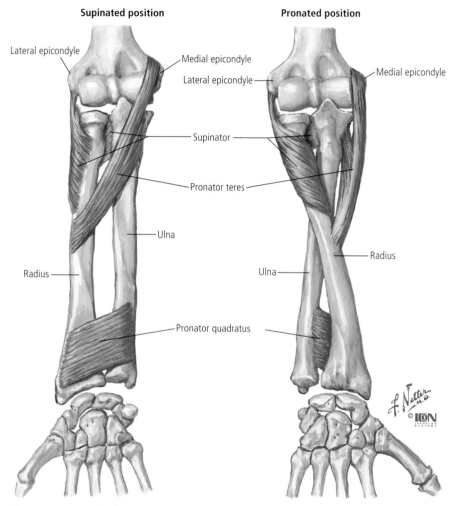

Figure 11-7: *Right forearm: anterior view*

Muscle	Proximal Attachment	Distal Attachment	Nerve and Segmental Level	Action
Supinator	Lateral epicondyle of humerus, supinator fossa, and crest of ulna	Proximal aspect of radius (C5, C6)	Deep branch of radial nerve	Supinate forearm
Pronator teres	Medial epicondyle of humerus and coronoid process of ulna	Lateral aspect of radius	Median nerve (C6, C7)	Pronate forearm and flex elbow
Pronator quadratus	Distal anterior aspect of ulna	Distal anterior aspect of radius	Anterior interosseous nerve (C8, T1)	Pronate forearm

Anterior Nerves of Forearm

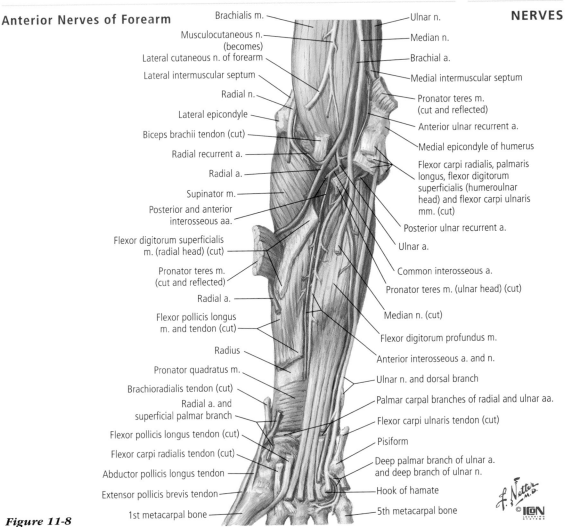

Brachialis m.
Musculocutaneous n. (becomes)
Lateral cutaneous n. of forearm
Lateral intermuscular septum
Radial n.
Lateral epicondyle
Biceps brachii tendon (cut)
Radial recurrent a.
Radial a.
Supinator m.
Posterior and anterior interosseous aa.
Flexor digitorum superficialis m. (radial head) (cut)
Pronator teres m. (cut and reflected)
Radial a.
Flexor pollicis longus m. and tendon (cut)
Radius
Pronator quadratus m.
Brachioradialis tendon (cut)
Radial a. and superficial palmar branch
Flexor pollicis longus tendon (cut)
Flexor carpi radialis tendon (cut)
Abductor pollicis longus tendon
Extensor pollicis brevis tendon
1st metacarpal bone

Ulnar n.
Median n.
Brachial a.
Medial intermuscular septum
Pronator teres m. (cut and reflected)
Anterior ulnar recurrent a.
Medial epicondyle of humerus
Flexor carpi radialis, palmaris longus, flexor digitorum superficialis (humeroulnar head) and flexor carpi ulnaris mm. (cut)
Posterior ulnar recurrent a.
Ulnar a.
Common interosseous a.
Pronator teres m. (ulnar head) (cut)
Median n. (cut)
Flexor digitorum profundus m.
Anterior interosseous a. and n.
Ulnar n. and dorsal branch
Palmar carpal branches of radial and ulnar aa.
Flexor carpi ulnaris tendon (cut)
Pisiform
Deep palmar branch of ulnar a. and deep branch of ulnar n.
Hook of hamate
5th metacarpal bone

Figure 11-8

Nerves	Segmental Levels	Sensory	Motor
Musculocutaneous	C5, C6, C7	Lateral antebrachial cutaneous nerve	Coracobrachialis, biceps brachii, brachialis
Lateral cutaneous of forearm	C5, C6, C7	Lateral forearm	No motor
Median	C6, C7, C8, T1	Palmar and distal dorsal aspects of lateral 3½ digits and lateral palm	Flexor carpi radialis, flexor digitorum superficialis, lateral ½ of flexor digitorum profundus, flexor pollicis longus, pronator quadratus, pronator teres, most thenar muscles, and lateral lumbricales
Anterior interosseous	C6, C7, C8, T1	No sensory	Flexor digitorum profundis, flexor pollicis longus, pronator quadratus
Ulnar	C7, C8, T1	Medial hand, including medial ½ of 4th digit	Flexor carpi ulnaris, medial ½ of flexor digitorum profundus, and most small muscles in hand
Radial	C5, C6, C7, C8, T1	Posterior aspect of forearm	Triceps brachii, anconeus, brachioradialis, extensor muscles of forearm
Posterior interosseous	C5, C6, C7, C8, T1	None	Abductor pollicis longus, extensor pollicis brevis and longus, extensor digitorum communis, extensor indicis, extensor digiti minimi

EXAMINATION: HISTORY

Initial Hypotheses Based on History

History	Initial Hypothesis
Pain over lateral elbow during gripping activities	Possible lateral epicondylitis[1-4] Possible radial tunnel syndrome[5-7]
Pain over medial elbow during wrist flexion and pronation	Possible medial epicondylitis[8, 9]
Reports of numbness and tingling in ulnar nerve distribution distal to elbow	Possible cubital tunnel syndrome[9, 10]
Pain in anterior aspect of elbow and forearm that is exacerbated by wrist flexion combined with elbow flexion and forearm pronation	Possible pronator syndrome[11]
Reports of pain during movement with sensations of catching or instability	Possible rotatory instability[11]
Reports of posterior elbow pain during elbow hyperextension	Possible valgus extension overload syndrome[11]

Range-of-Motion Measurements: Elbow Flexion and Extension

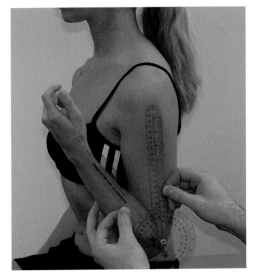

Figure 11-9: *Measurement of elbow flexion*

Test and Measure	Instrumentation	Population	Reliability ICC	
			Intra-examiner	Inter-examiner
AROM elbow flexion	12-in metal goniometer	24 patients referred to PT in which ROM measurements of elbow were appropriate	.94	.89
	10-in plastic goniometer		.97	.96
	6-in plastic goniometer		.96	.90
AROM elbow extension Rothstein et al.[12]	12-in metal goniometer		.86	.96
	10-in plastic goniometer		.96	.94
	6-in plastic goniometer		.99	.93
AROM elbow flexion/extension Boone et al.[13]	Plastic goniometer	12 asymptomatic subjects	.94	.87
AROM elbow flexion	Universal standard goniometer	38 patients who had undergone a surgical procedure for injury at elbow, forearm, or wrist	.55–.98	.58–.62
AROM elbow extension Armstrong et al.[14]			.45–.98	.58–.87
AROM elbow flexion Petherick et al.[15]	Universal plastic goniometer	30 healthy subjects	NR	.53
	Fluid-filled bubble inclinometer		NR	.92

ICC, Intraclass correlate coefficient; AROM, active range of motion; PT, physical therapy; ROM, range of motion.

Range-of-Motion Measurements: Forearm Supination and Pronation

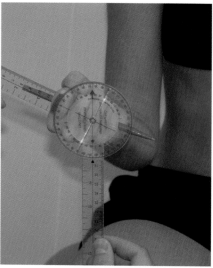

Figure 11-10A: *Measurement of forearm supination*

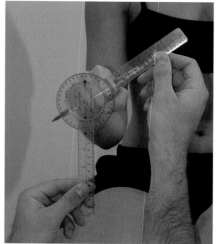

Figure 11-10B: *Measurement of forearm pronation*

Test and Measure		Instrumentation	Population		Reliability ICC	
					Intra-examiner	Inter-examiner
AROM *Armstrong et al.*[14]	Supination	Universal standard goniometer	38 patients who had undergone a surgical procedure for elbow, forearm, or wrist injury		.96–.99	.90–.93
	Pronation				.96–.99	.83–.86
AROM *Karagiannopoulos et al.*[16]	Supination	14.5-cm plastic goniometer	40 subjects, 20 injured and 20 non-injured	Injured	.98	.96
				Non-injured	.96	.94
	Pronation			Injured	.95–.97	.95
				Non-injured	.86–.98	.92
	Supination	Plumb line goniometer—a 14.5-cm single-arm plastic goniometer with a plumb line attached to the center of its 360°		Injured	.98	.96
				Non-injured	.94–.98	.96
	Pronation			Injured	.96–.98	.92
				Non-injured	.95–.97	.91
AROM Supination/pronation *Gajdosik*[17]		8-in steel goniometer	31 asymptomatic subjects		.81–.97	NR
PROM *Flowers et al.*[18]	Supination	Plumb line goniometer	30 hand therapy patients		.95	NR
	Pronation				.87	NR
	Supination	Standard goniometer			.95	NR
	Pronation				.79	NR

PROM, passive range of motion.

Elbow Strength Measurements Using Dynamometry

Procedure Performed	Population	Reliability ICC	
		Intra-examiner	Inter-examiner
Flexion Extension Agre et al.[19]	4 healthy subjects	Flexion .93–.98 Extension .88–.89	Flexion .93 Extension .89
Extension Wadsworth et al.[20]	13 patients receiving PT for orthopaedic and neuromuscular diagnoses	.90	NR
Flexion Extension Bohannon[21]	27 healthy subjects	Flexion .90–.92 (Pearson correlation coefficient*)	NR
Flexion Bohannon and Andrews[22]	30 patients with neurologic disorders	NR	.94 (Pearson correlation coefficient*)
Flexion Surburg et al.[23]	20 healthy volunteers and 10 patients with mild cognitive disabilities	.84–.99	.89–.97
Flexion Wikholm and Bohannon[24]	27 healthy subjects	NR	.78

*Authors used a Pearson correlation coefficient to determine the relationship between the forces captured during each test.

RELIABILITY OF THE CLINICAL EXAMINATION

Grip Strength Testing in Patients With Lateral Epicondylalgia

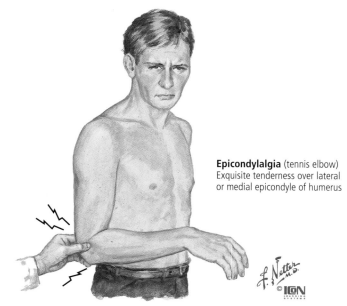

Epicondylalgia (tennis elbow)
Exquisite tenderness over lateral
or medial epicondyle of humerus

Figure 11-11: Palpation of lateral epicondyle

Grip Strength	Test Procedure	Population	Reliability ICC
Pain-free Smidt et al.[25]	Patient is standing with elbow extended and forearm in neutral. Patient is instructed to squeeze dynamometer until discomfort is felt	50 patients diagnosed with lateral epicondylalgia on clinical examination	Inter-examiner .97
Maximum Smidt et al.[25]	As above, except patient is instructed to squeeze dynamometer as hard as possible		Inter-examiner .98
Pain-free Stratford et al.[26]	As pain-free described above	35 consecutive patients with lateral epicondylalgia diagnosed on clinical examination	Inter-repetition .95–.99* Inter-occasion .92–.97*
Maximum Stratford et al.[26]	As maximum described above		Inter-repetition .97–.99* Inter-occasion .95–.98*
Pain-free Stratford et al.[27]	As pain-free described above	32 patients with signs and symptoms indicative of lateral epicondylalgia	Inter-occasion .87*
Maximum Stratford et al.[27]	As maximum described above		Inter-occasion Uninvolved arm .98* Involved arm .60*

*In these studies, researchers investigated the reliability of measurements performed during the same session and between two sessions, the second of which was completed within 7 days of the first. Reported ICCs are for intra-rater reliability.

Classification on End-Feel for Elbow Flexion and Extension

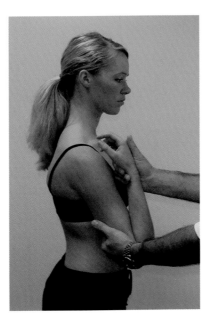

Figure 11-12A: Assessment of flexion end-feel

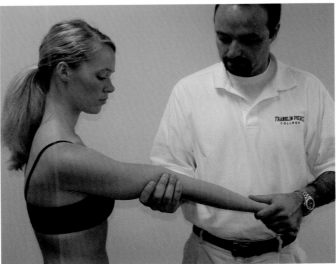

Figure 11-12B: Assessment of extension end-feel

Test and Measure	Test Procedure	Population	Inter-examiner Reliability Kappa Values
Flexion Extension *Patla and Paris*[28]	Patient is standing. Examiner stabilizes humerus with one hand and maintains forearm in neutral with other hand. Examiner extends or flexes elbow and assesses end-feel. End-feel is graded as soft tissue approximation—muscle, cartilage, capsule, or ligament	20 asymptomatic subjects	Flexion .40 Extension .73

RELIABILITY OF THE CLINICAL EXAMINATION

Detecting Cubital Tunnel Syndrome

Test and Measure	Test Procedure	Determination of Positive Findings	Population	Reference Standard	Sens	Spec	+LR	−LR
Pressure provocative test	Patient's elbow is in 20° of flexion and forearm supination. Examiner applies pressure to ulnar nerve just proximal to cubital tunnel for 60 sec	Positive if patient reports symptoms in distribution of ulnar nerve	55 subjects— 32 with cubital tunnel syndrome and 33 asymptomatic subjects	Electro-diagnostically proven cubital tunnel syndrome	.89	.98	44.5	.11
Flexion test	Patient's elbow is placed in maximum flexion with full supination of forearm and wrist in neutral. Position is held for 60 sec				.75	.99	75	.25
Combined pressure and flexion provocative test	Patient's arm is in maximum elbow flexion and forearm supination. Examiner applies pressure on ulnar nerve just proximal to cubital tunnel. Pressure is held for 60 sec				.98	.95	19.6	.02
Tinel sign Novak et al.[29]	Examiner applies 4–6 taps to patient's ulnar nerve just proximal to cubital tunnel	Positive if tingling sensation in distribution of ulnar nerve			.70	.98	35	.31
Tinel sign Kingery et al.[10]			50 patients with ulnar mono-neuropathies and 70 controls	Electro-diagnostic confirmation of ulnar nerve neuropathy at elbow	.68	.76	2.8	0.42
Side pinch strength Strength of the 5th digit abduction Nakazumi and Hamasaki[30]	NR	NR	21 patients with cubital tunnel syndrome and 60 patients with carpal tunnel syndrome	Nerve conduction velocity across the elbow	Not enough data were provided for calculation of sensitivity and specificity. It was reported that side pinch strength measurements exhibited a 70% false-negative rate, and manual muscle testing exhibited a 43% false-negative rate			

Sens, sensitivity; Spec, specificity; LR, likelihood ratio; NR, not reported.

Detecting Cubital Tunnel Syndrome (cont.)

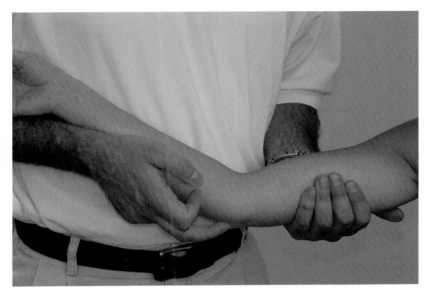

Figure 11-13: *Tinel sign*

DIAGNOSTIC UTILITY OF THE CLINICAL EXAMINATION

Elbow Flexion Test

Rayan and colleagues[31] investigated the elbow flexion test commonly used for diagnosing ulnar neuropathy in the cubital tunnel. Working with 102 asymptomatic volunteers, they performed the elbow flexion test as described here. Patients were seated and instructed to fully flex the elbow with wrist and shoulder in a neutral position. This position was held for 60 seconds. Full elbow flexion was again performed for 60 seconds with the wrist in full extension, and again with the shoulder abducted 90°. Finally, patients completed the test with wrist in full extension and shoulder abducted 90° at the same time. The test was positive if paresthesias were detected in the ulnar nerve distribution. Results of each test are shown below.

Position	Asymptomatic Volunteers With a Positive Test
Elbow flexion only	15%
Elbow flexion and wrist extension	13%
Elbow flexion and 90° of shoulder abduction	19%
Elbow flexion with wrist extension and 90° of elbow flexion	22%

Elbow Flexion Test (cont.)

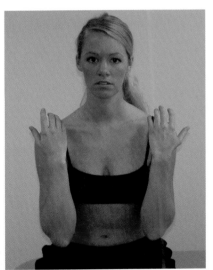

Figure 11-14A: Elbow flexion test with shoulders and wrists in neutral

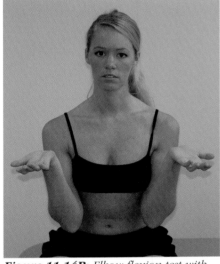

Figure 11-14B: Elbow flexion test with shoulders in neutral and wrists in extended

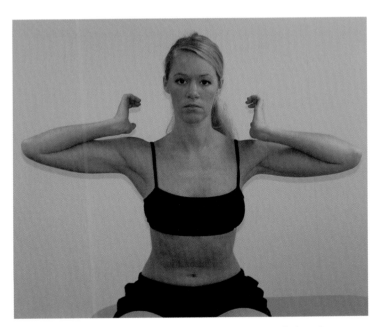

Figure 11-14C: Elbow flexion test with wrists extended and shoulders abducted to 90°

DIAGNOSTIC UTILITY OF THE CLINICAL EXAMINATION

Indication of Bony or Joint Injury: Elbow Extension Test

Test and Measure	Test Procedure	Determination of Findings	Population	Reference Standard	Sens (95% CI)	Spec (95% CI)	+LR	−LR
Elbow extension test *Docherty et al.[32]*	Patient is supine and is asked to fully extend elbow	Positive if patient is unable to fully extend elbow	114 patients with acute elbow injuries	Radiographic evaluation	.97	.69	3.13	.04
Elbow extension test *Hawksworth and Freeland[33]*	As above, except patient is standing		100 patients presenting to an emergency department with elbow		.91 (.81, 1.0)	.70 (.61, .78)	3.03	.13

CI, confidence interval.

Radial Head Fractures: Fat-Pad Sign

Test and Measure	Test Procedure	Determination of Positive Findings	Patient Population	Reference Standard	Sens	Spec	+LR	−LR
Fat-pad sign *Irshad et al.[35]*	Radiologists reviewed radiographs to determine if positive anterior fat-pad sign was noted	Positive if the radiologist noted anterosuperior displacement of the soft tissue shadow of the capsule	181 radiographs	Radiographic confirmation	.85	.50	1.7	.30

Posterolateral Rotatory Instability

O'Driscoll and colleagues[34] treated five patients with operatively confirmed posterolateral rotatory instability of the elbow. They reported that all five patients exhibited a positive posterolateral rotatory instability test of the elbow. The test is performed with the patient supine. The examiner flexes the patient's arm so it is above the head. One of the examiner's hands prevents external rotation (ER) of the humerus. The examiner's other hand grasps the patient's forearm in full supination. The examiner then brings the patient's elbow from a position of full extension slowly into flexion while applying a supinatory force at the forearm and a valgus stress and axial compression at the elbow. The test is considered positive if posterolateral rotatory displacement of the radius occurs followed by a reduction as elbow flexion progresses to 90°.

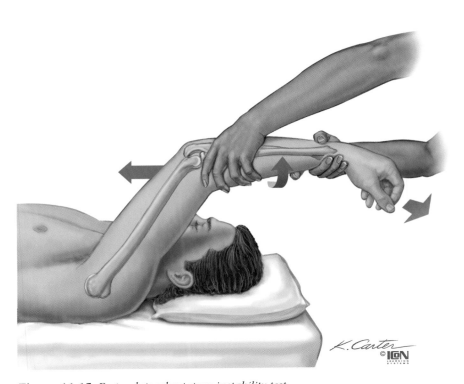

Figure 11-15: Posterolateral rotatory instability test

REFERENCES

1. Baquie P. Tennis elbow. Principles of ongoing management. *Aust Fam Physician.* 1999;28:724-725.

2. Borkholder CD, Hill VA, Fess EE. The efficacy of splinting for lateral epicondylitis: a systematic review. *J Hand Ther.* 2004;17:181-199.

3. Vicenzino B. Lateral epicondylalgia: a musculoskeletal physiotherapy perspective. *Man Ther.* 2003;8:66-79.

4. Vicenzino B, Wright A. Lateral epicondylalgia I: epidemiology, pathophysiology, etiology and natural history. *Phys Ther Rev.* 1996;1:23-34.

5. Pecina MM, Bojanic I. *Overuse Injuries of the Musculoskeletal System.* Boca Raton: CRC Press; 1993.

6. Ellenbecker TS, Mattalino AJ. *The Elbow in Sport.* Champaign: Human Kinetics; 1997.

7. Ekstrom R, Holden K. Examination of and intervention for a patient with chronic lateral elbow pain with signs of nerve entrapment. *Phys Ther.* 2002;82:1077-1086.

8. Pienimaki TT, Siira PT, Vanharanta H. Chronic medial and lateral epicondylitis: a comparison of pain, disability, and function. *Arch Phys Med Rehabil.* 2002;83:317-321.

9. Hertling D, Kessler RM. The elbow and forearm. In: *Management of Common Musculoskeletal Disorders: Physical Therapy Principles and Methods.* 3rd ed. Philadelphia: Lippincott; 1990:217-242.

10. Kingery WS, Park KS, Wu PB, Date ES. Electromyographic motor Tinel's sign in ulnar mononeuropathies at the elbow. *Am J Phys Med Rehabil.* 1995;74:419-426.

11. Ryan J. Elbow. In: *Current Concepts of Orthopaedic Physical Therapy.* La Crosse: Orthopaedic Section, American Physical Therapy Association; 2001.

12. Rothstein J, Miller P, Roettger R. Goniometric reliability in a clinical setting. Elbow and knee measurements. *Phys Ther.* 1983;63:1611-1615.

13. Boone DC, Azen SP, Lin CM, Spence C, Baron C, Lee L. Reliability of goniometric measurements. *Phys Ther.* 1978;58:1355-1390.

14. Armstrong AD, MacDermid JC, Chinchalkar S, Stevens RS, King GJ. Reliability of range-of-motion measurement in the elbow. *J Shoulder Elbow Surg.* 1998;7:573-580.

15. Petherick M, Rheault W, Kimble S, Lechner C, Senear V. Concurrent validity and intertester reliability of universal and fluid-based goniometers for active elbow range of motion. *Phys Ther.* 1988;68:966-969.

16. Karagiannopoulos C, Sitler M, Michlovitz S. Reliability of 2 functional goniometric methods for measuring forearm pronation and supination active range of motion. *J Orthop Sports Phys Ther.* 2003;33:523-531.

17. Gajdosik RL. Comparison and reliability of three goniometric methods for measuring forearm supination and pronation. *Percept Mot Skills.* 2001;93:353-355.

18. Flowers KR, Stephens-Chisar J, LaStayo P, Galante BL. Intrarater reliability of a new method and instrumentation for measuring passive supination and pronation. *J Hand Ther.* 2001;14:30-35.

19. Agre JC, Magness JL, Hull SZ, et al. Strength testing with a portable dynamometer: reliability for upper and lower extremities. *Arch Phys Med Rehabil.* 1987;68:454-458.

20. Wadsworth CT, Krishnan R, Sear M, Harrold J, Nielsen DH. Intrarater reliability of manual muscle testing and hand-held dynametric muscle testing. *Phys Ther.* 1987;9:1342-1347.

21. Bohannon RW. Make tests and break tests of elbow flexor muscle strength. *Phys Ther.* 1988;68:193-194.

REFERENCES

22. Bohannon RW, Andrews AW. Interrater reliability of hand-held dynamometry. *Phys Ther.* 1987;67:931-933.
23. Surburg PR, Suomi R, Poppy WK. Validity and reliability of a hand-held dynamometer with two populations. *Arch Phys Med Rehabil.* 1992;73:535-539.
24. Wikholm JB, Bohannon RW. Hand-held dynamometer measurements: tester strength makes a difference. *J Orthop Sports Phys Ther.* 1991;13:191-198.
25. Smidt N, van der Windt DA, Assendelft WJ, et al. Interobserver reproducibility of the assessment of severity of complaints, grip strength, and pain pressure threshold in patients with lateral epicondylitis. *Arch Phys Med Rehabil.* 2002;83:1145-1150.
26. Stratford PW, Norman GR, McIntosh JM. Generalizability of grip strength measurements in patients with tennis elbow. *Phys Ther.* 1989;69:276-281.
27. Stratford PW, Levy D, Gauldie S, Levy K, Miseferi D. Extensor carpi radialis tendonitis: a validation of selected outcome measures. *Physiother Can.* 1987;39:250-254.
28. Patla C, Paris S. Reliability of interpretation of the Paris classification of normal end feel for elbow flexion and extension. *Man Ther.* 1993;1:60-66.
29. Novak CB, Lee GW, Mackinnon SE, Lay L. Provocative testing for cubital tunnel syndrome. *J Hand Surg Am.* 1994;19:817-820.
30. Nakazumi Y, Hamasaki M. Electrophysiological studies and physical examinations in entrapment neuropathy: sensory and motor function compensation for the central nervous system in cases with peripheral nerve damage. *Electromyogr Clin Neurophysiol.* 2001;41:345-348.
31. Rayan GM, Jensen C, Duke J. Elbow flexion test in the normal population. *J Hand Surg Am.* 1992;17:86-89.
32. Docherty MA, Schwab R, Ma O. Can elbow extension be used as a test of clinically significant injury? *South Med J.* 2002;95:539-541.
33. Hawksworth CR, Freeland P. Inability to fully extend the injured elbow: an indicator of significant injury. *Arch Emerg Med.* 1991;8:253-256.
34. O'Driscoll SW, Bell DF, Morrey BF. Posterolateral rotatory instability of the elbow. *J Bone Joint Surg Am.* 1991;73:440-446.
35. Irshad F, Shaw NJ, Gregory RJ. Reliability of fat-pad sign in radial head/neck fractures of the elbow. *Injury.* 1997;28:433-435.

Wrist and Hand

Chapter 12

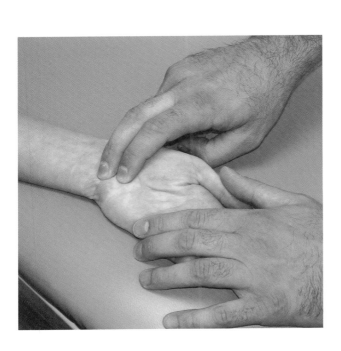

OSTEOLOGY   Bones of Wrist and Hand

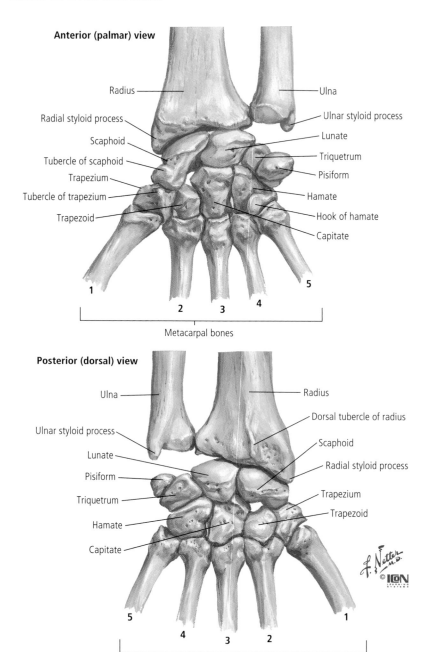

Anterior (palmar) view

Radius —
Ulna

Radial styloid process
Ulnar styloid process

Scaphoid
Lunate

Tubercle of scaphoid
Triquetrum

Trapezium
Pisiform

Tubercle of trapezium
Hamate

Trapezoid
Hook of hamate

Capitate

1
5

2   3   4

Metacarpal bones

Posterior (dorsal) view

Ulna
Radius

Dorsal tubercle of radius

Ulnar styloid process
Scaphoid

Lunate
Radial styloid process

Pisiform
Trapezium

Triquetrum
Trapezoid

Hamate

Capitate

5
1

4   3   2

Metacarpal bones

Figure 12-1

Bones of Wrist and Hand (cont.)

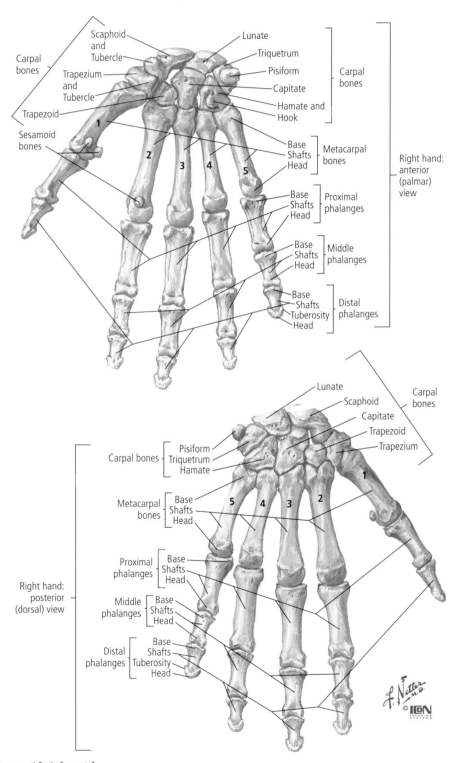

Figure 12-1 (cont.)

ARTHROLOGY Wrist Joint

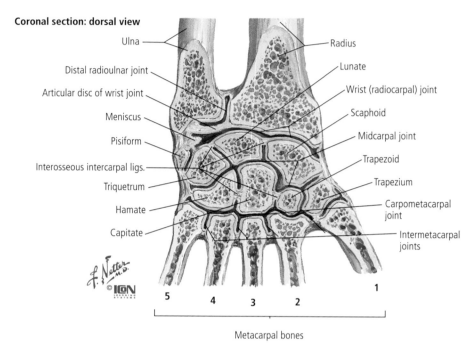

Coronal section: dorsal view

Ulna — Radius
Distal radioulnar joint — Lunate
Articular disc of wrist joint — Wrist (radiocarpal) joint
Meniscus — Scaphoid
Pisiform — Midcarpal joint
Interosseous intercarpal ligs. — Trapezoid
Triquetrum — Trapezium
Hamate — Carpometacarpal joint
Capitate — Intermetacarpal joints

5 4 3 2 1

Metacarpal bones

Figure 12-2

Joints	Type and Classification	Closed Packed Position	Capsular Pattern
Radiocarpal	Synovial: condyloid	Full extension	Limitation equal in all directions
Intercarpal	Synovial: plane	Extension	Limitation equal in all directions
Carpometacarpal (CMC)	Synovial: plane, except for first CMC, which is sellar	Full opposition	Limitation equal in all directions
Metacarpophalangeal (MCP)	Synovial: condyloid	Extension except for 1st digit	Limitation equal in all directions
Interphalangeal (IP)	Synovial: hinge	Extension	Flexion greater than extension

Wrist Joint (cont.)

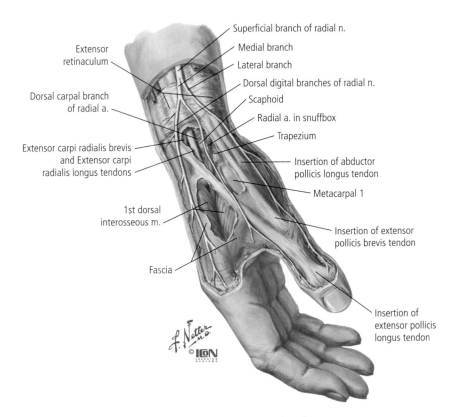

Superficial branch of radial n.

Medial branch

Lateral branch

Dorsal digital branches of radial n.

Scaphoid

Radial a. in snuffbox

Trapezium

Insertion of abductor pollicis longus tendon

Metacarpal 1

Insertion of extensor pollicis brevis tendon

Insertion of extensor pollicis longus tendon

Extensor retinaculum

Dorsal carpal branch of radial a.

Extensor carpi radialis brevis and Extensor carpi radialis longus tendons

1st dorsal interosseous m.

Fascia

Figure 12-3: *Sagittal sections through wrist and first finger*

LIGAMENTS   **Palmar Ligaments of Wrist**

Ligaments	Attachments	Function
Transverse carpal	Hamate and pisiform medially, and scaphoid and trapezium laterally	Prevent bowstringing of finger flexor tendons
Palmar radiocarpal (radioscapholunate and radiocapitate portions)	Distal radius to both rows of carpal bones	Reinforce fibrous capsule of wrist volarly
Palmar ulnocarpal (ulnolunate and ulnotriquetral portions)	Distal ulna to both rows of carpal bones	Reinforce fibrous capsule of wrist volarly
Palmar radioulnar	Distal radius to distal ulna	Reinforce volar aspect of distal radioulnar joint
Radial collateral	Radial styloid process to scaphoid	Reinforce fibrous capsule of wrist laterally
Ulnar collateral	Ulnar styloid process to triquetrum	Reinforce fibrous capsule of wrist medially
Pisometacarpal	Pisiform to base of 5th metacarpal	Reinforce 5th carpometacarpal joint
Pisohamate	Pisiform to hook of hamate	Maintain proximity of pisiform and hamate
Capitotriquetral	Capitate to triquetrum	Maintain proximity of captitate and triquetrum
Palmar carpometacarpal	Palmar aspect of carpals to bases of metacarpals 2–5	Reinforce volar aspect of carpometacarpal joints 2–5
Palmar metacarpal	Attaches bases of metacarpals 2–5	Maintain proximity between metacarpals

Palmar Ligaments of Wrist (cont.)

Carpal tunnel: palmar view

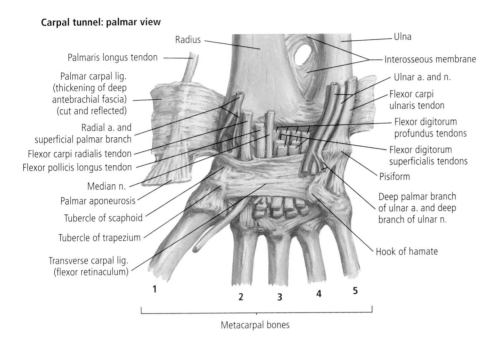

- Radius
- Palmaris longus tendon
- Palmar carpal lig. (thickening of deep antebrachial fascia) (cut and reflected)
- Radial a. and superficial palmar branch
- Flexor carpi radialis tendon
- Flexor pollicis longus tendon
- Median n.
- Palmar aponeurosis
- Tubercle of scaphoid
- Tubercle of trapezium
- Transverse carpal lig. (flexor retinaculum)
- Ulna
- Interosseous membrane
- Ulnar a. and n.
- Flexor carpi ulnaris tendon
- Flexor digitorum profundus tendons
- Flexor digitorum superficialis tendons
- Pisiform
- Deep palmar branch of ulnar a. and deep branch of ulnar n.
- Hook of hamate

1   2   3   4   5

Metacarpal bones

Flexor retinaculum removed: palmar view

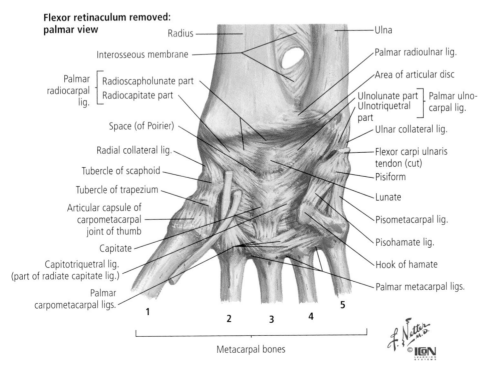

- Radius
- Interosseous membrane
- Palmar radiocarpal lig.
  - Radioscapholunate part
  - Radiocapitate part
- Space (of Poirier)
- Radial collateral lig.
- Tubercle of scaphoid
- Tubercle of trapezium
- Articular capsule of carpometacarpal joint of thumb
- Capitate
- Capitotriquetral lig. (part of radiate capitate lig.)
- Palmar carpometacarpal ligs.
- Ulna
- Palmar radioulnar lig.
- Area of articular disc
- Ulnolunate part / Ulnotriquetral part — Palmar ulno-carpal lig.
- Ulnar collateral lig.
- Flexor carpi ulnaris tendon (cut)
- Pisiform
- Lunate
- Pisometacarpal lig.
- Pisohamate lig.
- Hook of hamate
- Palmar metacarpal ligs.

1   2   3   4   5

Metacarpal bones

Figure 12-4

LIGAMENTS   Posterior Ligaments of Wrist

Posterior (dorsal) view

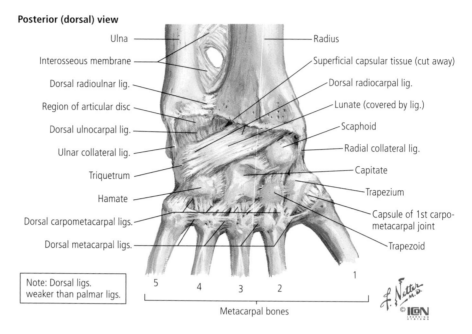

Ulna
Interosseous membrane
Dorsal radioulnar lig.
Region of articular disc
Dorsal ulnocarpal lig.
Ulnar collateral lig.
Triquetrum
Hamate
Dorsal carpometacarpal ligs.
Dorsal metacarpal ligs.

Radius
Superficial capsular tissue (cut away)
Dorsal radiocarpal lig.
Lunate (covered by lig.)
Scaphoid
Radial collateral lig.
Capitate
Trapezium
Capsule of 1st carpo-metacarpal joint
Trapezoid

Note: Dorsal ligs. weaker than palmar ligs.

5   4   3   2   1
Metacarpal bones

f. Netter M.D.
©ICN

Figure 12-5

Ligaments	Attachments	Function
Dorsal radioulnar	Distal radius to distal ulna	Reinforce dorsal aspect of distal radioulnar joint
Dorsal radiocarpal	Distal radius to both rows of carpal bones	Reinforce fibrous capsule of wrist dorsally
Dorsal carpometacarpal	Dorsal aspect of carpals to bases of metacarpals 2–5	Reinforce dorsal aspect of carpometacarpal joints 2–5
Dorsal metacarpal	Attaches bases of metacarpals 2–5	Maintain proximity between metacarpals

Metacarpophalangeal and Interphalangeal Ligaments   **LIGAMENTS**

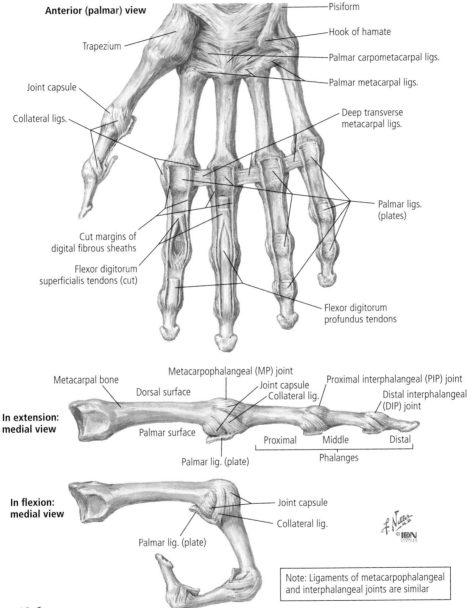

Figure 12-6

Ligaments	Attachments	Function
Collateral ligaments of IP joints	Sides of distal aspect of proximal phalanx to proximal aspect of distal phalanx	Reinforce medial and lateral capsules of IP joints
Deep transverse metacarpal ligaments	Connects adjacent MCP joints	Reinforce MCP joints
Palmar ligament (volar plate)	Individual plates attach to palmar aspect of MCP and IP joints	Reinforce palmar aspect of MCP and IP joints

MUSCLES   Extensors of Wrist and Digits

Muscles	Proximal Attachments	Distal Attachments	Nerve and Segmental Level	Action
Extensor carpi radialis longus	Lateral supracondylar ridge of humerus	Base of 2nd metacarpal	Radial nerve (C6, C7)	Extend and radially deviate wrist
Extensor carpi radialis brevis	Lateral epicondyle of humerus	Base of 3rd metacarpal	Deep branch of radial nerve (C7, C8)	Extend and radially deviate wrist
Extensor carpi ulnaris	Lateral epicondyle of humerus	Base of 5th metacarpal	Radial nerve (C6, C7, C8)	Extend and ulnarly deviate wrist
Extensor digitorum	Lateral epicondyle of humerus	Extensor expansions of digits 2–5	Posterior interosseous nerve (C7, C8)	Extend digits 2–5 at MCP and IP joints
Extensor digiti minimi	Lateral epicondyle of humerus	Extensor expansion of 5th digit	Posterior interosseous nerve (C7, C8)	Extend 5th digit at MCP and IP joints
Extensor indicis	Posterior aspect of ulna and interosseous membrane	Extensor expansion of 2nd digit	Posterior interosseous nerve (C7, C8)	Extend 2nd digit and assist with wrist extension
Abductor pollicis longus	Posterior aspect of ulna, radius, and interosseous membrane	Base of 1st metacarpal	Posterior interosseous nerve (C7, C8)	Abduct and extend thumb
Extensor pollicis brevis	Posterior aspect of radius and interosseous membrane	Base of proximal phalanx of thumb	Posterior interosseous nerve (C7, C8)	Extend thumb
Extensor pollicis longus	Posterior aspect of ulna and interosseous membrane	Base of distal phalanx of thumb	Posterior interosseous nerve (C7, C8)	Extend distal phalanx of thumb at MCP and IP joints

Extensors of Wrist and Digits (cont.)   **MUSCLES**

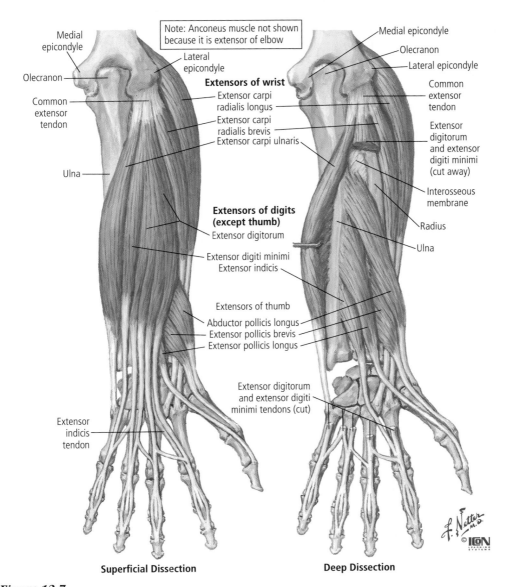

Note: Anconeus muscle not shown because it is extensor of elbow

Medial epicondyle
Olecranon
Common extensor tendon
Ulna

Lateral epicondyle
Extensors of wrist
Extensor carpi radialis longus
Extensor carpi radialis brevis
Extensor carpi ulnaris

Extensors of digits (except thumb)
Extensor digitorum
Extensor digiti minimi
Extensor indicis

Extensors of thumb
Abductor pollicis longus
Extensor pollicis brevis
Extensor pollicis longus

Extensor indicis tendon

Medial epicondyle
Olecranon
Lateral epicondyle
Common extensor tendon
Extensor digitorum and extensor digiti minimi (cut away)
Interosseous membrane
Radius
Ulna

Extensor digitorum and extensor digiti minimi tendons (cut)

Superficial Dissection   **Deep Dissection**

Figure 12-7

MUSCLES   **Flexors of Wrist and Digits**

Muscles		Proximal Attachments	Distal Attachments	Nerve and Segmental Level	Action
Flexor carpi radialis		Medial epicondyle of humerus	Base of 2nd metacarpal bone	Median nerve (C6, C7)	Flex and radially deviate hand
Flexor carpi ulnaris		Medial epicondyle of humerus and olecranon and posterior border of ulna	Pisiform, hook of hamate and 5th metacarpal	Ulnar nerve (C7, C8)	Flex and ulnarly deviate hand
Palmaris longus		Medial epicondyle of humerus	Distal aspect of flexor retinaculum and palmar aponeurosis	Median nerve (C7, C8)	Flex hand and tighten palmar aponeurosis
Flexor digitorum superficialis	Humeroulnar head	Medial epicondyle of humerus, ulnar collateral ligament, coronoid process of ulna	Bodies of middle phalanges of digits 2–5	Median nerve (C7, C8, T1)	Flex digits at proximal IP joints 2–5 and at MCP joints 2–5
	Radial head	Superoanterior border of radius			
Flexor digitorum profundus	Median portion	Proximal anteromedial aspect of ulna and interosseous membrane	Bases of distal phalanges of digits 2–5	Ulnar nerve (C8, T1)	Flex digits at distal IP joints 2–5 and assist with flexion of hand
	Lateral portion			Median nerve (C8, T1)	
Flexor pollicis longus		Anterior aspect of radius and interosseous membrane	Base of distal phalanx of thumb	Anterior interosseous nerve (C8, T1)	Flex phalanges of 1st digit

Flexors of Wrist and Digits (cont.)

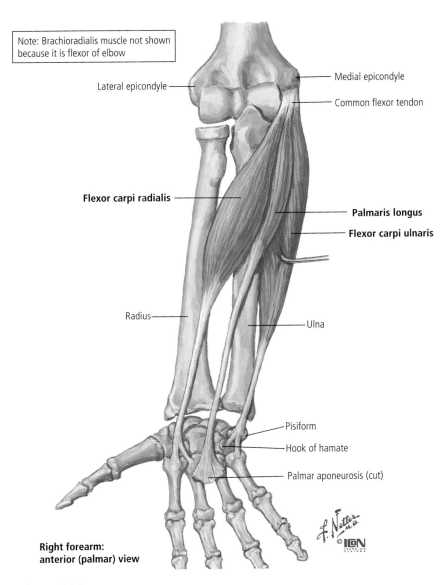

Note: Brachioradialis muscle not shown because it is flexor of elbow

Lateral epicondyle

Medial epicondyle

Common flexor tendon

Flexor carpi radialis

Palmaris longus

Flexor carpi ulnaris

Radius

Ulna

Pisiform

Hook of hamate

Palmar aponeurosis (cut)

Right forearm: anterior (palmar) view

Figure 12-8

MUSCLES   Flexors of Wrist and Digits (cont.)

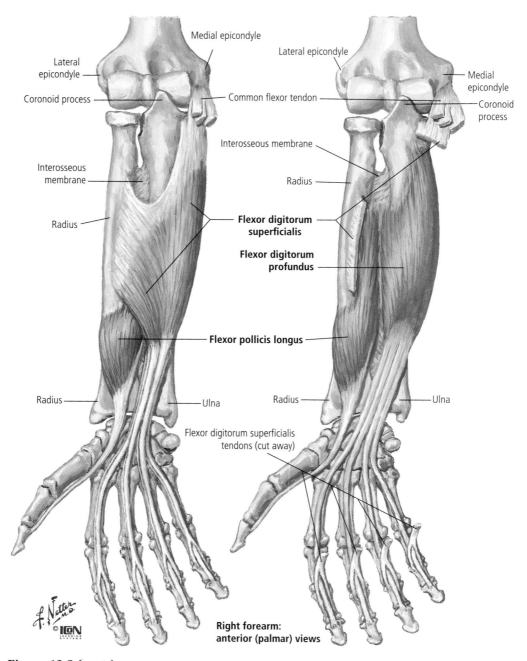

Right forearm: anterior (palmar) views

Figure 12-8 (cont.)

Intrinsic Muscles of Hand

Muscles		Proximal Attachments	Distal Attachments	Nerve and Segmental Level	Action
Opponens pollicis		Flexor retinaculum, scaphoid, and trapezium	Lateral aspect of 1st metacarpal	Median nerve (C8, T1)	Oppose and medially rotate thumb
Abductor pollicis brevis			Lateral aspect of base of proximal phalanx of thumb		Abduct thumb and assist in thumb opposition
Flexor pollicis brevis					Flex thumb
Adductor pollicis	Oblique head	Bases of metacarpals 2 and 3 and capitate	Medial aspect of base of proximal phalanx of thumb	Deep branch of ulnar nerve (C8, T1)	Adduct thumb
	Transverse head	Anterior aspect of 3rd metacarpal			
Abductor digiti minimi		Pisiform	Medial aspect of base of proximal phalanx of 5th digit		Abduct 5th digit
Flexor digiti minimi		Hook of hamate and flexor retinaculum			Flex proximal phalanx of 5th digit
Opponens digiti minimi			Medial aspect of 5th metacarpal		Draw 5th digit into opposition of thumb
Lumbricals	Lateral	Tendons of flexor digitorum profundus	Lateral sides of extensor expansions 2–5	Median nerve (C8, T1)	Flex digits at MCP joints, and extend IP joints
	Medial			Deep branch of ulnar nerve (C8, T1)	
Doral interosseous		Adjacent sides of two metacarpals	Bases of proximal phalanges 2–4 and extensor expansion	Deep branch of ulnar nerve (C8, T1)	Abduct digits and assist with action of lumbricals
Palmar interosseous		Palmar aspect of metacarpals 2, 4, and 5	Bases of proximal phalanges 2, 4, and 5 and extensor expansion		Adduct digits and assist with action of lumbricals

MUSCLES   Intrinsic Muscles of Hand (cont.)

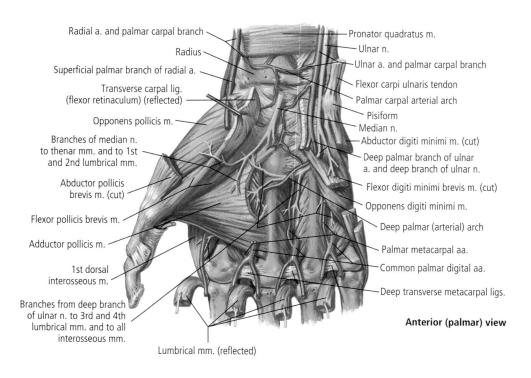

Radial a. and palmar carpal branch

Radius

Superficial palmar branch of radial a.

Transverse carpal lig.
(flexor retinaculum) (reflected)

Opponens pollicis m.

Branches of median n.
to thenar mm. and to 1st
and 2nd lumbrical mm.

Abductor pollicis
brevis m. (cut)

Flexor pollicis brevis m.

Adductor pollicis m.

1st dorsal
interosseous m.

Branches from deep branch
of ulnar n. to 3rd and 4th
lumbrical mm. and to all
interosseous mm.

Lumbrical mm. (reflected)

Pronator quadratus m.

Ulnar n.

Ulnar a. and palmar carpal branch

Flexor carpi ulnaris tendon

Palmar carpal arterial arch

Pisiform

Median n.

Abductor digiti minimi m. (cut)

Deep palmar branch of ulnar
a. and deep branch of ulnar n.

Flexor digiti minimi brevis m. (cut)

Opponens digiti minimi m.

Deep palmar (arterial) arch

Palmar metacarpal aa.

Common palmar digital aa.

Deep transverse metacarpal ligs.

Anterior (palmar) view

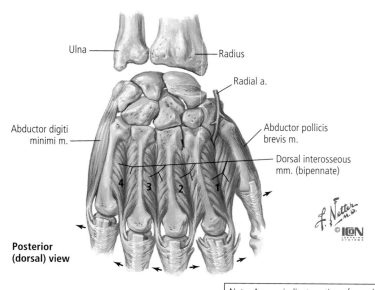

Ulna

Radius

Radial a.

Abductor digiti
minimi m.

Abductor pollicis
brevis m.

Dorsal interosseous
mm. (bipennate)

4   3   2   1

**Posterior
(dorsal) view**

Note: Arrows indicate action of muscles

Figure 12-9

Intrinsic Muscles of Hand (cont.)

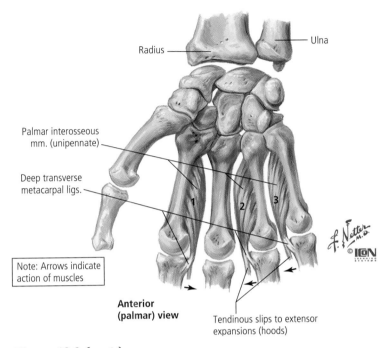

Radius — Ulna

Palmar interosseous mm. (unipennate)

Deep transverse metacarpal ligs.

1   2   3

Note: Arrows indicate action of muscles

Anterior (palmar) view

Tendinous slips to extensor expansions (hoods)

Figure 12-9 (cont.)

NERVES   Median Nerve

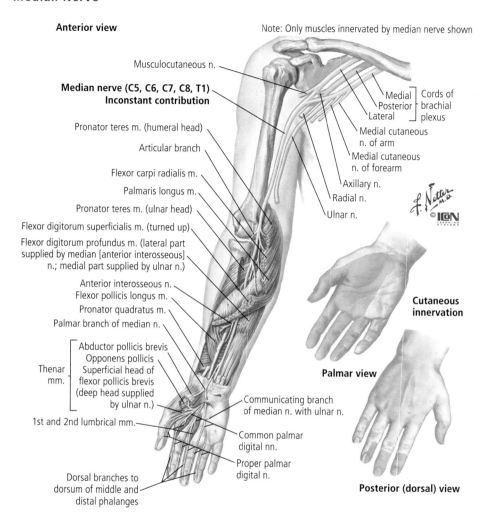

Anterior view   Note: Only muscles innervated by median nerve shown

Musculocutaneous n.

Median nerve (C5, C6, C7, C8, T1)
Inconstant contribution

Medial ⎤ Cords of
Posterior ⎬ brachial
Lateral ⎦ plexus

Pronator teres m. (humeral head)

Medial cutaneous
n. of arm

Articular branch

Medial cutaneous
n. of forearm

Flexor carpi radialis m.

Palmaris longus m.

Axillary n.

Pronator teres m. (ulnar head)

Radial n.

Flexor digitorum superficialis m. (turned up)

Ulnar n.

Flexor digitorum profundus m. (lateral part
supplied by median [anterior interosseous]
n.; medial part supplied by ulnar n.)

Anterior interosseous n.
Flexor pollicis longus m.
Pronator quadratus m.
Palmar branch of median n.

Cutaneous
innervation

Abductor pollicis brevis
Opponens pollicis
Thenar   Superficial head of
mm.   flexor pollicis brevis
(deep head supplied
by ulnar n.)

Palmar view

1st and 2nd lumbrical mm.

Communicating branch
of median n. with ulnar n.

Common palmar
digital nn.

Proper palmar
digital n.

Dorsal branches to
dorsum of middle and
distal phalanges

Posterior (dorsal) view

Figure 12-10

Nerves	Segmental Level	Sensory	Motor
Median nerve	C6, C7, C8, T1	Palmar and distal dorsal aspects of lateral 3½ digits and lateral palm	Abductor pollicis brevis, opponens pollicis, flexor pollicis brevis, lateral lumbricals

Ulnar Nerve

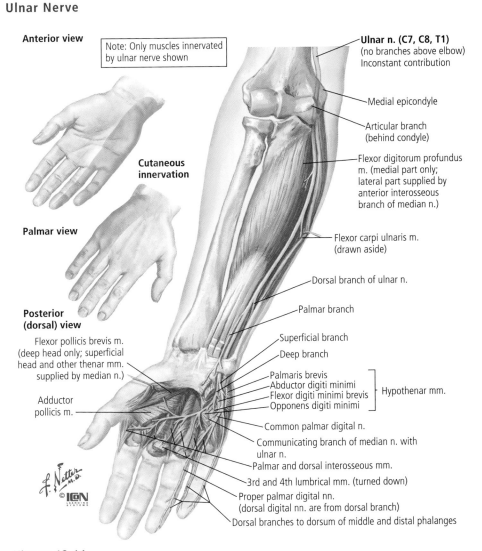

Anterior view

Note: Only muscles innervated by ulnar nerve shown

Ulnar n. (C7, C8, T1)
(no branches above elbow)
Inconstant contribution

Medial epicondyle

Articular branch
(behind condyle)

Flexor digitorum profundus
m. (medial part only;
lateral part supplied by
anterior interosseous
branch of median n.)

**Cutaneous
innervation**

Flexor carpi ulnaris m.
(drawn aside)

Palmar view

Dorsal branch of ulnar n.

Palmar branch

**Posterior
(dorsal) view**

Superficial branch

Deep branch

Flexor pollicis brevis m.
(deep head only; superficial
head and other thenar mm.
supplied by median n.)

Palmaris brevis
Abductor digiti minimi
Flexor digiti minimi brevis
Opponens digiti minimi

Hypothenar mm.

Adductor
pollicis m.

Common palmar digital n.

Communicating branch of median n. with
ulnar n.

Palmar and dorsal interosseous mm.

3rd and 4th lumbrical mm. (turned down)

Proper palmar digital nn.
(dorsal digital nn. are from dorsal branch)

Dorsal branches to dorsum of middle and distal phalanges

Figure 12-11

Nerves	Segmental Level	Sensory	Motor
Ulnar nerve	C7, C8, T1	Palmar and distal dorsal aspects of medial 1½ digits and medial palm	Interosseous, adductor pollicis, flexor pollicis brevis, medial lumbricals, abductor digiti minimi, flexor digiti minimi brevis, opponens digiti minimi

NERVES   **Radial Nerve in Forearm**

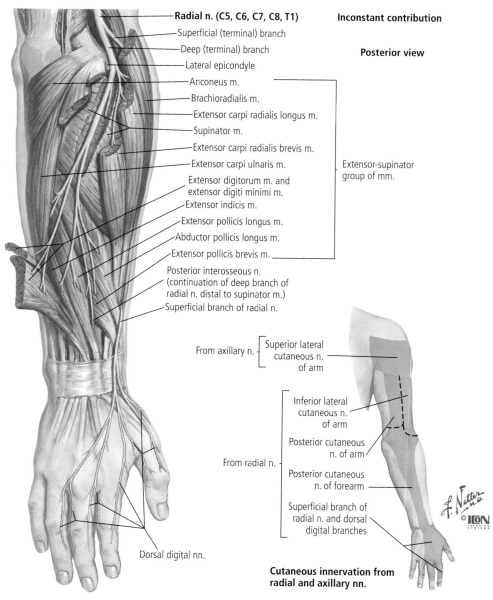

Radial n. (C5, C6, C7, C8, T1)
Superficial (terminal) branch
Deep (terminal) branch
Lateral epicondyle
Anconeus m.
Brachioradialis m.
Extensor carpi radialis longus m.
Supinator m.
Extensor carpi radialis brevis m.
Extensor carpi ulnaris m.
Extensor digitorum m. and extensor digiti minimi m.
Extensor indicis m.
Extensor pollicis longus m.
Abductor pollicis longus m.
Extensor pollicis brevis m.
Posterior interosseous n. (continuation of deep branch of radial n. distal to supinator m.)
Superficial branch of radial n.

Inconstant contribution

Posterior view

Extensor-supinator group of mm.

From axillary n. — Superior lateral cutaneous n. of arm

From radial n. —
Inferior lateral cutaneous n. of arm
Posterior cutaneous n. of arm
Posterior cutaneous n. of forearm
Superficial branch of radial n. and dorsal digital branches

Dorsal digital nn.

Cutaneous innervation from radial and axillary nn.

Figure 12-12

Nerves	Segmental Level	Sensory	Motor
Radial nerve	C5, C6, C7, C8, T1	Dorsal aspect of lateral hand, excluding digits	No motor in hand

Initial Hypotheses Based on Patient History

History	Initial Hypothesis
Pain over radial styloid process with gripping activities	Possible DeQuervain syndrome[1]
Reports of an insidious onset of numbness and tingling in 1st three fingers; possible report of worse pain at night	Possible carpal tunnel syndrome[2-4]
Reports of paresthesias over dorsal aspect of ulnar border of hand and fingers 4–5	Possible ulnar nerve compression at canal of Guyon[1, 5, 6]
Patient reports inability to extend MCP or IP joint	Possible Dupuytren[5] Possible trigger finger[7]
Reports of falling on hand with wrist hyperextended; reports of pain with loading of wrist	Possible scaphoid fracture[8, 9] Possible carpal instability[10]

Range-of-Motion Measurements of Wrist

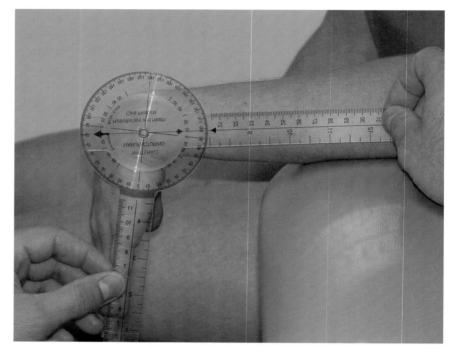

Figure 12-13A: *Measurement of wrist flexion*

Test and Measure	Instrumentation	Population	Reliability ICC			
			Intra-examiner		**Inter-examiner**	
Active ulnar deviation *Boone et al.[11]*	Plastic goniometer	12 asymptomatic. subjects	76		.72	
AROM	8-in plastic goniometer	48 patients in whom measurements of the wrist would routinely be included in the examination	Wrist flexion	.96	Wrist flexion	.90
			Wrist extension	.96	Wrist extension	.85
			Radial deviation	.90	Radial deviation	.86
			Ulnar deviation	.92	Ulnar deviation	.78
PROM *Horger[12]*			Wrist flexion	.96	Wrist flexion	.86
			Wrist extension	.96	Wrist extension	.84
			Radial deviation	.91	Radial deviation	.66
			Ulnar deviation	.94	Ulnar deviation	.83
Passive ROM *LaStayo and Wheeler[13]*	Alignment of plastic 6-in goniometer	140 patients in whom PROM of wrist would be included in standard evaluation	Radial flexion	.86	Radial flexion	.88
			Ulnar flexion	.87	Ulnar flexion	.89
			Dorsal flexion	.92	Dorsal flexion	.93
			Radial extension	.80	Radial extension	.80
			Ulnar extension	.80	Ulnar extension	.80
			Dorsal extension	.84	Dorsal extension	.84

ICC, Intraclass correlation coefficient; AROM, active range of motion; PROM, passive range of motion; ROM, range of motion.

Range-of-Motion Measurements of Wrist (cont.)

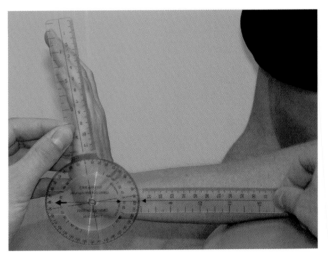

Figure 12-13B: *Measurement of wrist extension*

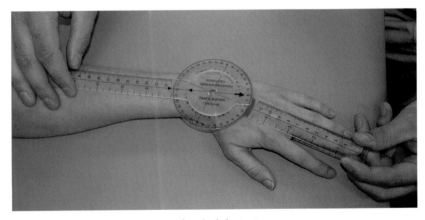

Figure 12-13C: *Measurement of radial deviation*

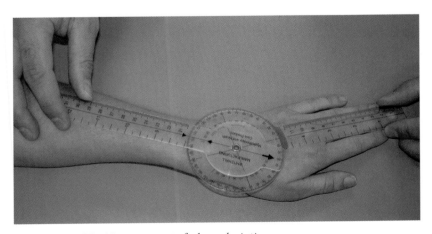

Figure 12-13D: *Measurement of ulnar deviation*

RELIABILITY OF THE CLINICAL EXAMINATION

Range-of-Motion Measurements of Fingers

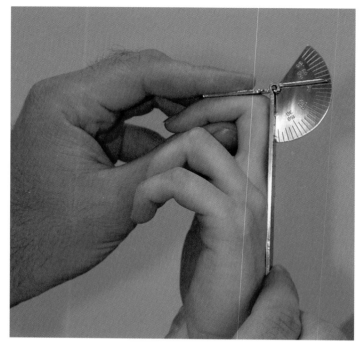

Figure 12-14: *Measurement of proximal interphalangeal joint flexion*

Test and Measure	Instrumentation	Population	Reliability ICC	
			Intra-examiner	Inter-examiner
Total AROM of IP flexion and extension *Brown et al.*[14]	Finger goniometer	30 patients with hand injuries	.97–.98	.97

Hand-Held Dynamometry

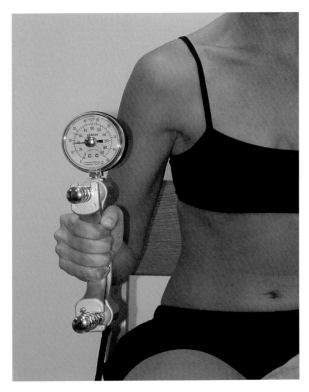

Figure 12-15: *Measurement of grip strength*

Test and Measure	Population	Reliability ICC
Wrist extensors *Bohannon and Andrews[15]*	30 patients presenting to a PT clinic	Inter-examiner .94
Wrist flexion Wrist extension *Rheault et al.[16]*	20 healthy subjects	Inter-examiner Wrist flexion .85 Wrist extension .91
Wrist extensors *Wadsworth et al.[17]*	13 patients receiving PT care for orthopaedic and neuromuscular diagnoses of upper extremity	Intra-examiner .88

PT, physical therapy.

Grip and Pinch Grip Testing

Procedure Performed	Instrumentation	Population	ICC (95% CI)	
Lateral pinch Agre et al.[18]	Dynamometer	8 healthy volunteers	Intra-examiner .93–.97	Inter-examiner .93
Grip Palmer pinch Key pinch Tip pinch Mathiowetz et al.[19]	Pinch gauge	27 healthy volunteers	Inter-examiner	
			Right .99 .98 .99 .99	Left .99 .99 .98 .99
Grip Tip pinch Key pinch Schreuders et al.[20]	Hand and pinch grip dynamometers	33 patients with a unilateral hand injury	Inter-examiner	
			Injured .93–.97 .89 .94	Non-injured .92–.94 .84 .86
Grip Tip pinch Jaw pinch Brown et al.[14]	Grip dynamometer and pinch gauge	30 patients with hand injuries	Intra-examiner .96 .86–.94 .88–.93	Inter-examiner .95 .91 .89
Grip	Dynamometer and pinch gauge	38 patients receiving PT for hand impairments	Symptomatic = .93 (.86, .96) Asymptomatic = .94 (.89, .97)	
Tripod			Symptomatic = .88 (.78, .96) Asymptomatic = .87 (.74, .93)	
Key pinch MacDermid et al.[21]			Symptomatic = .94 (.88, .97) Asymptomatic = .93 (.86, .96)	

CI, confidence interval.

Grip and Pinch Grip Testing (cont.)

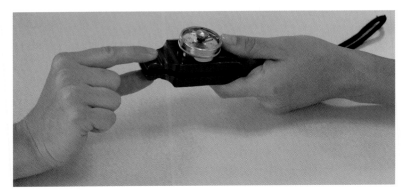

Figure 12-16A: Measurement of tip pinch strength

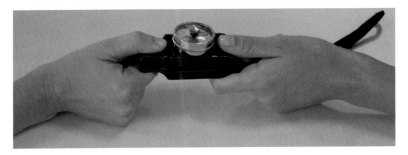

Figure 12-16B: Measurement of key pinch strength

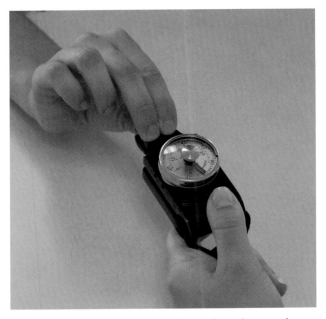

Figure 12-16C: Measurement of tripod pinch strength

RELIABILITY OF THE CLINICAL EXAMINATION

Figure-of-Eight and Volumetric Measurements of Hand

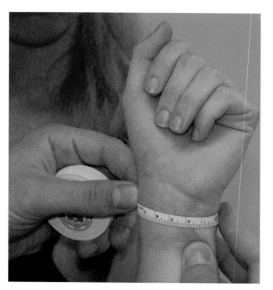

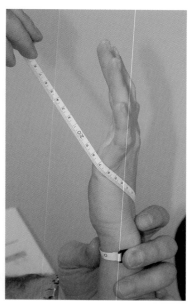

Figure 12-17A: *Start of figure-of-eight measurement*

Figure 12-17B: *Figure-of-eight measurement, continued*

Test and Measure	Test Procedure	Population	Reliability ICC	
			Intra-examiner	Inter-examiner
Figure-of-eight	Examiner places zero mark on distal aspect of ulnar styloid process. Tape measure is then brought across ventral surface of wrist to most distal aspect of radial styloid process. Next, tape is brought diagonally across dorsum of hand and over 5th MCP joint line, is brought over ventral surface of MCP joints, and is wrapped diagonally across dorsum to meet start of tape	24 persons (33 hands) with disease affecting the hand	.99	.99
Volumetric *Leard et al.*[22]	Hand is placed vertically in standard volumeter		.99	NR

NR, not reported.

Figure-of-Eight and Volumetric Measurements of Hand (cont.)

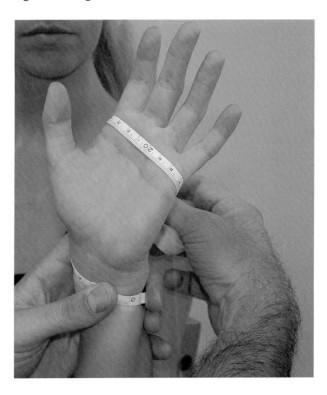

Figure 12-17C: *Figure-of-eight measurement, continued*

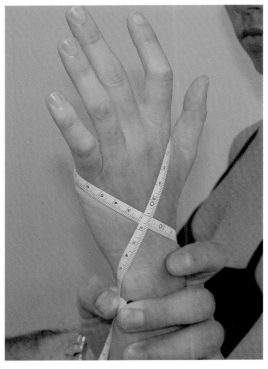

Figure 12-17D: *Completed figure-of-eight measurement*

Carpal Tunnel Syndrome: Historical Examination

History	Population	Reliability Kappa Values (95% CI)
Most bothersome symptom pain, numbness, tingling, loss of sensation?		$\kappa = .74\ (.55, .93)$
Location of most bothersome symptom?	82 patients presenting to primary care clinic, orthopaedic department, or electrophysiology laboratory with suspected cervical radiculopathy or carpal tunnel syndrome	$\kappa = .82\ (.68, .96)$
Symptoms intermittent, variable, constant?		$\kappa = .57\ (.35, .79)$
Hand swollen?		$\kappa = .85\ (.68, 1.0)$
Dropping objects?		$\kappa = .95\ (.85, 1.0)$
Entire limb goes numb?		$\kappa = .53\ (.26, .81)$
Nocturnal symptoms wake patient?		$\kappa = .83\ (.60, 1.0)$
Shaking the hand improves symptoms?		$\kappa = .90\ (.75, 1.0)$
Symptoms exacerbated with activities that require gripping? *Wainner et al.*[23]		$\kappa = .72\ (.49, .95)$

Carpal Tunnel Syndrome

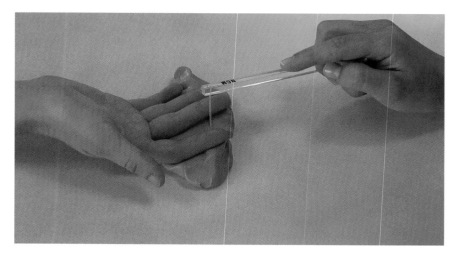

Figure 12-18: *Semmes-Weinstein monofilament testing*

Carpal Tunnel Syndrome (cont.)

Test and Measure	Test Procedure and Determination of Positive Findings	Population	Reliability Kappa Values and ICC (95% CI)	
			Intra-examiner	Inter-examiner
Two-point discrimination	NR	12 patients with carpal tunnel symptoms	Moving ICC = .58 Static ICC = .77	Moving ICC = .45 Static ICC = .66
Semmes-Weinstein monofilament testing			ICC = .71	ICC = .15
Vibration sense			κ = 1.0	κ = .40
Motor power			κ = 1.0	κ = .25
Phalen test			κ = .53	κ = .65
Tinel Test Marx et al.[24]			κ = .80	κ = .77
Wrist extension	Patient places palmar aspects of hands together, maintaining maximal wrist extension for 60 sec. Positive if symptoms are elicited in distribution of median nerve	36 hands with carpal tunnel syndrome	Inter-examiner κ = .72 (.55, .88)	
Phalen	Patient places dorsal aspects of hands together, maintaining maximal wrist flexion for 60 sec. Positive if symptoms are elicited in distribution of median nerve		κ = .88 (.77, .98)	
Tinel	Examiner percusses over palm from proximal palmar crease to distal wrist crease. Positive if symptoms are elicited in distribution of median nerve		κ = .81 (.66, .98)	
Semmes-Weinstein monofilament test	Sensory test is performed on pulp of thumb and index, long, and small fingertips		κ = .22 (.26, .42)	
Tethered median nerve test	Examiner passively extends patient's index finger while forearm is in supination and wrist is in full extension. Position is maintained for 15 sec. Positive if symptoms are elicited in distribution of median nerve		κ = .49 (.26, .71)	
Pinch test MacDermid et al.[25]	Patient actively pinches a piece of paper between tip of thumb and index and long fingers, using MCP flexion and IP extension. Positive if symptoms are elicited in distribution of median nerve		κ = .76 (.62, .91)	

Carpal Tunnel Syndrome (cont.)

Test and Measure	Test Procedure and Determination of positive Findings	Population	Reliability Kappa Values and ICC (95% CI)	
			Intra-examiner	Inter-examiner
Phalen test	Patient seated with elbow flexed 30° and forearm supinated. Examiner places the wrist in maximal flexion for 60 sec. Positive if patient experiences exacerbation of symptoms in median nerve distribution		κ = .79 (.59. 1.0)	
Tinel A	Patient seated with elbow flexed 30°, forearm supinated, and wrist in neutral. Examiner allows a reflex hammer to fall from a height of 6 in along median nerve between tendons at proximal wrist crease. Positive if patient reports a nonpainful tingling sensation along course of median nerve		κ = .47 (.21, .72)	
Tinel B	As Tinel A above, except examiner attempts to elicit symptoms using mild to moderate force with reflex hammer. Positive if pain is exacerbated along course of median nerve	82 patients presenting to a primary care clinic, orthopaedic department, or electrophysiology laboratory with suspected cervical radiculopathy or carpal tunnel syndrome	κ = .35 (.10, .60)	
Carpal compression test	Patient seated with elbow flexed 30°, forearm supinated, and wrist in neutral. Examiner places both thumbs over transverse carpal ligament and applies 6 lb pressure for 30 sec maximum. Positive if patient experiences exacerbation of symptoms in median nerve distribution		κ = .77 (.58, .96)	
Upper limb tension test A Wainner et al.[23]	Patient is supine. Examiner performs scapular depression, shoulder abduction, forearm supination, wrist and finger extension, shoulder lateral rotation, elbow extension, and contralateral/ipsilateral cervical side bending. Positive if symptoms are reproduced, side-to-side difference in elbow extension is 10°, contralateral neck side bending increases symptoms, or ipsilateral side bending decreases symptoms		κ = .76 (.51, 1.0)	

Carpal Tunnel Syndrome (cont.)

Test and Measure	Test Procedure and Determination of positive Findings	Population	Reliability Kappa Values and ICC (95% CI)	
			Intra-examiner	Inter-examiner
Upper limb tension test B	Patient supine with shoulder abducted 30°. Examiner performs scapular depression, shoulder medial rotation, full elbow extension, wrist and finger flexion, and contralateral/ipsilateral cervical side bending. Positive if symptoms are reproduced, side-to-side difference in wrist flexion >10°, contralateral neck side bending increases symptoms, or ipsilateral side bending decreases symptoms	82 patients presenting to a primary care clinic, orthopaedic department, or electrophysiology laboratory with suspected cervical radiculopathy or carpal tunnel syndrome	κ = .83 (.65, 1.0)	
Abductor pollicis strength	Examiner performs manual muscle testing of abductor pollicis. Graded as markedly reduced, reduced, or normal compared with contralateral extremity		κ = .39 (.00, .80)	
Median sensory field deficit of thumb pad	Sensation is tested with straight end of paper clip. Graded as absent, reduced, normal, or hyperesthetic		κ = .48 (.23, .73)	
Median sensory field deficit of index finger pad			κ = .50 (.25, .75)	
Median sensory field deficit of middle finger pad			κ = .40 (.12, .68)	
Wrist anterior-posterior width	Width of wrist is measured in centimeters with pair of calipers		ICC = .77 (.62, .87)	
Wrist medial-lateral width Wainner et al.[23]			ICC = .86 (.75, .92)	

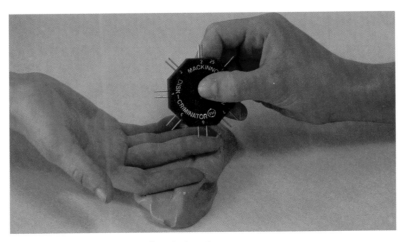

Figure 12-19: *Two-point discrimination*

DIAGNOSTIC UTILITY OF THE CLINICAL EXAMINATION

Detecting Scaphoid Fractures

Test and Measure	Test Procedure	Determination of Positive Findings	Population	Reference Standard	Sens (95% CI)	Spec (95% CI)	+LR	−LR
Scaphoid fracture test Powell et al.[26]	Examiner exerts passive overpressure into ulnar deviation of wrist while forearm is pronated	Positive if patient reports pain in anatomical snuff box	73 consecutive patients presenting to emergency department with wrist injury requiring x-rays		1.0	.34	1.52	0.00
Anatomical snuff box tenderness	Examiner palpates anatomical snuff box		221 patients with a suspected scaphoid injury		1.0	.29 (.23, .35)	1.41	0.0
Scaphoid tubercle tenderness	Examiner applies pressure to scaphoid tubercle				.83 (.70, .96)	.51 (.44, .58)	1.69	.33
Scaphoid compression tenderness Grover[27]	Examiner holds patient's thumb and applies long axis compression through metacarpal bone into scaphoid			Radiographic confirmation	1.0	.80 (.74, .86)	5.0	0.0
Snuff box tenderness	As anatomical snuff box tenderness above	Positive if pain is elicited	85 patients presenting to emergency department with mechanism of injury suggesting possible scaphoid fracture		1.0	.98	50.0	0.0
Pain with supination against resistance	Examiner holds patient's hand in handshake position and directs patient to resist supination of forearm				1.0	.98	50.0	0.0
Pain with longitudinal compression of thumb Waeckerle[28]	Examiner holds patient's thumb and applies long axis compression through metacarpal bone into scaphoid				.98	.98	49.0	.02

Sens, sensitivity; Spec, specificity; LR, likelihood ratio.

Detecting Scaphoid Fractures (cont.)

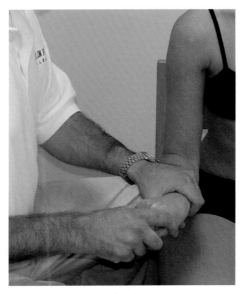

Figure 12-20: *Scaphoid fracture test*

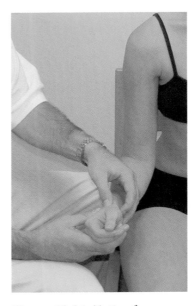

Figure 12-21: *Testing for tenderness of anatomical snuff box*

DIAGNOSTIC
UTILITY OF
THE CLINICAL
EXAMINATION

Acute Pediatric Wrist Fractures: Clinical Prediction Rule

Pershad and colleagues[29] developed a clinical prediction rule for use in identifying acute pediatric wrist injuries. Predictor variables included reduction in grip strength ≥20% as compared with the opposite side and distal radius point tenderness. The rule exhibited a sensitivity of 79%, a specificity of 63%, a +LR of 2.14 and a −LR of 0.33.

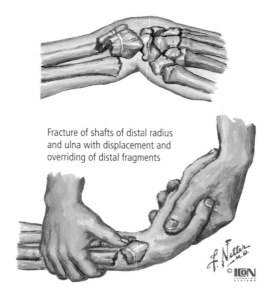

Fracture of shafts of distal radius
and ulna with displacement and
overriding of distal fragments

Figure 12-22: *Wrist fracture in a child*

Carpal Tunnel Syndrome: Tinel Sign

Test and Measure	Test Procedure	Determination of Positive Findings	Population	Reference Standard	Sens (95% CI)	Spec (95% CI)	+LR	−LR
Ahn[33]	Examiner taps median nerve at wrist 4–6 times	Positive if patient reports pain or paresthesias in distribution of median nerve	400 hands (200 symptomatic) of female patients	Electrophysiologic confirmation	.68	.90	6.80	.36
Hansen et al.[34]			142 patients referred for electrodiagnostic testing	Electrodiagnostic testing	.27 (.18, .36)	.91 (.84, 1.0)	3.0	.80
Heller et al.[35]			60 patients with suspected carpal tunnel syndrome referred for electrodiagnostic testing		.60	.77	2.61	.52
Williams et al.[36]			30 patients with carpal tunnel syndrome and 30 asymptomatic subjects	Clinical diagnosis of carpal tunnel syndrome based on symptomatology, symptoms presenting for ≥6 months, and absence of evidence of nerve compression proximal to carpal tunnel	.67	1.0	NA	.33
Tetro et al.[37]			71 patients presenting with clinical symptoms indicative of median nerve compression and 50 asymptomatic volunteers	Nerve conduction tests	.74 (.66, .81)	.91 (.86, .95)	8.22	.29
Durkan[38]			31 patients (46 hands) with symptoms characteristic of carpal tunnel syndrome		.56	.80	2.8	.55
Szabo et al.[3]			100 patients evaluated for hand, wrist, and forearm problems	Motor and sensory nerve conduction tests	.64 (.53, .75)	.83 (.77, .87)	3.76	.43

Carpal Tunnel Syndrome: Tinel Sign (cont.)

Test and Measure	Test Procedure	Determination of Positive Findings	Population	Reference Standard	Sens (95% CI)	Spec (95% CI)	+LR	−LR
Gellman et al.[39]	Examiner taps median nerve at wrist 4-6 times	Positive if patient reports pain or parathesis in distribution of median nerve	84 patients presenting with symptoms indicative of median nerve compression	Electrodiagnostic testing	.44	.94	7.33	.60
Katz et al.[31]	Examiner drops square end of reflex hammer on distal wrist crease from height of 12 cm	Positive if patient reports pain or paresthesias in at least one finger innervated by median nerve	110 patients referred to laboratory for electrophysiologic examination	Nerve conduction tests	.60	.67	1.82	.60
Gunnarsson et al.[32]	NR	NR	100 patients referred to laboratory for neurophysiologic examination of ulnar or median nerves		.62 (.48, .73)	.57 (.45, .69)	1.44	.67
Mondelli et al.[40]	Examiner taps median nerve over distal wrist crease with reflex hammer three times	NR	179 patients with suspected carpal tunnel syndrome	Electrodiagnostic testing	.41	.56	.93	1.05
Kuhlman and Hennessey[41]	Examiner taps firmly with index and middle fingers over area of median nerve	NR	228 hands referred for electrodiagnostic consultation with suspected carpal tunnel syndrome	Nerve conduction studies	.23	.87	1.77	.89
Gonzalez et al.[42]	Examiner gently percusses over median nerve in forearm and over flexor retinaculum 4–6 times with reflex hammer	NR	200 hands with clinical diagnosis of carpal tunnel syndrome and 200 asymptomatic hands	Clinical diagnosis of carpal tunnel syndrome, including pain at night, paresthesias, numbness, or sensory deficits in distribution of median nerve and weakness of abductor pollicis brevis	.33	.97	11.0	.69

Carpal Tunnel Syndrome: Tinel Sign (cont.)

Test and Measure	Test Procedure	Determination of Positive Findings	Population	Reference Standard	Sens (95% CI)	Spec (95% CI)	+LR	−LR
Tinel A	Patient seated with elbow flexed 30°, forearm supinated, and wrist in neutral. Examiner allows reflex hammer to fall from height of 6 in along median nerve between tendons at proximal wrist crease	Positive if patient reports nonpainful tingling sensation along course of median nerve	82 patients presenting to a primary care clinic, orthopaedic department, or electrophysiology laboratory with suspected cervical radiculopathy or carpal tunnel syndrome	Needle electromyography and nerve conduction studies	.41 (.22, .59)	.58 (.45, .72)	.98 (.56, 1.7)	1.0 (.69, 1.5)
Tinel B *Wainner et al.*[23]	As Tinal A above, except examiner attempts to elicit symptoms using mild to moderate force with reflex hammer	Positive if pain is exacerbated along course of median nerve			.48 (.29, .67)	.67 (.54, .79)	1.4 (.84, 2.5)	.78 (.52, 1.2)

NA, not available.

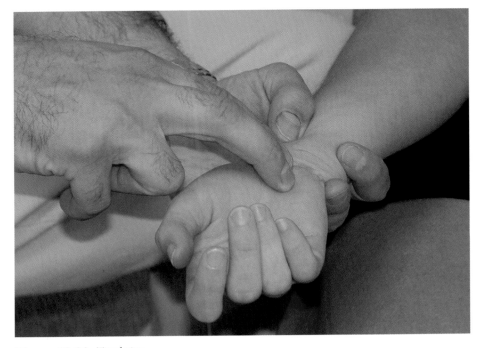

Figure 12-23: *Tinel sign*

DIAGNOSTIC UTILITY OF THE CLINICAL EXAMINATION

Detecting Carpal Instability

Test and Measure	Test Procedure	Determination of Positive Findings	Population	Reference Standard	Sens	Spec	+LR	−LR
Scaphoid shift test *LaStayo and Howell*[30]	Patient's elbow is stabilized on table with forearm in slight pronation. With one hand, examiner grasps radial side of patient's wrist with thumb on the palmar prominence of scaphoid. With other hand, examiner grasps patient's hand at metacarpal level to stabilize wrist. Examiner maintains pressure on scaphoid tubercle and moves patient's wrist into ulnar deviation with slight extension, then radial deviation with slight flexion. Examiner releases pressure on scaphoid while wrist is in radial deviation and flexion	Positive for instability of scaphoid if scaphoid shifts, test elicits a "thunk," or patient's symptoms are reproduced when scaphoid is released	50 painful wrists undergoing arthroscopy	Arthroscopic visualization	.69	.66	2.03	.47
Ballottement test	Examiner stabilizes patient's lunate bone between thumb and index finger of one hand while other hand moves piso-triquetral complex in a palmar and dorsal direction	Positive for instability of luno-triquetral joint if patient's symptoms are reproduced or excessive laxity of joint is revealed			.64	.44	1.14	.82
Ulnomenisco-triquetral dorsal glide *LaStayo and Howell*[30]	Patient is seated with elbow on table, forearm neutral. Examiner places thumb over head of distal ulna. Examiner then places radial side of index proximal interphalangeal (PIP) joint over palmar surface of patient's pisotriquetral complex. Examiner squeezes thumb and index finger together, creating a dorsal glide of pisotriquetral complex	Considered positive for ulnomenisco-triquetral complex instability if the patient's symptoms are reproduced or excessive laxity of the joint is revealed			.66	.64	1.69	.56

Detecting Carpal Instability (cont.)

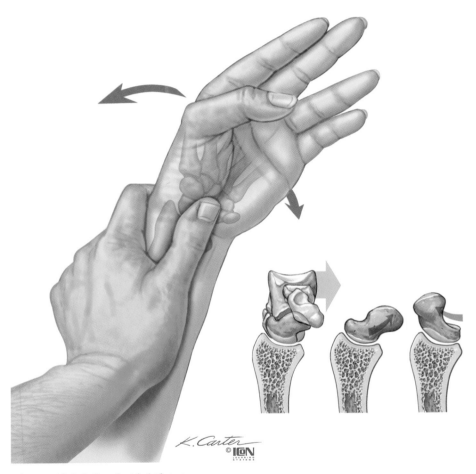

Figure 12-24: *Scaphoid shift test*

DIAGNOSTIC UTILITY OF THE CLINICAL EXAMINATION

Detecting Carpal Tunnel Syndrome

History	Population	Reference Standard	Sens (95% CI)	Spec (95% CI)	+LR (95% CI)	−LR (95% CI)
Age ≥40 years	110 patients referred to laboratory for electrophysiologic examination	Nerve conduction tests	.80	.42	1.38	.48
Nocturnal symptoms			.77	.28	1.07	.82
Bilateral symptoms *LeStayo and Howell[30]* *Katz et al.[31]*			.61	.58	1.45	.67
Numbness in thumb and index and long fingers	100 patients referred to laboratory for a neurophysiologic examination of ulnar or median nerves		.95 (.87, .98)	.26 (.16, .37)	1.28	.19
Numbness disappears when shaking hands			.90 (.80, .96)	.30 (.20, .42)	1.29	.33
Reports of reduced sensation of touch in thumb and index and long fingers *Katz et al.[31]* *Gunnarsson et al.[32]*			.39 (.30, .52)	.67 (.54, .78)	1.18	.91
Night pain *Szabo et al.[3]*	100 patients evaluated for hand, wrist, and forearm problems	Motor and sensory nerve conduction tests	.96 (.87, .98)	.59 (.48, .69)	2.34	.07
Age >45	82 patients presenting to a primary care clinic, orthopaedic department, or electrophysiology laboratory with suspected cervical radiculopathy or carpal tunnel syndrome	Needle electromyography and nerve conduction studies	.64 (.47, .82)	.59 (.47, .72)	1.58 (.46, 2.4)	.60 (.35, 1.0)
Most bothersome symptom pain, numbness, tingling, loss of sensation			.04 (−.04, .11)	.91 (.83, .98)	.42 (.05, .34)	1.1 (.94, 1.2)
Location of most bothersome symptom			.35 (.16, .53)	.40 (.27, .54)	.58 (.33, 1.0)	1.6 (1.1, 2.5)
Symptoms intermittent, variable, or constant			.23 (.07, .39)	.89 (.81, .97)	2.1 (.74, .58)	.87 (.69, 1.4)
Reports of hand becoming swollen			.38 (.20, .57)	.63 (.50, .76)	1.0 (.57, 1.9)	.98 (.68, 1.4)
Dropping of objects			.73 (.56, .90)	.57 (.44, .71)	1.7 (1.2, 2.5)	.47 (.24, .92)
Entire limb goes numb			.38 (.20, .57)	.80 (.69, .90)	1.9 (.92, 3.9)	.77 (.55, 1.1)
Nocturnal symptoms wake patient			.73 (.56, .90)	.31 (.19, .44)	1.1 (.79, 1.4)	.86 (.41, 1.8)
Shaking hand improves symptoms			.81 (.66, .96)	.57 (.43, .70)	1.9 (13, 2.7)	.34 (.15, .77)
Symptoms exacerbated with activities that require gripping *Wainner et al.[23]*			.77 (.61, .93)	.37 (.24, .50)	1.2 (.91, 1.6)	.62 (.28, 1.4)

Detecting Carpal Tunnel Syndrome (cont.)

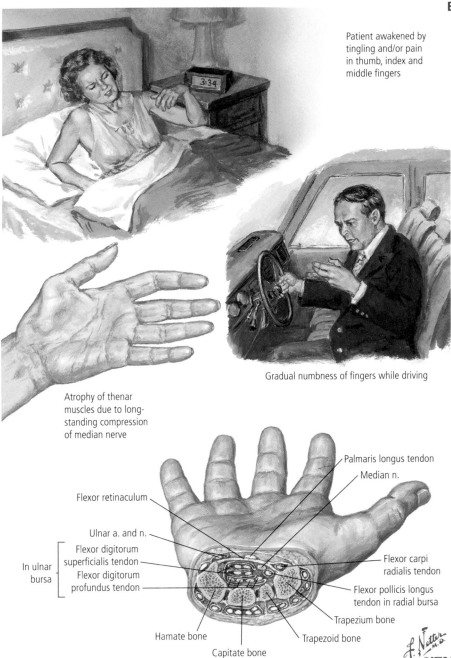

Patient awakened by
tingling and/or pain
in thumb, index and
middle fingers

Gradual numbness of fingers while driving

Atrophy of thenar
muscles due to long-
standing compression
of median nerve

Palmaris longus tendon

Median n.

Flexor retinaculum

Ulnar a. and n.

In ulnar
bursa

Flexor digitorum
superficialis tendon

Flexor digitorum
profundus tendon

Flexor carpi
radialis tendon

Flexor pollicis longus
tendon in radial bursa

Trapezium bone

Hamate bone

Trapezoid bone

Capitate bone

Section through wrist at distal row of carpal bones shows carpal tunnel. Increase in
size of tunnel structures caused by edema (trama), inflammation (rheumatoid disease);
ganglion, amyloid deposits, or diabetic neuropathy may compress median nerve

Figure 12-25: *Carpal tunnel syndrome*

DIAGNOSTIC UTILITY OF THE CLINICAL EXAMINATION

Carpal Tunnel Syndrome: Phalen Sign

Test and Measure	Test Procedure	Determination of Positive Findings	Population	Reference Standard	Sens (95% CI)	Spec (95% CI)	+LR	−LR
Katz et al.[31]	Examiner instructs patient to flex both wrists to 90° with dorsal aspects of held in opposition for 60 sec	Positive if patient reports pain or paresthesias in at least one finger nnervated by median nerve	110 patients referred to laboratory for electrophysiologic examination	Nerve conduction tests	.74	.47	1.4	.55
Gunnarsson et al.[32]	NR	NR	100 patients referred to laboratory for neurophysiologic examination of ulnar or median nerves		.86 (.75, .93)	.48 (.37, .60)	1.65	.29
Ahn[33]	Patient is asked to hold wrist in complete flexion with elbow extended and forearm pronated for 60 sec	Positive if symptoms are produced	400 hands (200 symptomatic) of female patients	Electrophysiologic confirmation	.68	.91	1.15	.78
Williams et al.[36]	Patient is instructed to perform maximum wrist flexion with elbow extended and forearm pronated for 60 sec		30 patients with carpal tunnel syndrome and 30 asymptomatic subjects	Clinical diagnosis of carpal tunnel syndrome based on symptoma-tology, symptoms presenting for ≥6 months, and absence of evidence of nerve compression proximal to carpal tunnel	.88	1.0	NA	.12
Szabo et al.[3]	Patient rests elbow on examination table with wrist over edge. Patient is instructed to let wrist flex over edge of table for 60 sec		100 patients evaluated for hand, wrist, and forearm problems	Motor and sensory nerve conduction tests	.75 (.62, .82)	.71 (.62, .77)	2.59	.35

Carpal Tunnel Syndrome: Phalen Sign (cont.)

Test and Measure	Test Procedure	Determination of Positive Findings	Population	Reference Standard	Sens (95% CI)	Spec (95% CI)	+LR	−LR
Gonzalez et al.[42]	Patient rests elbow on examination table with forearm supinated. Examiner maintains wrist in flexion for 60 sec	100 patients evaluated for hand, wrist, and forearm problems	200 hands with clinical diagnosis of carpal tunnel syndrome and 200 asymptomatic hands	Clinical diagnosis of carpal tunnel syndrome, including pain at night, paresthesias, numbness, or sensory deficits in distribution of median nerve and weakness of abductor pollicis brevis	.87	.90	8.7	.14
Fertl et al.[43]	Patient holds forearms in pronation with elbows resting on examination table, forearms vertical, and wrists in gravity-assisted flexion		132 patients with pain of upper limb	Electrophysiologic confirmation	.79	.92	9.88	.23
Hansen et al.[34]	Patient is instructed to maximally flex wrist and hold position for 60 sec	Positive if symptoms are produced	142 patients referred for electrodiagnostic testing	Electrodiagnostic testing	.34 (.24, .43)	.74 (.62, .87)	1.31	.89
Durkan[38]			31 patients (46 hands) with symptoms characteristic of carpal tunnel syndrome	Nerve conduction tests	.70	.84	4.38	.36
Tetro et al.[37]			71 patients presenting with clinical symptoms indicative of median nerve compression and 50 asymptomatic subjects		.61 (.53, .69)	.83 (.77, .89)	3.59	.47
Gellman et al.[39]			84 patients presenting with symptoms indicative of median nerve compression	Electrodiagnostic testing	.71	.80	3.55	.36

DIAGNOSTIC UTILITY OF THE CLINICAL EXAMINATION

Carpal Tunnel Syndrome: Phalen Sign (cont.)

Test and Measure	Test Procedure	Determination of Positive Findings	Population	Reference Standard	Sens (95% CI)	Spec (95% CI)	+LR	−LR
Kuhlman and Hennessey[41]	Patient is instructed to maximally flex wrist and hold position for 60 sec.	Positive if symptoms are are produced	228 hands referred for electrodiagnostic consultation with suspected carpal tunnel syndrome	Nerve conduction studies	.51	.76	2.13	.64
Mondelli et al.[40]			179 patients with expected carpal tunnel syndrome	Electrodiagnostic testing	.59	.72	2.11	.57
Heller et al.[35]			60 patients with suspected carpal tunnel syndrome referred for electrodiagnostic testing		.67	.59	1.63	.56
Wainner et al.[23]	Patient seated with elbow flexed 30° and forearm supinated. Examiner places wrist in maximal flexion for 60 sec	Positive if patient experiences an exacerbation of symptoms in median nerve distribution	82 patients presenting to a primary care clinic, orthopaedic department, or electrophysiology laboratory with suspected cervical radiculopathy or carpal tunnel syndrome	Needle electromyography and nerve conduction studies	.77 (.61, .93)	.40 (.26, .53)	1.3 (.94, 1.7)	.58 (.27, 1.3)

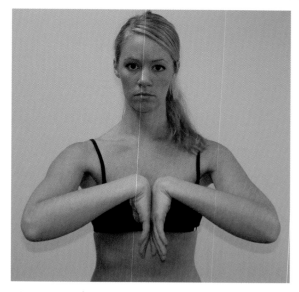

Figure 12-26: Phalen sign

Carpal Tunnel Syndrome: Clinical Prediction Rule

Wainner and colleagues[23] developed a clinical prediction rule for detecting carpal tunnel syndrome. Results of their study demonstrated that if five variables (a Brigham and Women's Hospital Hand Severity Scale[47] score >1.9, a wrist ratio index >.67, a patient report of shaking the hand for symptom relief, diminished sensation on the thumb pad, and age >45) were present, the +LR was 18.3 (95% CI:1.0, 328.3). This clinical prediction rule results in a posttest probability of 90% that the patient has carpal tunnel syndrome. If 415 variables were present the TLR was 4.6 (95% CI 2.5-8.7) resulting in a positive posttest probability of 70%.

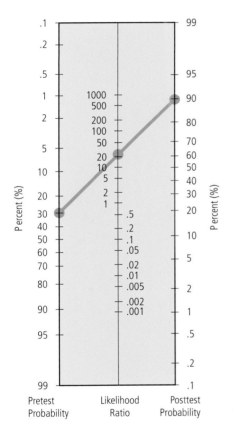

Figure 12-27: Nomogram representing the change in pretest (34% in this study) to posttest probability given the clinical prediction rule. (Nomogram adapted with permission, Massachusetts Medical Society, Copyright © 2005.)

DIAGNOSTIC UTILITY OF THE CLINICAL EXAMINATION

Carpal Tunnel Syndrome: Sensory Loss

Test and Measure	Test Procedure	Determination of Positive Findings	Population	Reference Standard	Sens (95% CI)	Spec (95% CI)	+LR	−LR
Moving two-point discrimination Katz et al.[31]	Examiner strokes tip of index and 5th fingers five times with one or two caliber tips	Positive if patient is unable to identify number of tips performed on at least one stroke	110 patients referred to laboratory for electrophysiologic examination	Nerve conduction tests	.32	.81	1.68	.84
Semmes-Weinstein test—wrist flexed Koris et al.[44]	Monofilament pressure is applied perpendicular to palmar digital surface in position of wrist flexion	Positive if patient is not able to determine when monofilament contacts skin	21 patients (33 symptomatic hands) with numbness in median nerve distribution	Electrical confirmation	.82	.86	5.86	.21
Semmes-Weinstein neutral	Monofilament is applied three times to each digit and palm with wrist in neutral	Positive if patient cannot determine when monofilament contacts skin two out of three times	100 patients evaluated for hand, wrist, and forearm problems	Motor and sensory nerve conduction tests	.65 (.52, .75)	.70 (.62, .75)	2.17	.50
Semmes-Weinstein—Phalen Szabo et al.[45]	As above, with the wrist flexed				.83 (.69, .88)	.70 (.63, .76)	2.77	.24
Semmes-Weinstein test	NR	NR	84 patients presenting with symptoms indicative of median nerve compression	Electrodiagnostic testing	.91	.80	4.55	.11
Two-point discrimination Gellman et al.[39]	NR	NR			.33	1.0	NA	.67
Sensory loss at pad of thumb	Sensation is tested with straight end of paper clip	Positive if sensation is absent or reduced	82 patients presenting to a primary care clinic, orthopaedic department, or electrophysiology laboratory with suspected cervical radiculopathy or carpal tunnel syndrome	Needle electromyography and nerve conduction studies	.65 (.47, .84)	.70 (.47, 84	2.2 (1.3, 3.6)	.49 (.28, 46)
Sensory loss at pad of index finger					.52 (.32, .72)	.67 (.32, .72)	1.6 (.92, 2.7)	.72 (.86, 1.1)
Sensory loss at pad of medial finger Wainner et al.[23]					.44 (.26, .63)	.74 (.26, .63)	1.7 (.58, .52)	.75 (.86, 1.1)

Carpal Tunnel Syndrome: Sensory Loss (cont.)

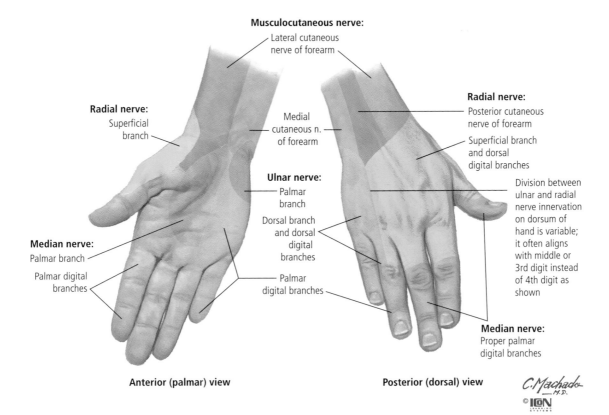

Musculocutaneous nerve:
Lateral cutaneous
nerve of forearm

Radial nerve:
Superficial
branch

Medial
cutaneous n.
of forearm

Radial nerve:
Posterior cutaneous
nerve of forearm

Superficial branch
and dorsal
digital branches

Ulnar nerve:
Palmar
branch

Dorsal branch
and dorsal
digital
branches

Division between
ulnar and radial
nerve innervation
on dorsum of
hand is variable;
it often aligns
with middle or
3rd digit instead
of 4th digit as
shown

Median nerve:
Palmar branch

Palmar digital
branches

Palmar
digital branches

Median nerve:
Proper palmar
digital branches

Anterior (palmar) view

Posterior (dorsal) view

C.Machado
—M.D.

© ICN

Figure 12-28: Cutaneous innervation of the wrist and hand

DIAGNOSTIC UTILITY OF THE CLINICAL EXAMINATION

Carpal Tunnel Syndrome: Carpal Compression Test

Test and Measure	Test Procedure	Determination of Positive Findings	Population	Reference Standard	Sens (95% CI)	Spec (95% CI)	+LR	−LR
Tetro et al.[37]	Examiner applies compression over median nerve at carpal tunnel with two fingers for 30 sec		71 patients presenting with clinical symptoms indicative of median nerve compression and 50 asymptomatic volunteers	Nerve conduction tests	.75 (.67, .82)	.93 (.88, .97)	10.71	.93
Durkan[38]	As above, except pressure is applied with specialized instrument that applied a pressure of 150 mm Hg to the carpal tunnel for 30 sec		31 patients (46 hands) with symptoms characteristic of carpal tunnel syndrome		.87	.90	8.7	.14
Szabo et al.[3]	As above		100 patients evaluated for hand, wrist, and forearm problems	Motor and sensory nerve conduction tests	.89 (.76, .93)	.84 (.77, .88)	5.56	.13
Mondelli et al.[40]	Examiner applies manual pressure to palmar aspect of carpal tunnel for 60 sec	Considered positive if pain, paresthesia, or numbness is reproduced	179 patients with expected carpal tunnel syndrome	Electrodiagnostic testing	.42	.95	8.4	.61
Kuhlman and Hennessey[41]	Examiner applies moderate pressure over median nerve just distal to distal flexor wrist crease for 5 sec		228 hands referred for electro-diagnostic consultation with suspected carpal tunnel syndrome	Nerve conduction studies	.28	.74	1.08	.97
Gonzalez et al.[42]	The examiner applies moderate pressure with thumbs over transverse carpal ligament with wrist in neutral for 30 sec		200 hands with a clinical diag-nosis of carpal tunnel syndrome and 200 asymptomatic hands	Clinical diagnosis of carpal tunnel syndrome, including pain at night, paresthesias, numbness, or sensory deficits in distribution of median nerve and weakness of abductor pollicis brevis	.87	.95	17.4	.14
Fertl et al.[43]			132 patients with pain of upper limb	Electrophysiological confirmation	.83	.92	10.38	.18

Carpal Tunnel Syndrome: Carpal Compression Test (cont.)

Test and Measure	Test Procedure	Determination of Positive Findings	Population	Reference Standard	Sens (95% CI)	Spec (95% CI)	+LR	−LR
Wainner et al.[23]	Patient seated with elbow flexed 30°, forearm supinated, and wrist in neutral. Examiner places both thumbs over transverse carpal ligament and applies 6 lb pressure for 30 sec maximum	Positive if patient experiences exacerbation of symptoms in median nerve distribution	82 patients presenting to a primary care clinic, orthopaedic department, or electrophysiology laboratory with suspected cervical radiculopathy or carpal tunnel syndrome	Needle electromyography and nerve conduction studies	.64 (.45, .83)	.30 (.17, .42)	.91 (.65, 1.3)	1.2 (.62, 2.4)

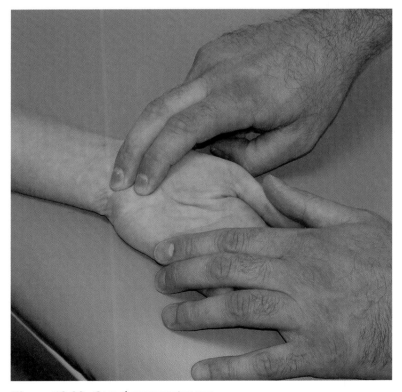

Figure 12-29: *Carpal compression test*

DIAGNOSTIC UTILITY OF THE CLINICAL EXAMINATION

Carpal Tunnel Syndrome: Miscellaneous Special Tests

Test and Measure	Test Procedure	Determination of Positive Findings	Population	Reference Standard	Sens (95% CI)	Spec (95% CI)	+LR	−LR
Wrist extension test *Mondelli et al.*[40]	Patient is instructed to extend wrist and hold position for 60 sec	Considered positive if the patient reports paresthesia in the distribution of the median nerve	179 patients with expected carpal tunnel syndrome	Electro-diagnostic testing	.55	.82	3.06	.55
Lumbrical provocation test *Karl et al.*[46]	Patient is instructed to make a fist for 60 sec		96 consecutive patients referred for electrodiagnostic testing	Electro-diagnostic consultation	.37	.71	1.28	.89
Flick maneuver *Hansen et al.*[34]	Patient is instructed to demonstrate hand motions or positions patient uses when pain is most severe	Positive if patient demonstrates a flicking down of hands similar to shaking a thermometer	142 patients referred for electrodiagnostic testing	Electro-diagnostic testing	.37 (.27, .46)	.74 (.62, .87)	1.42	.85
Wrist/ratio index greater than .67	Anterior-posterior width of wrist is measured and divided by medial-lateral width	Positive if ratio is greater than .67	82 patients presenting to a primary care clinic, orthopaedic department, or electrophysiology laboratory with suspected cervical radiculopathy or carpal tunnel syndrome	Needle electro-myography and nerve conduction studies	.93 (.83, 1.0)	.26 (.14, .38)	1.3 (1.0, 1.5)	.29 (.07, 1.2)
Strength of abductor pollicis brevis	Strength of abductor pollicis brevis is tested by placing thumb in a position of abduction and applying a force in direction of adduction at proximal phalanx	Positive if strength is reduced or markedly reduced compared with contralateral extremity			.19 (.04, .34)	.89 (.81, .90)	1.7 (.58, 5.2)	.91 (.74, 1.1)
Upper limb tension test A	As above (pg. 476)				.75 (.58, .92)	13. (.04, .22)	.86 (.67, 1.1)	1.9 (.72, 5.1)
Upper limb tension test B *Wainner et al.*[23]	As above (pg. 477)				.64 (.45, .83)	.30 (.17, .42)	.91 (.65, 1.3)	1.2 (.62, 2.4)
Abductor pollicis brevis weakness	Patient is instructed to touch pads of thumb and 5th digit together. Examiner applies posteriorly directed force over thumb IP joint toward palm	Positive if weakness is detected	228 hands referred for electrodiagnostic consultation with suspected carpal tunnel syndrome	Nerve conduction studies	.66	.66	1.94	.52

Carpal Tunnel Syndrome: Miscellaneous Special Tests (cont.)

Test and Measure	Test Procedure	Determination of Positive Findings	Population	Reference Standard	Sens (95% CI)	Spec (95% CI)	+LR	−LR
Square-shaped wrist *Kuhlman and Hennessey*[41]	Anteroposterior and mediolateral dimensions of wrist are measured at distal flexor wrist crease with the use of standard calipers	Positive if wrist ratio (anteroposterior dimension divided by mediolateral dimension) is ≥.70	228 hands referred for electrodiagnostic consultation with suspected carpal tunnel syndrome	Nerve conduction studies	.69	.73	2.56	.42
Hand elevation test *Ahn*[33]	Patient is instructed to elevate both hands above the head and hold position for 2 min	Positive if patient reports pain or paresthesias in distribution of median nerve	400 hands (200 symptomatic) of female patients	Electro-physiologic confirmation	.76	.99	76.0	.24
Grip strength	Grip and pinch strength measurements are recorded with dynamometer	Positive if affected side demonstrated strength deficit >12% compared with the unaffected side	100 patients evaluated for hand, wrist, and forearm problems	Motor and sensory nerve conduction tests	.48 (.26, .70)	.38 (.26, .49)	.77	1.37
Key pinch					.33 (.14, .52)	.52 (.39, .63)	.69	1.29
Three-jaw pinch					.43 (.24, .62)	.49 (.36, .60)	.84	1.16
Tip pinch *Szabo et al.*[3]					.65 (.41, .88)	.38 (.25, .50)	1.05	.92

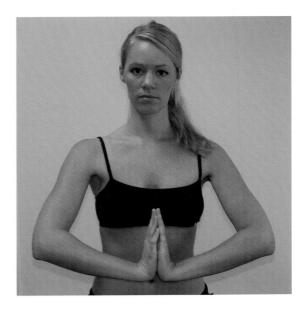

Figure 12-30: *Wrist extension test*

REFERENCES

1. Wadsworth C. Cumulative trauma disorders of the wrist and hand. In: *The Wrist and Hand*. La Crosse: Orthopaedic Section, American Physical Therapy Association; 1995.

2. D'Arcy C, McGee S. Does this patient have carpal tunnel syndrome? *JAMA*. 2000;283:3110-3117.

3. Szabo RM, Slater RR Jr, Farver TB, Stanton DB, Sharman WK. The value of diagnostic testing in carpal tunnel syndrome. *J Hand Surg Am*. 1999;24:704-714.

4. MacDermid JC, Wessel J. Clinical diagnosis of carpal tunnel syndrome: a systematic review. *J Hand Ther*. 2004;17:309-319.

5. Wadsworth C. Current concepts in orthopaedic physical therapy. In: *The Wrist and Hand*. La Crosse: Orthopaedic Section, American Physical Therapy Association; 2001.

6. Skirven T. Tendon and nerve injuries of the wrist and hand. In: *The Wrist and Hand*. La Crosse: Orthopaedic Section, American Physical Therapy Association; 1995.

7. Wolff TW, Hodges A. Common orthopaedic dysfunction of the wrist and hand. In: Placzek JD, Boyce DA, eds. *Orthopaedic Physical Therapy Secrets*. Philadelphia: Hanley and Belfus; 2001:315-321.

8. Cole IC. Fractures and ligament injuires of the wrist and hand. In: *The Wrist and Hand*. La Crosse: Orthopaedic Section, American Physical Therapy Association; 1995.

9. Hartley A. *Practical Joint Assessment*. St. Louis: Mosby; 1995.

10. O'Brien MP. Fractures and dislocations of the wrist and hand. In: Placzek JD, Boyce DA, eds. *Orthopaedic Physical Therapy Secrets*. Philadelphia: Hanley and Belfus; 2001:322-326.

11. Boone DC, Azen SP, Lin CM, Spence C, Baron C, Lee L. Reliability of goniometric measurements. *Phys Ther*. 1978;58:1355-1360.

12. Horger MM. The reliability of goniometric measurements of active and passive wrist motions. *Am J Occup Ther*. 1990;44:342-348.

13. LaStayo PC, Wheeler DL. Reliability of passive wrist flexion and extension goniometric measurements: a multicenter study. *Phys Ther*. 1994;74:162-174.

14. Brown A, Cramer LD, Eckhaus D, Schmidt J, Ware L, MacKenzie E. Validity and reliability of the Dexter hand evaluation and therapy system in hand-injured patients. *J Hand Ther*. 2000;13:37-45.

15. Bohannon RW, Andrews AW. Interrater reliability of hand-held dynamometry. *Phys Ther*. 1987;67:931-933.

16. Rheault W, Beal JL, Kubik KR, Nowak TA, Shepley JA. Intertester reliability of the hand-held dynamometer for wrist flexion and extension. *Arch Phys Med Rehabil*. 1989;70:907-910.

17. Wadsworth CT, Krishnan R, Sear M, Harrold J, Nielsen DH. Intrarater reliability of manual muscle testing and hand-held dynametric muscle testing. *Phys Ther*. 1987;9:1342-1347.

18. Agre JC, Magness JL, Hull SZ, et al. Strength testing with a portable dynamometer: reliability for upper and lower extremities. *Arch Phys Med Rehabil*. 1987;68:454-458.

19. Mathiowetz V, Weber K, Volland G, Kashman N. Reliability and validity of grip and pinch strength evaluations. *J Hand Surg Am*. 1984;9:222-226.

20. Schreuders TA, Roebroeck ME, Goumans J, van Nieuwenhuijzen JF, Stijnen TH, Stam HJ. Measurement error in grip and pinch force measurements in patients with hand injuries. *Phys Ther*. 2003;83:806-815.

21. MacDermid JC, Kramer JF, Woodbury MG, McFarlane RM, Roth JH. Interrater relia-bility of pinch and grip strength measurements in patients with cumulative trauma disorders. *J Hand Ther.* 1994;7:10-14.

22. Leard J, Breglio L, Fraga L, et al. Reliability and concurrent validity of the figure-of-eight method of measuring hand size in patients with hand pathology. *J Orthop Sports Phys Ther.* 2004;24:335-340.

23. Wainner RS, Fritz JM, Irrgang JJ, Delitto A, Allison S, Boninger ML. Development of a clinical prediction rule for the diagnosis of carpal tunnel syndrome. *Arch Phys Med Rehabil.* 2005;86:609-618.

24. Marx RG, Hudak PL, Bombardier C, Graham B, Goldsmith C, Wright JG. The relia-bility of physical examination for carpal tunnel syndrome. *J Hand Surg Br.* 1998;23:499-502.

25. MacDermid JC, Kramer JF, McFarlane RM, Roth JH. Inter-rater agreement and accu-racy of clinical tests used in diagnosis of carpal tunnel syndrome. *Work.* 1997;8:37-44.

26. Powell JM, Lloyd GJ, Rintoul RF. New clinical test for fracture of the scaphoid. *Can J Surg.* 1988;31:237-238.

27. Grover R. Clinical assessment of scaphoid injuries and the detection of fractures. *J Hand Surg Br.* 1996;21:341-343.

28. Waeckerle JF. A prospective study identifying the sensitivity of radiographic findings and the efficacy of clinical findings in carpal navicular fractures. *Ann Emerg Med.* 1987;16:733-737.

29. Pershad J, Monroe K, King W, Bartle S, Hardin E, Zinkan L. Can clinical parameters predict fractures in acute pediatric wrist injuries? *Acad Emerg Med.* 2000;7:1152-1155.

30. LaStayo P, Howell J. Clinical provocative tests used in evaluating wrist pain: a de-scriptive study. *J Hand Ther.* 1995;8:10-17.

31. Katz J, Larson M, Sabra A, et al. The carpal tunnel syndrome: diagnostic utility of the history and physical examination findings. *Ann Intern Med.* 1990;112:321-327.

32. Gunnarsson LG, Amilon A, Hellstrand P, Leissner P, Philipson L. The diagnosis of carpal tunnel syndrome. Sensitivity and specificity of some clinical and electrophys-iological tests. *J Hand Surg Br.* 1997;22:34-37.

33. Ahn DS. Hand elevation: a new test for carpal tunnel syndrome. *Ann Plast Surg.* 2001;46:120-124.

34. Hansen PA, Micklesen P, Robinson LR. Clinical utility of the flick maneuver in diag-nosing carpal tunnel syndrome. *Am J Phys Med Rehabil.* 2004;83:363-367.

35. Heller L, Ring H, Costeff PS. Evaluation of Tinel's and Phalen's sign in diagnosis of the carpal tunnel syndrome. *Eur Neurol.* 1986;25:40-42.

36. Williams TM, Mackinnon SE, Novak CB, McCabe S, Kelly L. Verification of the pres-sure provocative test in carpal tunnel syndrome. *Ann Plast Surg.* 1992;29:8-11.

37. Tetro AM, Evanoff BA, Hollstien SB, Gelberman RH. A new provocative test for carpal tunnel syndrome. Assessment of wrist flexion and nerve compression. *J Bone Joint Surg Br.* 1998;80:493-498.

38. Durkan JA. A new diagnostic test for carpal tunnel syndrome. *J Bone Joint Surg Am.* 1991;73:535-538.

REFERENCES

REFERENCES

39. Gellman H, Gelberman RH, Tan AM, Botte MJ. Carpal tunnel syndrome. An evaluation of the provocative diagnostic tests. *J Bone Joint Surg Am.* 1986;68:735-737.

40. Mondelli M, Passero S, Giannini F. Provocative tests in different stages of carpal tunnel syndrome. *Clin Neurol Neurosurg.* 2001;103:178-183.

41. Kuhlman KA, Hennessey WJ. Sensitivity and specificity of carpal tunnel syndrome signs. *Am J Phys Med Rehabil.* 1997;76:451-457.

42. Gonzalez del Pino J, Delgado-Martinez AD, Gonzalez I, Lovic A. Value of the carpal compression test in the diagnosis of carpal tunnel syndrome. *J Hand Surg Br.* 1997;22:38-41.

43. Fertl E, Wober C, Zeitlhofer J. The serial use of two provocative tests in the clinical diagnosis of carpal tunnel syndrome. *Acta Neurol Scand.* 1998;98:328-332.

44. Koris M, Gelberman RH, Duncan K, Boublick M, Smith B. Carpal tunnel syndrome. Evaluation of a quantitative provocational diagnostic test. *Clin Orthop.* 1990;157-161.

45. Szabo RM, Gelberman RH, Dimick MP. Sensibility testing in patients with carpal tunnel syndrome. *J Bone Joint Surg Am.* 1984;66:60-64.

46. Karl AI, Carney ML, Kaul MP. The lumbrical provocation test in subjects with median inclusive paresthesia. *Arch Phys Med Rehabil.* 2001;82:935-937.

47. Levine D, Simmons B, Koris M, et al. A self-administered questionnaire for the assessment of severity of symptoms and functional status in carpal tunnel syndrome. *J Bone Joint Surg Am.* 1993;75:1585-1592.

Additional Orthopaedic Physical Therapy Examination Tests

Test	Description	Positive Findings
Cervical Spine		
Rhomberg test[1]	While standing, patient is asked to close eyes for 20–30 sec	Positive for upper motor neuron lesion if patient sways excessively or loses balance
Vertebral artery test[2]	Examiner passively rotates, extends, and side-bends head to each side, holding each position for 1 min	Positive for vertebral artery involvement if nystagmus, slurring of speech, blurry vision, dizziness, or unconsciousness occurs
Transverse ligament stress test[1]	Patient is supine. Examiner supports occiput with both hands, with index fingers between occiput and C2. Examiner translates occiput anteriorly, avoiding cervical flexion or extension	Positive for atlantoaxial hypermobility if soft end-feel, muscle spasm, dizziness, nausea, or paresthesias are present
Alar ligament stress test[1]	Patient is supine. Examiner stabilizes axis with one hand and attempts to side-bend head on axis	Positive for ligamentous instability if excessive motion or soft end-feel is present
Shoulder		
Sulcus sign[3]	Patient is seated with arm in neutral. Examiner applies distraction force to humerus	Positive for multidirectional instability of glenohumeral joint if examiner notes excessive inferior translation of humeral head and a sulcus defect just superior to humeral head
Acromioclavicular shear test[4]	Examiner cups both hands over shoulder, one hand on clavicle, the other over scapular spine. Examiner then compresses hands, producing shearing motion at AC joint	Positive for AC joint involvement if pain or excessive movement is noted
Wright test[4]	Patient is supine. Examiner palpates patient's pulse at radial artery and hyperabducts shoulder	Positive for thoracic outlet syndrome if pulse dissipates or is absent as examiner abducts arm
Adson maneuver[5]	Examiner palpates radial pulse while abducting, extending, and externally rotating arm. Patient is instructed to take a deep breath and turn head toward arm being tested	Positive for compression of subclavian artery if examiner notes a marked decrease or absence of radial pulse during maneuver
Allen test[5]	Examiner instructs patient to open and close the fist quickly several times, then squeeze the fist tightly to force venous blood out of the hand. Examiner then occludes radial and ulnar arteries using index and middle fingers. Patient is instructed to open hand, and examiner releases pressure on one artery. This process is repeated for the contralatered extremity	Positive for impaired blood supply to hand if patient's hand does not flush or flushes very slowly after artery is released
Halstead maneuver[4]	Examiner palpates radial pulse while applying distraction to upper extremity. Examiner then instructs patient to extend neck and rotate to contralateral side	Positive for thoracic outlet syndrome if examiner detects absence of pulse during maneuver

APPENDIX Additional Orthopaedic Physical Therapy Examination Tests (cont.)

Test	Description	Positive Findings
Elbow		
Wartenberg sign[1]	Patient is seated with hands on table. Patient is asked to separate fingers, then bring them together	Positive for ulnar neuropathy if patient is unable to bring 5th digit toward 4th digit
Test for pronator teres syndrome[1]	Patient is seated with elbow flexed to 90° while examiner resists pronation and extends elbow	Positive for median nerve involvement if tingling or paresthesia is present in distribution of median nerve
Wrist and Hand		
Thumb ulnar collateral ligament instability test[1]	Examiner stabilizes patient's hand while taking thumb into extension and applying a valgus stress	Positive for ruptured ulnar collateral or accessory collateral ligament if laxity is >30°–35°, and positive for partial tear if laxity is greater than contralateral side, but <30°
Lunotriquetral ballottement test[1]	Examiner grasps triquetrum with one hand and lunate with the other hand. Examiner then translates lunate anteriorly and posteriorly	Positive for lunotriquetral instability if laxity, crepitus, or pain is present
Scaphoid stress test[1]	Patient is seated. Examiner applies pressure over palmar aspect of scaphoid. Patient is asked to perform radial deviation of wrist	Positive for scaphoid instability if excessive laxity is present, or if examiner feels a "clunk" as scaphoid shifts out of its fossa
Axial load test[1]	Patient is seated. Examiner applies axial compression to thumb	Positive for metacarpal or adjacent carpal fracture if pain and/or crepitus is present

Additional Orthopaedic Physical Therapy Examination Tests (cont.)

Test	Description	Positive Findings
Thoracolumbar Spine		
Slump test[6]	Patient is seated, hands behind back. Examiner asks patient to slump forward, rounding back, then bring chin to chest, then extend knee of symptomatic side. Examiner adds overpressure into slump until patient reports symptoms. Examiner then asks patient to look up, extending cervical spine	Positive for neural involvement if symptoms are increased or peripheralized during slump, and decreased or centralized during cervical extension
Straight-leg-raise test[7]	Patient is supine. Examiner elevates leg with knee extended. If patient experiences symptoms, examiner lowers leg slightly and dorsiflexes foot, noting symptoms, then returns ankle to neutral, noting symptoms	Positive for neural involvement if symptoms increase with dorsiflexion and decrease with neutral ankle position
Prone knee-bend test[7]	Patient is prone while examiner stabilizes over ischium, fully flexes knee, and, if possible, extends hip	Positive for femoral nerve involvement if symptoms are reproduced
Yeoman sign[7]	Patient is prone. Examiner stabilizes sacrum with one hand and extends hip with other hand. Examiner overextends hip to produce anterior innominate rotation	Positive for sacroiliac dysfunction if patient's pain is reproduced at sacroiliac joint
Hoover test[1]	Patient is supine while examiner grasps each calcaneus. Patient is instructed to lift one leg off table, knees straight	Positive for nonorganic influence if patient does not lift leg, or if examiner does not feel pressure from contralateral heel as leg is attempting to lift
Burns test[5]	Patient is instructed to kneel on stool, bend over, and attempt to touch floor	Positive for nonorganic influence if patient cannot attempt task secondary to significant pain

APPENDIX   **Additional Orthopaedic Physical Therapy Examination Tests (cont.)**

Test	Description	Positive Findings
Pelvis		
Sacrotuberous ligament stress test[2]	Patient is supine. Examiner fully flexes and adducts hip with knee in flexion. Examiner then applies longitudinal force through femur	Positive for sacrotuberous ligament involvement if maneuver reproduces patient's symptoms
Torsion stress test[2]	Patient is prone. Examiner stabilizes apex of sacrum and applies downward pressure at contralateral posterior superior iliac spine	Positive for sacroiliac joint involvement if symptoms are reproduced
Femoral shear test[2]	Patient is supine with hip in flexion, abduction, and external rotation. Examiner applies axial force through femur	Positive for sacroiliac involvement if patient's symptoms are reproduced
Leg-length test[7]	Patient is prone as examiner compares levels of medial malleoli. Patient's knees are then flexed to 90°, and examiner again compares levels of medial malleoli	Positive for leg-length discrepancy if one malleolus is at a different level than another in the prone position. Positive for shortened tibia if malleolus is also lower in 90° of knee flexion
Hip		
Craig test[7]	Patient is prone with knee flexed to 90°. Examiner internally and externally rotates hip while palpating greater trochanter to determine point at which it is most lateral	Positive for femoral anteversion if angle is >15° of internal rotation
Sign of the buttock[8]	Patient is supine while examiner passively performs a unilateral straight-leg raise. If unilateral restriction is noted, examiner then repeats leg raise with knee in flexion and notes whether hip flexion increases	Positive if hip flexion does not increase with knee flexion. A positive test is indicative of disease in the buttock region
Piriformis test[8]	Patient is supine while examiner performs passive internal rotation of extended hip	Positive for sacroiliac or piriformis involvement if patient's symptoms are reproduced
Scour test[8]	Patient is supine. Examiner applies overpressure while passively circumducting thigh through extremes of motion	Gross clearing test; positive if pain, intermittent locking, joint sounds, snapping tendon, and/or limitation of range of motion is present

Additional Orthopaedic Physical Therapy Examination Tests (cont.)

Test	Description	Positive Findings
Knee		
Sag sign[9]	Patient is supine with knee and hip flexed to 90°	Positive for posterior cruciate ligament instability if examiner notes a "sag" just superior to tibial tubercle
Slocum test[7]	Patient is supine, with knee flexed to 90° and hip flexed to 45°. Foot is taken to 30° of internal rotation. Examiner stabilizes foot and pulls tibia anteriorly. Test is repeated with foot in 15° of external rotation	Positive for rotary instability of knee if examiner notes excessive translation on medial or lateral tibia
Bounce home test[5]	Patient is supine. Examiner passively fully flexes knee, then allows knee to fall into extension	Positive for torn meniscus, loose body, or intracapsular joint swelling if knee does not extend fully with a firm end point upon release
O'Donohue test[7]	Patient is supine, knee flexed to 90°. Examiner stabilizes at thigh and rotates tibia medially and laterally. Examiner repeats this test with knee in full flexion	Positive for meniscal tear or capsular irritation if test elicits pain
Plica test[2]	Patient is supine. Examiner passively flexes and extends knee 30°–90° while applying pressure to patella medially and medially rotating tibia	Positive for plica syndrome if maneuver reproduces patient's symptoms, including a painful popping sensation
Foot and Ankle		
Thompson test[7]	Patient is prone with feet over edge of plinth. Examiner squeezes at mid calf	Positive for Achilles tendon rupture if no plantarflexion is associated with squeezing calf
Tinel test[7]	Examiner taps over anterior branch of fibular nerve at anterior ankle or posterior tibial nerve behind medial malleolus	Positive for nerve involvement if patient reports tingling or paresthesia when examiner taps over nerve
Morton test[7]	Patient is supine. Examiner grasps foot at level of metatarsal heads and applies medial-lateral pressure	Positive for stress fracture or neuroma if symptoms are reproduced

REFERENCES

1. Magee D. *Orthopedic Physical Assessment*. 4th ed. Philadelphia, Pa: WB Saunders; 2002.
2. Hertling D, Kessler RM. *Management of Common Musculoskeletal Disorders*. 3rd ed. Pennsylvania, Pa: Lippincott Williams & Wilkins; 1996.
3. Donatelli R. *Physical Therapy of the Shoulder*. Philadelphia, Pa: Churchill Livingstone; 1997.
4. Tovin BJ, Greenfield BH. *Evaluation and Treatment of the Shoulder*. Philadelphia, Pa: FA Davis Company; 2001.
5. Hoppenfeld S. *Physical Examination of the Spinal Extremities*. East Norwalk: Appleton-Century-Crofts; 1976.
6. Butler DS. *The Sensitive Nervous System*. Unley DC, Australia: Noigroup Publications; 2000.
7. Dutton M. *Orthopaedic Examination, Evaluation, & Intervention*. New York, NY: McGraw-Hill Companies; 2004.
8. Fagerson TL. *The Hip Handbook*. Boston, Mass: Butterworth-Heinemann; 1997.
9. Ellenbecker TS. *Knee Ligament Rehabilitation*. Philadelphia, Pa: Churchill Livingstone; 2000.

Frank H. Netter was born in 1906 in New York City. He studied art at the Art Student's League and the National Academy of Design before entering medical school at New York University, where he received his MD degree in 1931. During his student years, Dr. Netter's notebook sketches attracted the attention of the medical faculty and other physicians, allowing him to augment his income by illustrating articles and textbooks. He continued illustrating as a sideline after establishing a surgical practice in 1933, but he ultimately opted to give up his practice in favor of a full-time commitment to art. After service in the United States Army during World War II, Dr. Netter began his long collaboration with the CIBA Pharmaceutical Company (now Novartis Phamaceuticals). This 45-year partnership resulted in the production of the extraordinary collection of medical art so familiar to physicians and other medical professionals worldwide.

Icon Learning Systems acquired the Netter Collection in July 2000 and continues to update Dr. Netter's original paintings and to add newly commissioned paintings by artists trained in the style of Dr. Netter.

Dr. Netter's works are among the finest examples of the use of illustration in the teaching of medical concepts. The 13-book *Netter Collection of Medical Illustrations*, which includes the greater part of the more than 20,000 paintings created by Dr. Netter, became and remains one of the most famous medical works ever published. *The Netter Atlas of Human Anatomy*, first published in 1989, presents the anatomical paintings from the Netter Collection. Now translated into 11 languages, it is the anatomy atlas of choice among medical and health professions students the world over.

The Netter illustrations are appreciated not only for their aesthetic qualities, but more importantly, for their intellectual content. As Dr. Netter wrote in 1949, "…clarification of a subject is the aim and goal of illustration. No matter how beautifully painted, how delicately and subtly rendered a subject may be, it is of little value as a *medical illustration* if it does not serve to make clear some medical point." Dr. Netter's planning, conception, point of view, and approach are what inform his paintings and what make them so intellectually valuable.

Frank H. Netter, MD, physician and artist, died in 1991.

INDEX

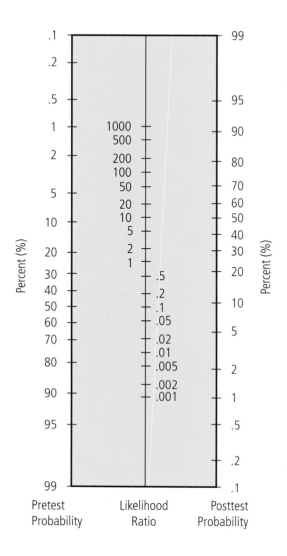

Pretest
Probability

Likelihood
Ratio

Posttest
Probability